Contents

Bold type indicates author gave oral presentation.

PREFACE

Process Tomography was evolving in the late 1980's to meet a widespread need for the direct analysis of the internal characteristics of process plants in order to improve the design and operation of equipment. The measuring instruments for such applications must use robust non-invasive sensors which, if required, can operate in aggressive and fast moving fluids and multiphase mixtures. Process Tomography thus involves using tomographic imaging methods to manipulate data from remote sensors in order to obtain precise quantitative methods to manipulate data from inaccessible locations. The need for tomography is analogous to the medical need for body scanners, which has been met by the development of computer-aided tomography.

For instance process tomography will improve the operation and design of processes handling multi-compound mixtures by enabling boundaries between different components in a process to be imaged in real-time using non-intrusive sensors. Information of the flow regime, vector velocity, and component size distributions and concentrations in process vessels and pipelines will be determined from the images.

The basic idea is to install a number of sensors around the pipe or vessel to be imaged. The sensor output signals depend on the position of the component boundaries within their sensing zones. A computer is used to reconstruct a tomographic image of the cross section being observed by the sensors. This will provide, for instance, identification of the distribution of mixing zones in stirred reactors, interface measurement in complex separation processes and measurements of two-phase flow boundaries in pipes with applications to multi-phase flow measurement.

By 1990 it was felt that Process Tomography was maturing as a potentially useful technique for application to industrial process design and operation, although the effort was somewhat fragmented and dispersed. Therefore it was timely to establish a four year programme for a European Concerted Action on Process Tomography (proposal reference BE-4015-90) within the framework of the Brite Euram scheme. This resulted in the first workshop on the subject, held during March 1992 in Manchester, England.

The main objective of the Concerted Action is to improve the design and operation of industrial process plants by tomographically imaging the distribution of material in process vessels and pipelines. The tomographically derived data may be used for:

(i) process model verification (to design improved equipment),

(ii) process operation and control (*internal measurements* by tomography will give better information on process behaviour than will *external measurements*),

(iii) multi-component flow measurement (e.g. oil/gas mixtures, pneumatic conveyors).

This Concerted Action harnesses together a range of projects by:

(i) holding annual meetings of workers from European industrial research institutes and universities, in order to:

    a) monitor and encourage the success of their projects in Process Tomography

    b) facilitate transferring tomographic technology from medicine to process plants and

    c) develop a longer term strategy for ensuring the success of Process Tomography in improving industrial productivity and safety,

(ii) preparing an annual report of progress in process tomography, including papers from each contributor to the annual meeting,

(iii) supporting a database of EC and international progress in process tomography which will be accessible through the Joint Academic Network (JANET) to members of the co-ordinated activity and other appropriate groups (Appendix 1).

This Concerted Action will ultimately improve the efficiency of a wide spectrum of process operations including the chemical, mineral, biochemical, paper, ceramic, pharmaceutical and food industries. The most recent reports of the European Communities Chemistry Committee show the European chemical industry alone to have a turnover of 236 billion ECU per annum. Even a small improvement in the operating efficiency of such a major industry can result in a substantial saving in costs, with obvious financial advantages. It is the purpose of the Concerted Action to make this possible. A second less quantifiable benefit is improved safety resulting from better knowledge of the *internal* situation of a process. A third most desirable benefit is the reduction of environmental pollution. This uses the ability of tomographic techniques to locate specific contaminants in a large area, while needing only a few strategically placed sensors. Possible applications include the detection of fugitive emissions from a factory site and the location of groundwater leakages from a landfill site.

The major aim of the Manchester Workshop was to provide a forum whereby researchers from European industry, and research institutes and universities who have an interest in developing and applying tomographic techniques could meet. Invited research and applications papers were solicited and these form part of the book.

The topics covered in the Workshop, defined by the management committee, spanned a wide range including:

i)   sensors
ii)   image reconstruction and analysis
iii)   process model verification
iv)   applications
v)   international standards for performance assessment
vi)   CAD of process tomography systems
vii)   data processing hardware
viii) PT for process operation and control

The first two themes of sensors and image reconstruction and analysis cover the basic techniques necessary to obtain a tomographic image of a process. A primary use of tomographic image information is to verify the models of process systems, so that processes can be better designed on the basis of more accurate models (Theme iii). The fourth theme on 'applications' is initially concerned with the use of tomography on unit processes in a laboratory situation, but great emphasis is being placed on extending this to industrial processes as our work develops. Several groups in different countries are developing systems for tomographic imaging, so it is necessary to have a standard for performance assessment and comparison of results, thus the fifth theme involves consideration of using standard test objects (referred to as phantoms in medical tomograpy), the construction of these will involve careful consideration of geometry and materials in order to generate realistic and reproducible physical simulations of processes. The sixth theme concerns computer-aided design. The electrode systems used for process tomography require careful design to optimise the field which interrogates the process, and data on the field geometry must be incorporated in the reconstruction algorithm. In addition to this sensing aspect of CAD, some groups may investigate the total design of PT systems using CAD. Low-cost computed tomography is now possible because of recent developments in digital data processing systems. The PT activity should carefully monitor other developments in data processing relevant to our subject and this is the seventh theme. At an early stage process tomography can be used for process model verification (Theme iii). However, as our subject develops it is likely that the 'internal' information available from a tomographic image will be useful for process operation and control; the development of this new type of measurement system is the subject of Theme viii.

A Workshop report is included and forms Part 1 of this book. This gives an overview of this current status of research in Process Tomography and proposes a strategy for industrial exploitation. The aim is to provide a sound basis from the European point of view, on specifying research needs and the areas where future collaboration should be sought. Specific recommendations are suggested and the means by which they can be achieved. A major review of the ensuing developments will take place at the second meeting of the Concerted Action which will be held at Universitat (TH) Karlsruhe, Germany in 1993.

Our heartfelt thanks are due to many people who contributed to the success of the Manchester Workshop. These include: Dorothy Denton for administrative and secretarial work; the deputy chairpersons E. Etuke, W. Tang, Z. Yu, X. Zhao and M. Wang for taking care of visual aids; W.Q. Yang for preparing the poster arrangements; the session reporters and chairpersons named in the following page; the demonstrators on the UMIST and industrial visits; C. Rowland for his overview of research funding arrangements; British Gas for supporting a special opening of the Manchester Museum of Science and Industry; ICI for the industrial visit which showed new horizons for some younger researchers.

M.S. Beck
E. Campogrande
Margaret Morris
R.A. Williams
R.C. Waterfall

Concerted Action on Process Tomography
Management Committee

Dr D.C. Barber	Royal Hallamshire Hospital, Sheffield
Prof M. Beck	UMIST - *Co-ordinating Editor of Annual Report*
Prof A. Borges	University of Aveiro
Mr E. Campogrande	Brite-Euram
Mr R.B. Edwards	Unilever Research
Prof E. Hammer	University of Bergen
Dr C.P. Lenn	Schlumberger Cambridge Research
Dr J. Morris	MIRO
Mrs M. Morris	UMIST - *Programme Administrator*
Prof F. Mesch	University of Karlsruhe
Prof A. Naylor	BNF plc/UMIST
Prof R. Pallas-Areny	University Polytechnic of Catalunya
Dr R.W. Taylor	University of York - *Database Manager*
Prof B. Scarlett	TU Delft
Dr R.W. Waterfall	UMIST - *Meetings Co-ordinator*
Dr R.A. Williams	UMIST - *Programme Manager*

Part I:

WORKSHOP REPORT AND RECOMMENDATIONS

by

M Z Abdullah, T Allen, M S Beck, R Brassington, E Campogrande, F J Dickin,
D G Hayes, E A Hammer, M Lee, S L McKee, A Naylor, J E Nordtvedt, S V Quick,
J D Tallantire, R C Waterfall, R A Williams, C G Xie

TECHNICAL SESSION: Sensors

<u>Session Chairman</u>: Prof E A Hammer (University of Bergen, Norway)
<u>Session Reporter</u>: Dr C G Xie (UMIST, UK)

1. Summary of papers

The keynote paper was delivered by Prof F Mesch from the University of Karlsruhe, Germany, entitled "Sensors - their interaction with the measurand". In his paper, sensors' interactions were classified into two categories: the scalar interaction and the vector interaction. The scalar interactions were further divided into the following: (i) absorption (e.g. gamma ray CT for flow pattern recognition); (ii) reflection (e.g. SAR radar on aeroplane; ultrasonic array transmitters/receivers for gas or vapour identification); (iii) scattering (e.g. acoustic diffraction tomography); and (iv) electrical impedance (e.g. the capacitance tomography for flow imaging). The vector interactions were typified by two examples: (i) flow velocity sensing from the time-of-flight measurements using ultrasonic sensors, where, to obtain a velocity vector, both the longitudinal interaction and the transversal interaction of the ultrasonic waves with the flow were measured. (ii) Schlieren method (optical) for flow measurement, where the transversal interaction of a laser beam with the flow was used to extract the flow information. Sensors based on magnetic-field sensing were also categorised as ones having vector interactions. In addition to the above two type of sensing techniques, Prof Mesch also gave an interesting example of an optical technique for obtaining a 3D image from a series of 2D images obtained at different focus depths (related to microscopy of 3D objects).

Other papers and posters presented in this session have covered the following sensing techniques for tomography:

(a) Optical:

In Bolton Institute of Higher Education, UK, up to two pairs of 16 infra-red emitters and 16 detectors were mounted outside a Perspex pipe of 120 mm diameter, projecting parallel beams (beam diameter 5 mm) (Dugdale et al). At present, two orthogonal projections (at 0° and 90°) were made to interrogate the flow. However, the transputer-based sensor hardware can accommodate two extra projections (e.g. at 45° and 135°). The data-capture speed is 200 μs.

(b) Electrical resistance:

Several papers and posters were presented relating to this area. A multi-frequency EIT system was proposed by Riu et al (from UPC, Spain) as an alternative to absolute imaging. Measurements are made at dual frequencies (e.g. 16 kHz and 125 kHz), those made at one frequency being taken as the reference, and those made at another frequency being used to extract the absolute-image information. The design of a 16-electrode EIT system and some experimental results were also described.

The design of a 32-electrode EIT data-collection system was presented by Wang *et al* (from UMIST, UK). In this improved design, programmable injection currents (0 to 30 mA) and excitation frequencies (75 Hz to 153.6 kHz) can be generated, making the system versatile for different industrial applications. The designs of the critical components of the system, such as the VCCS of high output impedance and the demodulation unit with high CMRR were described in detail.

A theoretical design of a DSP-based architecture for EIT data collection was proposed by Lyon and Oakley (from Manchester University, UK). They also studied, using the finite element method (FEM), the variations of the field sensitivity distributions due to the presence of a stirrer (insulating or conducting) inside a mixing vessel. The case when electrodes are mounted on the stirrer itself was also investigated. They concluded that the presence of the stirrer will have no detrimental effect on the image reconstruction.

The effects of electrode size and geometry with respect to the size of the process vessel to be interrogated were studied by Abdullah *et al* (from UMIST, UK). Small cyclonic separators (2") were used as a case study. Results (differential voltages made from all the electrode pairs) of experimental measurements and FE calculations were compared, indicating that rectangular electrodes are most suitable for imaging cyclonic separators.

In order to compare the performance of different EIT data collection systems, Zhao *et al* (from UMIST, UK) recommended some performance-evaluation criteria. They are mainly: accuracy, CMRR, SCIR (signal to common-mode interference ratio) and stability.

(c) Electrical capacitance:

The FE modelling (using PE2D package) of 12-electrode capacitance imaging systems was validated by Khan and Abdullah (from City University, UK), with the experimental data obtained at UMIST being used as the reference for comparison. In general, the sensitivity profiles calculated using the FEM have the same trend as those measured using the UMIST system. Closer agreement was obtained for the adjacent electrode pair than for the diagonally-separated electrode pair. The errors of discrepancy were analysed in detail, and they are mainly due to the measurement uncertainty of the transducer hardware when measuring very small capacitance change between the diagonally-separated electrode pair.

The design of a new capacitance transducer with potentially higher SNR and accuracy than that based on the charge/discharge method (used in the present 12-electrode capacitance flow imaging system at UMIST) was described by Yang and Stott (from UMIST, UK). The transducer is based on a stray-immune AC bridge with feedback balance and phase-sensitive demodulation. The projected measurement range of the new transducer is 0.1 fF to 10 pF (the range of the charge/discharge transducer is 0.3 fF to 2 pF). The transducer will operates at 500 kHz (sinewave), and will be used with a 16-electrode capacitance imaging system.

A comparison of electrode excitation methods for capacitance tomography system was made by Bair and Oakley (from Manchester University, UK), using the PE2D FE package. Single-excitation system (e.g. the UMIST one) and dual-excitation system (opposing pair of electrodes are excited with potentials of equal magnitude but opposite polarity) were studied. The sensitivity distributions of the two systems were analysed. The qualities of reconstructed images of the two systems, obtained using backprojection algorithm, were also compared and were found quite similar. The image reconstruction algorithm was identified as the limiting factor of the imaging system.

(d) Electrodynamic (charge):

Preliminary work was conducted by Bidin *et al* (from Sheffield Polytechnic, UK) on the use of an array of charge detecting electrodes mounted outside a pipe in which solids are conveyed pneumatically. By detecting charges carried by the solids, the solids distribution over the pipe cross-section can be determined. A mathematical model relating the induced voltages on the electrodes to the position of a single particle carrying certain charge was established, and was confirmed by experiments.

2. Discussion

The detailed answers by the author(s) of the papers to the questions and discussion points raised by the audience are given in an appendix.

Some general points raised during discussion are:

E A Hammer:	To industrialist: Is it worthwhile doing process tomography (PT)?
M S Beck:	Further pointed out the triangular relationship between university researchers designing PT systems, instrument manufacturers making the systems, and the industrial users using them. The Sheffield APT system was manufactured by an industrial firm. However, after some years bad sales, the firm had to cease to make them. The Sheffield University group are now manufacturing the APT system themselves. Should universities become the manufacturers themselves ?
C McLeod:	There are still some technical problems associated with the medical APT system. It is still some way from being used in routine medical care. The APT system is now back to the university for further improvement. The university research groups should push the technology to industry themselves.
D Holder:	User feedback is important: there are problems associated with the underlying physics and engineering of the technique; there are few worked images produced that convince industrialists; there are absence of studies of valid examples. As a result, the industrialists have, at present, shown no strong commitment to

investing money for making the PT systems.

R A Williams: I agree with David Holder. We now don't have good standard
                         regarding the sensitivity, accuracy and resolution of the
                         systems, i.e. no yardstick ! Most of the work have been done
                         with static phantoms, dynamic experiments are needed to
                         quantify the system. Are there any fundamental problems with
                         the technique ?

S M Huang: The methods to quantify the performance of a PT system are
                         to compare the image reconstruction algorithms, and maybe the
                         whole system (hardware and software). Initial efforts have been
                         made by Seagar *et al*. Image reconstruction errors, for
                         example, can be quantified by using static phantoms, and a
                         paper on this will be presented during this conference.
                         Dynamic performance evaluation is difficult to achieve because
                         of the lack of independent calibration techniques.

3. Implication for future development of process tomography

Process tomography is defined as measurement of different process variables in space
and time. When such measurements are achieved it often will result in a large amount
of data about the process and information saturation can easily occur.

Traditional control theory can handle the utilisation of the information about single
and multiple process variables to control the process if the transfer functions for the
different variables in the process are known in the frequency domain or in the time
domain. The process tomograph will contain information of the space distribution of
process variables but this information cannot be utilised for control purposes unless
we know the transfer functions between certain process input parameters and the
space distribution of the process variables.

Generally, such transfer functions are known for some processes in steady state, but
not dynamically. Therefore, all the information we can get from a process tomograph
cannot be fully utilised for many processes today. Obviously the development in
process tomography will increase the possibility to optimise processes with respect
to efficiency. It is therefore of great importance to work out theories and do
experimental work to optimise processes based on the information from tomographical
measurements.

Process tomography is the coming process information technology. The industry
which can utilise this technology will be the leading industry within process
instrumentation and control in the future.

We have seen during this conference that process tomography has been applied only
in very few industrial processes so far. One example is imaging of the component
distribution in cyclones used for separation. Obviously many other industrial
processes can benefit from using tomographic measurement systems.

One good example of this is level measurement in oil/gas/water-tank separators in the oil process industry. To optimise the efficiency of such separators the level of gas/oil and the oil/water interfaces have to be measured. Since these interfaces consist of a foam layer and a layer of oil/water emulsion, known tank level measurement techniques do not work satisfactorily. An image of the separator cross section will solve the problem if it is possible to achieve. Cross section image reconstruction of a separator might be possible by using multiple gamma ray absorption. This technique will have the feature that the equipment can be clamped on, thus making it more acceptable for the oil industry. Imaging using multiple ultrasonic transducers might also be possible. Thus the level of different interface layers and the thickness of these layers in a separator tank can be determined and the information can be used on line for controlling the input flow of the mixture in such a way that the separator can be run under an optimum condition.

Another important application of process tomography is within testing and calibration of multiphase flow meters. There are different meters on the market today intended for flow measurement in multiphase flows. All these meters will be influenced by the phase distribution (flow regime) of the flow. In testing or even calibration of these instruments in multiphase flow rigs it is of vital importance to know the phase distribution at the test site. Several such multiphase calibration rigs are going to be built around the world and all of them need a tomographic system to determine the different flow regimes occurring during the tests. Test rigs containing oil and gas can easily be imaged using multiple capacitance techniques and pipe imaging systems based on this technique are already on the market.

In the future process tomography techniques will be applied also in refinery processes and in the food industry to make the different processes more efficient and increase the quality of the product.

Today, the process industry does not realise the potential for using process tomography for measurement and control. However the different groups developing process tomography systems suffer from lack of practical knowledge about the different processes. Therefore, the ECAPT organisation should spend some time arranging workshops between selected groups of the process industry and research and development groups working with process tomography.

The possibilities and the needs should thus be clarified and research and development programs worked out. The funding of the different research and development programs will come partly from the process industry and partly from research councils if the different proposals worked out based on the workshop meetings contain the necessary convincing arguments, technical and economical benefits.

Cross-border research and development programs should be aimed at. The expertise within different subjects could be utilised and an international effort would have a greater possibility of obtaining technological success.

Appendix - Questions and Answers (Topic A - Sensors)

1. Keynote paper:

Title: *Sensors - their interaction with the measurand*
Presenter: Prof F Mesch, University of Karlsruhe, Germany

Q1:   Can electromagnetic fields be used to image 2D and 3D objects ? (M S Beck)

A1:   Not directly to my knowledge. But tomography can be used to compute field
       lines of, e.g. permanent magnets from measurements taken with specially
       shaped measuring coils.

       There was a pertinent paper at the last IMEKO congress in Beijing presented
       by a Japanese author.

2. Other Papers

Paper 1

Title: *Optical sensors for process tomography*
Authors: P Dugdale, R G Green, A J Hartley, R G Jackson and J Landauro
Presenter: Mr P Dugdale, Bolton Institute of Higher Education, United Kingdom

Q1:   What are the most critical factors limiting the use of this measuring device in
       an industrial context ? (R A Williams)

A1:   As well as optical access (e.g. chemical engineering - yeast vats), an increase
       in IR radiation intensity is necessary for industrial applications. This can be
       achieved using laser diodes. These also enable their radiation to be monitored,
       and thus controlled by feedback. In this way the sensors can be calibrated for
       given environments. (P Dugdale)

       Also we feel that both rectangular and polar arrays should be used in
       combination to see if the number of projections can be reduced - still
       providing a certain level of resolution and a large objects. (R G Green)

Q2:   The emitters in your study are placed in a rectangular fashion. Have you tried
       using polar placement to avoid the influence of different indexes ?
       (P Henriksson)

A2:   Yes. However this increases the spatial resolution at the centre, while
       reducing it at the edges.

Paper 2

Title: *Multifrequency EIT as an alternative to absolute imaging*
Authors: P Riu, J Rosell and R Pallas-Areny
Presenter: Dr P Riu, Universitat Politecnica de Catalunya, Barcelona, Spain

Q1: You have shown some sample images and claimed you can discern erector spinae, vertebrae and bowel. They do not exactly correspond to known anatomy and could be artefacts or other structures. Do you have any independent evidence for your claims ? (D Holder)

A1: We claim that our system allows us to visualise regions inside a body provided the frequency dependence of the impedance for each region is different. We also claim that according to biomedical data, a cross section at 10 cm below the sternum displays a frequency dependence that would provide images like the ones we have obtained. We believe a different imaging method with better resolution would provide images certainly better in detail but not in substance. Measurement in phantoms have not shown any gross error in our system.

Q2: Is the multi-frequency EIT system less sensitive to electrode-placement error than the adaptive current system ? Does the reconstruction not depend on the knowledge of the electrode positions ?

A2: We have not compared our system with the adaptive current system. Our system, being a relative imaging method, is less sensitive to electrode-position knowledge than absolute imaging systems.

Q3: Can the use of two frequencies lead to errors if the frequencies are harmonically related ? Is the measurement system non-linear (i.e. is the current proportional to voltage ?) (M S Beck)

A3: We use harmonically related frequencies because they are very easy to generate. In order to check whether or not there is any non-linearity that increases errors because of the relationship between the frequency pair being injected, we have measured the voltage errors when injecting each frequency alone and when injecting them simultaneously. No increase in error was detected.

Paper 3

Title: *Validation of FE modelling of multi-electrode capacitive system for process tomography flow imaging*
Authors: S H Khan and F Abdullah
Presenter: Dr S H Khan, City University, London, United Kingdom

Q1: Did you use only one test rod ? What happens with n objects so that the field for the nth object is distorted by the n-1 previous objects ? This question is practically relevant to sensing multiphase flow with non-uniform distribution of phases. Theoretically, this problem is related to the multiple scattering problem which is much more involved than fields for a uniform dielectric. (F Mesch)

A1:   Yes, we did. The main objective of this particular simulation study was to validate FE modelling of (capacitance) electrode systems by comparing results with corresponding experimental data obtained from UMIST. The experimental results were obtained from sensitivity studies for two different electrode systems using only one test rod. That is why we also used one test rod. In general I agree with Prof Mesch that field distortions do occur due to various ways of distributions of flow phases and these distortions should be taken into account while appropriate.

Q2:   Have you tried to measure the capacitances with a HP impedance bridge ? (Ø Isaksen)

A2:   All experiments were carried out by researchers at UMIST who used relevant electronics designed by themselves.

Paper 4

Title: *Improved EIT data collection system and measurement protocols*
Authors: M Wang, F J Dickin and M S Beck
Presenter: Mr M Wang, UMIST, United Kingdom

Q1:   What factors influence the choice of frequency for EIT in industry ? (J Oakley)

A1:   (i) for calibration; (ii) for separator studies; (iii) for comparison with the images obtained from high frequency and low frequency; (iv) for cancelling influence of stray capacitances and obtaining accurate measurements at low frequency although the collection speed will be slow.

Q2:   Why should frequencies only go down to 600 Hz ? Why not 1 Hz say ? Ion mobility velocities are more likely to show up at very low frequencies. (R G Green)

A2:   The specification of the system was decided arbitrarily - you are correct, if the process reaction or occurrence inside the vessel is sufficiently slow then there is no reason why 1 Hz could not be used.

Paper 5

Title: *High resolution EIT in stirred vessels*
Authors: G Lyon and J Oakley
Presenter: Mr G Lyon, Manchester University, United Kingdom

Q1: Why isn't the flow faster at the end of the paddle rather than at the centre near to the axis of the stirrer. (R G Green)

A1: (i) Flow rates ultimately dependent on flow regime within the vessel.
(ii) Speed of flow maybe great, but not in the imaging plane, but passing through it.
(iii) Key point not the relative speed of flow in the central region but the difficulty in producing: accurate EIT images, accurate CFD model results, both in the central region.

Q2: From the results, this paper has important implications for the process industries. How is the system 'excited' using sensors placed on the central impeller shaft. Would rotation of the sensors mounted on the shaft reduce the effective 'resolution' of the image obtained. (R A Williams)

A2: (i) Excitation on central electrodes no different to that on other electrodes. The use of an adaptive DAS would allow a wider range of possible excitation patterns by incorporating the central electrodes. (ii) Initial work would use fixed electrodes (not rotating) on a sleeve surrounding the rotating shaft. Have little effect on flow regime when using low viscosity liquids. (iii) Rotating electrodes/impellers would not reduce effective resolution providing sufficient knowledge of their geometry and position when measurement is made are used in image reconstruction.

Paper 6

Title: *A prototype electrodynamic tomographic imaging system for pneumatic conveyors*
Authors: A R Bidin, R G Green, R W Taylor and M E Shackleton
Presenter: Dr R G Green, Sheffield City Polytechnic, United Kingdom

Q1: (i) What are the relative merits of electrodynamic sensing methods over capacitance methods ?

(ii) Would you anticipate that all particles carry the same charge ? Would not the charge carried also depend on the flow rate, in which case it might be more difficult to reconstruct measured data to form an image in an independent fashion. (R.A. Williams)

A1: (i) The electrodynamic sensing volume is less than that for capacitance sensors so that the measurement bandwidth is greatest for the electrodynamic sensor. Capacitance method has a significant fringe field.

(ii) No particles are gaining or losing charge continuously. However, the maximum voltage on a particle is limited by its size and a lot of particles seem to have similar levels of charge. The maximum charge is independent of velocity, however slow particles will not get much charge.

Electrodynamic sensors are very useful for obtaining velocity information by cross-correlation - so that velocity information is fairly readily available. Our present aim is to produce images showing combined concentration and velocity.

TECHNICAL SESSION: Data processing, mathematical techniques & simulation

Session Chairman: Dr Fraser Dickin (UMIST, UK)
Session Reporter: Mr Derek Hayes   (UMIST, UK)

1.   Summary of papers and discussion

A total of seven papers (including the keynote paper) were presented in this session which was attended by the majority of the delegates. The keynote paper was delivered by Professor Antonio Rui Borges from the Electronic Engineering Department at the University of Aveiro in Portugal. Professor Borges' keynote paper was entitled "Strategies for parallelisation in MIMD-architectures" and gave a concise account of the mechanisms of exploiting concurrency present in a computational process in order to reduce its execution time. A comparison of MIMD machines versus SIMD machines was presented in terms of their efficiency, flexibility and financial cost. It was noted that MIMD machines were more suited to coarse-grained parallelism problems. Consequently strategies for developing parallel algorithms for data-driven problems were discussed followed by a description of a basic computational model to enhance coarse-grain parallelism in data-driven solutions. The final part of the presentation was given over to the characterisation of the filtered backprojection algorithm, in particular the filtering and backprojection operations in terms of partitioned matrix manipulation.

Professor Borges was asked a number of questions, the first was by Dr Brian Hoyle: "Spatial/temporal decomposition is clearly efficient for process tomography where data arrival rate is constant. These methods have been found less effective than process farming when time of arrival is variable, e.g. ultrasound. Please contrast your ideas with process farming."

Answer: "In the diagram shown during the presentation explaining the planar message passing topology, the processor allocation does not have to be completely static. Some of the processors may be assigned simultaneously to P tasks belonging to different stages and be triggered to execute a particular one according to load requirements. In this way the chain can be balanced dynamically".

Professor Maurice Beck asked the following: "Do you think that a uniform approach to data processing hardware is needed? How will this help with dual-modality imaging and could you suggest a suitable system?"

Answer: "Yes I believe this would be very important. Initially, it might not be possible to get everyone to agree on a common approach therefore some effort should be expended on developing data processing algorithms to run on a virtual machine which at a later date could be mapped onto specific hardware.

I think that could be very significant for an efficient and fast development of such systems. Work from different groups could be made portable and everybody could then benefit from this increased synergy in sharing information.

A possible way to start with, could be planar message-passing architectures based on transputer processors. They are flexible enough to be re-configured to emulate many different decomposition paradigms."

The first paper in session B was given by a colleague of the keynote speaker. The paper presented by Dr Antonio da Rocha focused on the implementations of iterative image reconstruction algorithms on parallel computer architectures. An evaluation of ART algorithms for both X-ray transmission tomography and single photon emission tomography was given. This was followed by a performance assessment detailing the relative rates of convergence to a final solution and the subsequent quality of the reconstructed images. Finally, a SIMD-parallel computer architecture based on arrays of GLITCH processors developed at Bristol University was described. Simulation results for a 128 x 128 image vector were shown vindicating the ability of general-purpose SIMD machines to reconstruct near real-time images.

Dr da Rocha was asked two questions, the first was by Dr Bob Green: "What happens as the number of projections is reduced and will the system work, with reduced resolution, with only 10 or so projections?"

Answer: "The reduction of the number of projections will reduce the reconstructed image quality, but the algorithm will continue to work."

Dr Tom Dyakowski asked the second question: "Could your technique be employed on an underdetermined as well as an overdetermined problem and what would happen to the stability?"

Answered by Professor Borges co-author: "When an undetermined system is considered, the direct application of ART (addictive ART) will make it converge to a region of the solution hyperspace whose dimensionality is equal to the number of degrees of freedom of the system.

To make it converge further some prior knowledge of the solution is required to get additional constraints similar to those described by Andreas Wernsdörfer. When the system is inconsistent due to noise and imperfections on the adopted model of data collection, it is necessary to impose an optimisation criterion for the solution to converge to a class with desirable features such as the maximum entropy criterion (multiplicative ART)."

The second paper given by Mr Andreas Wernsdörfer from the University of Karlsruhe in Germany was concerned with reconstruction from limited data with a-priori knowledge. The paper described the vectorised ART algorithm, an extension of the scalar ART method, used to reconstruct a two-dimensional velocity field from ultrasound transducer data. Continuing additional a-priori information from the laws of mass and momentum conservation governing fluid mechanics an iterative reconstruction/restoration procedure was successfully developed.

Dr Bob Green asked Mr Wernsdörfer the following question "For a-priori knowledge can one use a physical model of the section of a flow pipe and could one use this approach in a pneumatic conveyor with only approximately 10 projections?"

Answer: "Air is a compressive medium so no simple model is available which has a practicable number of parameters. I have investigated a model for a vortex of water and have identified the parameters from the measured projection data. The problem is that it is not possible to detect if the real flow field differs from the model. Thus, I have decided to incorporate the differential equations at local points of the image."

Dr Brian Hoyle asked "Is it possible to extend your method, perhaps through quasi-linearisation or other techniques, to situations such as two-phase flows where some of your assumptions do not hold true?"

Answer: "The method I proposed can be applied to any particular reconstruction process. To incorporate the conservation laws is only an example for the application. The only condition is that you can formulate your a-priori knowledge in such a way that it can be applied to a local point of your image. There is no limitation to linear or non-linear problems."

The third paper was given by Mr Zaid Abdullah a research student in the Process Tomography Unit at UMIST. Mr Abdullah's presentation concerned the reconstruction algorithm used in the UMIST EIT system, the hardware description of which had been given previously in session A. The algorithm developed by Abdullah is an enhanced version of the modified Newton-Raphson algorithm described in 1987 by Yorkey. A description of the forward and inverse problems in EIT was given and reconstructed images from the fully determined architecture being developed at UMIST to tackle the envisaged computational burden imposed by increasing the mesh size to 464 elements.

Dr S H Khan asked the following question: "Why do you have such a small number of finite elements in field solutions and does this consequently introduce errors into the reconstruction algorithm?"

Answer: "To ensure that the system of equations is always determined. Yes, it will introduce some errors in the reconstruction algorithm and this is why we seek an approximate solution."

Dr Øyvind Isaksen asked a similar question "If you used a larger number of elements in the finite element solution and afterwards performed a mapping to the 104 elements would the reconstruction be more accurate?"

Answer: "Not really, increasing the number of elements in the forward problem will improve the accuracy. However, in the inverse problem to ensure that the system of equations is always determined the number of elements cannot be greater than the number of independent measurements."

Professor Dieter Mewes asked: "The local position of the interface in the hydrocyclone is changing with time. How is it recognised in the calculation since the calculated pathways of the electrical currents according to the differential equation are dependent on the actual cross-section of the two phases which might not be axisymmetric?"

Answer: "In our measurement system, the measurements are taken quickly enabling any interface reactions to be detected. These changes can either be removed by filtering our averaged out which means that the algorithm is not affected."

The fourth paper was given by Mr Juan Landauro and was entitled "Algorithm for optical process tomography". The presentation covered the application of an ART-like algorithm based on Kaczmarz's method for a limited amount of projection data, the hardware for which was described by Paul Dugdale in Section A. A concise description of the algorithm was given with reference to a simple example based on a 2 x 2 grid of values. Results from a trial test model of a human face were shown and it was noted that the accuracy of the algorithm was better than 80%

Dr Jon Salkeld asked questions concerning the pre- and inversion of matrices before entering the iteration process.

The fifth presentation was by Ms. Qi Chen, a PhD student at Leeds University. Her talk was concerned with the development of an enhanced reconstruction algorithm for use in capacitance process tomography based on the linearised backprojection algorithm. Due to the significant field interaction between the sensing electrodes and the process material it is necessary to attempt to overcome the inherent limitations in linear backprojection. The methods of modifying the permittivity distribution and subsequently the sensitivity distribution used in the iterative reconstruction algorithms were described.

Ms Chen was asked the following questions by Dr Jon Salkeld: "1. Will the 'soft-field' effect be worse for stratified flow than for well dispersed flow, or vice versa? 2. Assuming that, for bubbly flow, the concentration profile is a parabola about the axis, could such a model be used for a one-off approximation to perform image correction?

Answered by co-author Dr Brian Hoyle: "We have only investigated a small number of examples of flow regimes. The present aim is to examine the viability of the basic method -we have chosen systems where a high 'soft-field' error would be expected using backprojection based upon a 'uniform' sensitivity matrix."

The final presentation was given by Dr Jan Erik Nordtvedt from the University of Bergen, Norway and was also concerned with the reconstruction algorithm for a capacitance process tomography system. The implementation of the algorithm was somewhat similar to the one described by Abdullah in a previous presentation in that a finite element model is iteratively employed to solve the forward problem after modifying the parameters characterising, in this case, the dielectric distribution. The updating of the dielectric distribution was performed using the Gauss-Newton technique along with the Levenberg-Marquardt algorithm: A number of comparisons of the output from this new quantitative algorithm were made with respect to the existing linearised backprojection algorithm. Despite the increasing computational complexity, the algorithm showed great promise.

No questions asked directly after Dr Nordtvedt's presentation.

2. **Implications for future development of process tomography**

The chairman, Fraser Dickin, summarised the applications and algorithms described in the six presentations given during the session in the following table:

	Electrical	3
	X-Ray/Photon	1
Application	Ultrasound	1
	Optical	1
	Qualitative	3
	Quantitative	3
Algorithm	Iterative	6
	Architecture	4
	Limited data	2

Following comments made during the question periods, it was noted that this area of process tomography has a number of common interests and goals unlike the sensors which are almost specific for each particular application. As can be seen from the table above, there is an interest in quantitative algorithms generated by motivation from the process engineers to receive data which can be used to improve computational fluid dynamics models and other previously empirical derived models. The requirement for faster and more efficient computer architectures was highlighted in four of the presentations. All of the image reconstruction algorithms described were of an iterative nature, reinforcing the need for better computer hardware. Optical and ultrasound tomography will be the first measurement techniques to benefit from limited data reconstruction algorithms and it remains to be seen if the same methods will be employed in capacitance and process tomography.

To assist the industrial attendees, the 'deliverables', with respect to presently available image reconstruction algorithms, were categorised as follows:-

1. Fast 'real-time' **qualitative** reconstruction algorithm for on-line monitoring and control.
   - Good range of suitable/adaptable algorithms *e.g.* ART, SART, SIRT, VART, LBP *etc.*

2. Accurate **quantitative** reconstruction algorithm to validate/update existing CFD models
   - At present this can only be performed off-line due to large computational burden.

A short discussion then ensued, the contributors were: Professor Franz Mesch, Professor Erling Hammer, Dr Bob Green, Dr Chris McLeod, Dr Richard Williams,

Professor Dieter Mewes, Dr Arthur Naylor and Dr Brian Hoyle. The initial discussion centred around the type of information needed to visualise the process application. It was agreed that a reconstructed image, inherent in medical systems, was initially necessary in process tomography to establish confidence but thereafter quantitative information should be supplied. Following this it was suggested that image interpretation algorithms could be employed to provide such quantitative information. Finally, in tandem with feelings expressed in session A, it was suggested that criteria be established to assess the quality of reconstruction algorithms and associated data processing techniques.

A summary of the future technical needs for data processing, mathematical techniques and simulations are listed below in no order of priority:-

1.　　Improved/faster **quantitative** algorithm
- Reduce number of iterations by employing output of qualitative algorithm as first guess.
- Better accuracy by using larger number of finite element mesh elements.
- Use of sparse/vector matrix factorisation methods.

2.　　Three-dimensional forward problem solvers
- Will mean more elements & more nodes per element, therefore more computationally intensive.

3.　　Image reconstruction from a limited number of projections
- Liaison with Professor Mesch's group in Karlsruhe (present leaders).

4.　　Definition of 'real-time' as applied to image reconstruction
- What is an acceptable frame rate?

5.　　Parallel computer architecture to perform matrix manipulations on large double precision floating-point matrices in real-time.
- Is the SIMD architecture optimal?

6.　　Suitable benchmark by which reconstruction algorithms can be compared with respect to accuracy and performance

7.　　Multi-modal imaging
- Implementation

TECHNICAL SESSION: Equipment Design and Modelling

Session Chairman: Dr T Allen (E.I. du Pont de Nemours and Company, USA)
Session Reporter: Mr M Z Abdullah (UMIST, UK)

Summary of papers and discussion

In his opening remarks the Chairman noted that ECAPT was organized to foster interaction between European academic and industrial groups working on process tomography. The conference also summarized development in this field.

Process Tomography provides cross-sectional images of the distribution of material in pipes, fluidized beds, and reactors. In some cases it can also provide flowrate and flow velocities. A variety of detection methods have been used, including: x-ray attenuation, sonic and ultasonic time-of-flight, impedance, capacitance and inductance sensors. Much of the work presented at this conference dealt with electrical impedance tomography (EIT) and electrical capacitance tomography (ECT).

Although Tomography is in an embryo stage, it already provides information about phase separation and material transport and shows great promise in process development.

The Keynote speaker was Dr J B Middleton from the Fluid Dynamic Group of ICI Chemicals, Runcorn, who spoke on applications of tomography to chemical process development.

The session proceedings opened with a presentation on the use of a gamma-ray scanner to obtain tomographic images of gas fluidized and spouted beds given by Dr S J Simons from the University of Surrey. The scanner consisted of a single collimated photon beam of 5 mm diameter together with a single NaI detector. By means of a stepper motor, the source and detector are rotated through 180 degrees in 100 steps, around the area of interest. The tomographic images are obtained from the filtered back-projection. Experiments were conducted on a 51 mm semi-cylindrical fluidized bed of quartz sand at several scan heights. Tomographic images were obtained from 35 and 70 mm orifices for both dry and sticky solids. A questioner asked about the practical implementation of this method, and Dr Simons stated that he was not sure what modification would be needed for real process applications of this system.

The second speaker, Dr D J Parker from the University of Birmingham, spoke on process engineering studies (PET) using positron-based imaging techniques. Reconstruction is based on the back-projection convolution. Data acquisition is less than 300 events per second and data collection takes an hour and noise contamination severely degrades the image quality. For high speed process applications, such as tracking a large particle in a mixer, positron emitting particle tracking is necessary.

This was followed by a talk on advances in and prospects for the use of electrical impedance tomography (EIT) for processes, presented by Dr R A Williams of UMIST. Mixing behaviour in a stirrer tank was studied by video-imaging after injecting a dye, and the results were validated by the use of EIT. Image capturing using video is not possible unless the walls of the tank are transparent, but EIT does not suffer from this limitation. Tomographic imaging using EIT measurement can also be used for modelling the stirrer tank, and fluid flow cross-verification can be carried out using the standard CFD package. In order to extend the use of tomographic imaging for process control image, quantification is necessary.

Mr S L McKee, also from UMIST, spoke on the use of resistance and capacitance technology for monitoring and modelling fluid-based conveying processes. A practical limitation, in hydraulic conveying, was explained graphically. A questioner asked about the particle trade-off size in this graph, and Mr McKee replied that it depended on the tomographic instrument used. A second questioner asked the speaker about the number of electrodes needed in this type of equipment, and he replied that one should use as many as possible.

Finally, Mr M Faraj from Sheffield Polytechnic, discussed initial results using a prototype sensor to measure the pressure distribution on either side of a phantom model. Since the pressure is related to impedance, the cross-section of interest can be visualised by the use of EIT. Asked about the typical frequency, the speaker replied that the optimum frequency is that at which the changes in voltage with pressure distribution is a maximum, and this needs to be determined experimentally.

TECHNICAL SESSION: Process Monitoring and Control

<u>Session Chairman:</u>   Dr J E Nordtvedt (University of Bergen, Norway)
<u>Session Reporter:</u>   Mr S Quick (UMIST, United Kingdon)

1.   **Summary of papers and discussion**

Dr Chris Lenn, in his comprehensive keynote lecture, highlighted the 'grand challenge' to process tomographers attempting to develop multiphase flow measurement instruments. The need for long-term production monitoring of oil reservoirs to permit more effective economic exploitation especially in the North Sea could potentially eliminate production platforms with their associated problems. The platforms are mainly concerned with separating the fluids, metering them and then pumping them ashore. For three phase component measurement ie gas, water and oil, the flow meter must measure nine variables. However by making some assumptions a minimum of four variables are essential. The present process tomography systems can only deliver an image across a single plane and do not take into account slip velocity. Dr Lenn stated that more than one tomographic image would be necessary to attempt to solve the multiphase flow measurement problem unambiguously. He then went on to quickly review a number of potential oil industry applications to which process tomography would be suited:

i)   void fraction measurement in metering systems,
ii) flow regime identification with its associated problem of slip velocity thereby requiring :-
iii) velocity measurement,
iv) well monitoring of flow rates over extended periods
v)   more precise fiscal metering,
vi) corrosion detection and monitoring.

Dr Lenn concluded his presentation with a slide of a goldfish bowl representing a typical three phase measurement problem: the bowl has a flow rate of gas going through it, the flow of water is zero but the holdup is extremely high necessitating the measurement of more than one variable and finally, the fish do not contribute to the net flow.

Professor Mesch was the only person to ask Dr Lenn a question and wanted to establish why the phases separated on the platform were not metered before being recombined for pumping ashore. Dr Lenn answered this by stating that several operating companies had shares in each field and ideally the combined outputs from wells, each metered by a sub sea meter, would make the problem of getting the fluid to shore much cheaper.

The other papers and posters in this session were mainly addressed towards the problem of process monitoring. We have categorized the papers by the technique applied in the data acquisition.

a) Electrical Impedance Tomography:

Henriksson *et al* (Lund University, Sweden) presented the paper "Development of an EIT System for Thermal Mapping and Process Control". In this paper the EIT method is used for monitoring the temperature changes in a phantom. A new EIT system is under development in Lund.

b) Capacitance Tomography:

A transputer-based electrical capacitance tomography system for real-time imaging of oilfield flow pipelines was presented by Xie *et al* (UMIST, Schlumberger Cambridge Research, and University of Leeds, United Kingdom). The system presented used 12 capacitance electrodes for imaging gas/oil flow in pipelines, and was capable of reconstructing and displaying the distribution of each component of a flow over the pipe cross-section at 40 frames per second. However, by using the new generation of transputers (T9000), a 100 frames per second imaging speed can readily be achieved.

An experimental method for evaluating the performance of capacitance tomographic flow imaging systems was presented by Huang *et al* (UMIST and Schlumberger Cambridge Research, United Kingdom, Tsinghua University, China). Static physical models simulating typical flow distribution patterns were used as standard phantoms. Several criteria were proposed for quantitatively describing the system performance; signal to noise and input signal resolution ratios, cross-sectional area error, spatial image error, permittivity error, and component fraction measurement error. It might be emphasised that for an object with a permittivity at about 3 in an empty pipe, the minimum size that the imaging system can resolve is 0.2% (of pipe cross-section) near the pipe wall and 2% at the pipe centre.

Hayes *et al* (UMIST, United Kingdom) addressed the problem of velocity profile measurements in two-phase flow in pipes. They propose to obtain the velocity profile by cross correlating images from two capacitance tomography systems placed a short distance apart along the pipe to be monitored. They investigated the computational requirements for performing the cross correlation and presented suitable algorithms.

Brodowicz *et al* (Warsaw University, Poland and UMIST, United Kingdom) contributed a paper entitled "Application of capacitance tomography to pneumatic conveying processes", in which results from experiments monitoring pneumatic processes (transportation of seeds in air) using an 8 electrode capacitance tomography system were presented. The analysis was capable of providing significant information about which part of the flow structure was in motion and which was stationary. The images also provided void fraction field information - important information for further modelling of pneumatic transport.

c) Optical Tomography

In the poster session, one paper was presented: "Application of the optical tomography for education and laboratory research", by Plaskowski *et al* (Micromath, Poland). The tomograph device construction, the measurement algorithms, technical parameters, and experimental results are described in the paper. The optical tomograph allows simulation of four kinds of field patterns: parallel, grid,polar, and grid-polar. At each projection 40 measurements can be made, and a total of 144 projections are possible.

2.   Discussion

Dr Nordtvedt began by asking the question "What is needed for process tomography in industrial applications? Dr Chris Lenn responded by picking up on a point made by Professor Mesch in the previous session namely 'what information is needed from an image?' Dr Lenn pointed out that although imaging techniques are useful for a variety of reasons, in many cases, for example in a metering system, only a single value indicating the holdup or void fraction measurement is required hence obviating the need for an image. However, to develop multiphase science, particularly those aspects exploiting CFD models images are vital to enable the CFD parameters to be validated.

Professor Erling Hammer felt that we were not able, at this point, to fully utilize all of the information from a tomographic system since efficient process control is only possible by controlling all of the parameters of the process.

Dr Richard Williams suggested two priorities for studying the behaviour of mixing processes. The first was to obtain a high-quality quantitative image over a short time period and the second was to obtain 3D measurements.

Dr John Oakley picked up a point made by Mr Barrie Edwards concerning the use of artificial intelligence to 'understand' images from process tomography systems and suggested that such techniques are already available. Computers could be 'trained' in the future to identify subtle information changes in reconstructed images and the information acted upon.

In a written question to Dr Henriksson, Dr Holder asked:-

"In your calibration experiments, it is unclear what the units of resistivity are. What was the relation between actual temperature (measured by thermocouple) and the resistivity change in the EIT image? Was it linear?"

Dr Henriksson's prepared reply is:-

"Up until today we have been been using the Sheffield system in most of our experiments. This systems presents data using "relative impedance units". In figure 7, the relationship between the recorded relative impedance units and temperature, measured with thermistors, can be studied.

In the report "Temperature Measuring in Hyperthermia using Electric Impedance Tomography" (Blad B, 1991, internal report 7/91, Dept of Electrical Measurements, Lund Institute of Technology, LUTEDX/(TEEM-1045)/1-10) a coefficient k (resistivity value change/temperature change) was estimated. This coefficient has different values depending upon the distance from center.

dist	k [ohm m / degr (Celsius)
10 mm	-0.008
15 mm	-0.005
20 mm	-0.020

Due to the rather poor spatial resolution and the change in sensitivity depending upon distance from center, it is not possible to calculate the coefficient exactly nor to make any precise conclusions about the dependence.   However, we will study this relationship further."

After Dr Cheng Gang Xie's presentation, Dr Roger Waterfall sought clarification of the construction of the transputer array used to perform the backprojection algorithm. With the help of Dr Brian Hoyle, a co-author, it was pointed out that it was a MIMD system but performs SIMD-type operations by splitting the data from the acquisition system into separate channels.   Mr Øyvind Isakson wanted to establish whether Dr Xie's algorithm employed a thresholding operation before displaying the image of the flow pattern and if so did it have to be adapted to the flow regime. Dr Xie indicated that a thresholding was performed and that an adaptation is made based on the average void fraction change in the flow regime. He also mentioned that the image could be improved by employing an iterative and more time consuming reconstruction algorithm.

Dr Bob Green asked a question after Dr Song Ming Huang's presentation concerning the non-linear sensitivity field of the capacitance measurements inside the vessel and whether this non-linear effect was taken into account in the reconstruction algorithm. Dr Huang responded by saying that the sensitivity map is built into the algorithm, which goes some way towards alleviating the problem, although this could be tackled more directly by employing an iterative reconstruction algorithm.

Professor Brodowicz was asked by Dr Bob Green "What was the lowest phase concentration (solid/air ratio) that could be measured?" Professor Brodowicz replied that their system could go as low as 10%. Dr Juan Landauro tried to establish if the diameter of the pipe had any effect on the accuracy of the measurement. Professor Brodowicz stated that the diameter of the pipe was an industry standard 80 mm and could handle objects of 1 mm diameter.

After Mr Derek Hayes paper Professor Erling Hammer asked whether it was possible to obtain any information from the 'containment' component. Mr Hayes replied that this problem was being addressed and would probably be solved by obtaining additional data from another measurement technique. Dr John Oakley suggested that a reduction in the overall number of 'view' pixels and hence an improvement in correlation speed could be achieved by some form of feature analysis to identify the 'useful' pixels.   Professor Franz Mesch proposed that the order in which the correlation and tomographic reconstructions were performed could be reversed and that a tracking correlator could be used to improve overall performance. Mr Hayes agreed that, in principle, the order could be reversed but cautioned against it on the grounds that flow components were likely to alter inside inclined vessels. He had tried the tracking correlator and found that there was a danger of following the wrong maximum.

3.   Implications for future development of process tomography

Tomography is a large and fast growing research field, still mainly due to the value of the technique within medical diagnostics. The branch of process tomography, however, has over the past few years experienced an increase in interest, mostly because it is now possible to *monitor* processes non-invasively in quasi "real-time". Unlike medical tomography systems, for which an accurate image is in itself a goal, process tomography systems have to be able to provide estimates of variables (scalar quantities) which could be included in the control algorithms in a production plant. This is an absolute necessity if the control engineer is to find process tomography valuable not only for monitoring but also for *control* purposes. At this conference many papers have been presented describing equipment and algorithms, which in turn make it possible to build instruments capable of monitoring processes. However, none have actually looked at the control engineering aspect of the problem.

The two most commonly used techniques for process imaging (or *monitoring*) today are capacitance tomography and Electrical Impedance Tomography (EIT). The UMIST groups (United Kingdom) have shown that capacitance tomography can be used for monitoring two-phase flow in pipes and that the EIT system can be used for studying stirring and separation processes in hydrocyclones. We have also learned that the capacitance system can be used in thermal mapping and that a range of other systems are under development for other applications.

The current position is that a lot of effort has been put into the development of sensor systems, computer hardware, and reconstruction algorithms. One may argue that this is because process tomography is a rather new research field, and indeed process tomography experiences some new and quite difficult and challenging problems:

1. For measuring the development of processes on site, sensors as well as sensor configuration are extremely important. The fact that the instruments are going to be used on industrial sites constrains the engineer quite severely with respect to for example sensor electronics. The measuring principle in itself may be quite different from a laboratory device. For instance, in a laboratory a perspex pipe is quite acceptable, but the oil industry would definitely not allow a perspex pipe in, for example, an instrument monitoring subsea wells.

2. The computer hardware has to be powerful, small in size, flexible, and preferably cheap, in order to meet, for example, the requirements of low cost and "real-time" imaging. This is a big challenge and one which really pushes the limit of the computer technology.

3. The problem of reconstruction is a difficult one for many reasons. One is the limited amount of data usually available (28 for an 8 electrode capacitance tomography system as opposed to about half a million for a traditional CAT scanner) and the non-linearities involved in the measuring process. So far research has concentrated on overcoming these very difficult and challenging electronic and

computational problems. The interpretation of the images into control variables has been a neglected topic and inclusion of control engineers into the ECAPT "community" should be a major concern for the management in the near future.

Since one cannot buy a process tomography unit, with the exception of the universities and research companies, it is only the research departments in the large industrial companies that have paid attention to the development of this field. Hence the knowledge of process tomography within industry is most probably slight. It might also be a reason why there are not a large number of industrial applications (in particular within control) for process tomography, making the funding situation, at least in the future, quite difficult for the universities. Therefore, the need for at least two directions within process tomography is apparent; one being to improve the process tomography systems already developed and to develop new ones; and the another being to interpret the images in new ways and deduce control parameters from complex images. This calls for a survey of processes in which the internal structure of the process, for example the flow pattern information is crucial for the process to be optimized. The latter direction also calls for joint projects between the universities and industry; projects which should be promoted through the ECAPT organization, its technical meetings and workshops.

TECHNICAL SESSION: Environmental Monitoring

Session Chairman: Prof A Naylor (BNF plc, UK)
Session Reporter: Mr M Lee (UMIST, UK)

1.   **Summary of Papers and Discussion**

The Chairman introduced the keynote speaker Mr R B Edwards (Unilever Research, Port Sunlight). The speech was entitled "Opportunity For Tomography Application in the Environment".

Opportunity for Tomography Application in the Environment

In Mr Edwards' speech he considered the industrial applications of tomography, looking at the general situation and, in particular, environmental engineering. Here he subdivided the topic into three main groups.

a. Process measurement and control

In this section Mr Edwards displayed an interest in a heterogenous interrogating system where knowledge of property distribution is essential to measurements. Examples are the mass flow of a single phase in a multiphase system, and the use of tomographic imaging in sewers (this is discussed later in a presentation by Dr R Green).

b. Process modelling

Here he discussed the strong synergy between tomography and the verification of Computational Fluid Dynamics (CFD) packages. He commented on the need for tremendous amounts of information necessary for CFD verification and how the use of tomography could provide this information in an efficient way.

The topic of environmental control was also discussed in this section. Here the imaging of emission plumes was under consideration. Although many models exist there is some difficulty in verifying such models and therefore, a good opportunity for the application of tomography.

An example is the temperature and velocity fields in furnaces which is addressed later. In gas plume imaging Mr Edwards expressed the need for greater resolution to verify the models. Because the gas plume is unbounded it is unlikely to have a monitoring system on one side and an excitation system on the other to monitor the plume. A solution to the problem is "Scanning LIDAR" (LIght Detection and Ranging). This is a light analogue to radar where a short laser shot is fired at the plume and the reflected spectrum gives information on the optical density and position.

c. Environmental monitoring

The key phrase in this section is "Fugitive emissions". These are emissions which arise in an unplanned and uncontrolled manner and can arise at any point over a large area. Mr Edwards commented that point source technology is not applicable in this situation and it is an opportunity for tomography to scrutinise a large area over a long time to pinpoint emission quickly.

Large sites need to be monitored continuously and near real-time imaging is very important. To combat the problem a system called OTIM (Optical Transform Image Modulation) is used. This looks at the passive emission spectrum which gives an integrated line signal. The system has a fast response and good sensitivity.

Next he moved on to the problem of "Fugitive liquid emissions" and the use of Electrical Impedance Tomography (EIT) to monitor ground water emission plumes. Aided by a matrix of sensors in the ground, an emission plume could be located, assuming that its electrical conductivity were different from that of the surrounding area.

Mr Edwards then discussed time frames and how they varied according to the appplication. The two time frames, which are very important, are:

i)   data capture time (or aperture time)
ii)   data processing time

For process measurement and control it is necessary to have fast data capture, in relation to transport kinetics, and fast data processing, so that the operator can respond to any deviation in control. In process modelling it is desirable to have a rapid capture time, but the data processing may be slow in comparison. The data capture time in environmental monitoring may be slow, but it is essential that the processing time is fast in order to respond quickly.

Concluding the session Mr Edwards set a challenge to all present. He wanted to link tomography to spectroscopic techniques. This would allow near real-time imaging and the production of concentration maps.

There was a brief question and answer session. The first question directed towards Mr Edwards was "Is OTIM purely emissive or does it work on absorption as well as light going through?"

Mr Edwards replied *"The system works on the way natural light is modified when passing through the plume. It will not work in darkness"*.

Another question from Prof A Naylor (BNF plc) was *"Can it measure hot clouds, and does different cloud humidity and formation affect the image?"*

The answer given by Mr Edwards was *"Hot clouds produce a better image as there is a better emission spectrum"*.

Prof Naylor then went on to introduce the next speaker, Mr A Schwarz (University of Karlsruhe, Germany) and his paper entitled "Acoustic Measurement of Temperature and Velocity Fields in Furnaces".

Acoustic Measurement of Temperature and Velocity Fields in Furnaces

Mr Schwarz began his presentation by describing how the changing temperature distribution within furnaces can affect safety, control, and efficiency as well as avoiding high air pollution. He proceeded to discuss the principal ideas of his work, the use of an acoustic time-of-flight measurement, and the reconstruction techniques, Algebraic Reconstruction Technique (ART), used to solve the tomographic problems. Also there was a review of the simulation of the furnace and the effect of ray bending. (This work is described in more detail in the paper presented at the ECAPT meeting).

Following the presentation a number of questions were raised, the first from Mr Θ Isaksen (University of Bergen, Norway). His question was *"Are these results based on simulation or experimental results?"*

Mr Schwarz's answer was *"The results shown are all simulation, but there have been real temperature and velocity measurements from power stations".*

The next query from Prof E Hammer (University of Bergen, Norway) was, *"What kind of ultrasonic transducers have been used to cope with those temperatures and what frequency is used when penetrating gaseous streams. Is the acoustic impedance between transducer and gaseous stream very high?"*

The reply was *"Transmitters using spark discharge; receivers using industrial microphones".*

Prof Hammer then asked *"Is it low frequency?"*

The answer was *"the frequency used is 2-4 Khz and is detected by a trigger level".* Prof Hammer then inquired *"What about the temperature and the microphone?"*

Mr Schwarz explained that *"The boundary temperature is approximately 800K. The microphone is mounted in holes in the wall and are protected."*

Dr R Williams (UMIST) probed *"What influence does the amount of dust in hot gases have on the measurements?"*

The answer was *"It is difficult to correct if the amount of dust suddenly varies. Calculation of all errors that may occur are considered and a 2% error in the reconstruction is incurred."*

The final question was from Dr R Jackson (Bolton Institute) who asked *"If the flame was to flicker whilst doing the experiment would the Fermat's principle correction that you apply run fast enough to cope with flicker or does it work on steady state?"*

Mr Schwarz's response was *"The results were averaged over 10 measurements. Each path was measured 10 times."*

Dr Jackson then asked *"What are the time intervals?"*

The reply *"5 - 7 minutes."*

Pursuing the matter further Dr Jackson then asked *"Can you watch the instability?"*

"It is difficult to get dynamic measurements" was the reply.

Prof. Naylor then introduced the next paper, presented by Dr R Green (Sheffield Polytechnic), entitled "Initial Findings on a Tomographic Imaging System for Sewers."

Initial Findings on a Tomographic Imaging System for Sewers

Dr Green reviewed the aim of his project which is to determine size and concentration of solids in stone sewers. He talked about how sewer designers had models, but needed on-line measurements to back-up the models and in the long term to improve the quality of water in rivers.

He discussed the current situation where the liquid level and flow rate may be measured using commercially available ultrasonic sensors. However, at present solids are determined by weighing dried solids collected in bags over a weir in the sewer and the aim is to eliminate this crude procedure. Another objective is to provide concentration and size profiles and to try and make them more specific.

The problems associated with the process were then discussed. These were:

Hazards   - the presence of poisonous and explosive gases which could disrupt instrument readings

Solids   - which can smear everything

Tissues   - which can stick and wrap round objects (ragging)

Level   - measurements depend on the level. As the boundaries are not fixed this causes a major problem in imaging

This is therefore a possible application for tomography. Dr Green suggested that he wanted to image the following: faeces, cellulose products (tissues and rags), rubber items and liquid. Looking at the sensors available he did not seem to be able to choose a single sensor, which could detect all the constituents. He found that ultrasound could detect faeces, liquid level and velocity, but not rubber and cellulose products. This led to his decision to use both impedance and infra-red sensors. By combining the two, (impedance can detect faeces, rubber and liquid conductivity while infra-red can detect solids and paper) all the constitutes may be measured. His reasons for using these sensors are that they are cheap and small and therefore many sensors can be used, with little effect on the sewer.

In the work Dr Green commented on aiming for a crude system. A dual modality problem arises as they do not know if the 2 sets of measurements when overlaid will assist or blur the image.

Next Dr Green went on to describe the system, the experimental work and the results. He found that the results were very repeatable. They wished to determine the voltage change from the phase shift variations, which were affected by the frequency values.

Following the session a number of questions were asked, the first from Dr R Waterfall (UMIST). *"It is known that electrodes are prone to contamination, aging and polarization and without conditioning and calibration, results can be variable, even meaningless. What sort of electrodes would be used in your sewer monitoring EIT equipment?"*

To which Dr Green replied, *"The system is meant for test purposes initially, so they are not left in for long periods. If the system is effective then we will develop for long periods."*

Dr Waterfall further commented *"Chemists use known solutions and look up tables to decide on an answer."*

Dr Green agreed that *"Electrodes are a problem at present"*.

Prof Hammer (University of Bergen, Norway) asked *"What is the number of degrees of phase shift measured?"*

Dr Green's answer *"About 10 degrees. They are low values and very repeatable"*.

Prof Hammer then further queried Dr Green by asking *"Though the current is conducted, doesn't it mean there is no phase shift?"*

His reply *"So I'm told, but there is"*.

The final question was from Mr E Etuke (UMIST) *"Does the concentration of the base solution affect the phase shift?"*

The answer *"Don't know. We need to find a range of conductivity in sewers"*.

Following the "question and answer" session there was a discussion on the whole session of ENVIRONMENTAL MONITORING. It began with Dr Waterfall (UMIST) asking the keynote speaker, Mr Edwards (Unilever Research) to comment on *"EC funding and funding as a whole"*.

Mr Edwards replied that *"There may be funding available from sensor companies."*

Prof Beck (UMIST) added *"We need to enlarge the number of people from different fields coming to the meeting to widen interest"*.

Prof Naylor (BNF plc) further commented *"We need to have complimenting schemes"* thus concluding the discussion session.

3.   **Implications for Future Development of Process Tomography**

With more attention being paid to the environment, industry continues to assess all aspects of pollution.

In general, the chemical industry examines environmental conditions and pollution mainly from three aspects:-

    i)   minimisation of waste streams by consideration of optimum design and effluent conditions
    ii)   evaluation of hazards and maloperation, where release of pollutants might occur.
    iii)   monitoring of waste streams to detect contaminents and ensure regulatory requirements have been met.

Process tomography can play a major role in the latter two cases, and in these cases it is important to develop sensor reliability and accuracy, and also fast response times rather than precise imaging of data.

As indicated, (Edwards lecture) optical tomography coupled with other analytical techniques, such as spectroscopy, could assist greatly the monitoring of gaseous emissions from many industrial processes. Similarly the environmental evaluation of land-fill sites could be carried out by the use of resistance tomography along with conventional analytical techniques to measure water concentration and model ground water flow.

Both in solid/liquid and liquid/liquid separation processes, tomography can prove of value in measurement of change in flow phase conditions and in determining concentration of solid particles for process control and detection of maloperation. In hydraulic and pneumatic conveying of solids and in the handling of slurries, again process tomography can play a valuable part in control systems.

The use of process tomography in the many fields of environmental monitoring will certainly increase over the next few years and it will be necessary to develop reliable sensors and encourage industry to carry out development tests on selected process cases where tomography can improve detection and measurement of contaminants in control equipment and waste streams.

TECHNICAL SESSION: Tomography in Perspective

Session Chairman: Mr J D Tallantire (SERC, UK - Co-ordinator control and instrumentation)

Session Reporter: Mr M Lee (UMIST, UK)

1.   Summary of papers and Discussion

Mr D Tallantire (SERC) as the chairman began by taking stock of "Where we have got to and where we are going".

As an aside, he then added that funding is available from SERC for academic/industrial collaboration on measurement research, as long as half the funds can be raised by the institute.

Mr Tallantire then introduced the first paper presented by Mr F McArdle (IBEES) entitled "Medical Application of Impedance Tomography".

Medical Applications of Impedance Tomography

Mr McArdle began his presentation by querying the need for another medical imaging technique such as EIT and listing the advantages of EIT such as the portability, size and cost of the system as well as being non-invasive.

He went on to discuss the main problem with the medical EIT system which was that the boundaries are not fixed but "squiggly". Small electrodes cannot be placed with any accuracy thus leading to the development of electrode bands. The latest development in this area is *screen printed electrodes* which allows electrodes to be in a single plane. Because the boundary is not circular the electrodes do not need to be equally spaced out, thus leading to the second development *hydrogel*. This is a conductive adhesive for the electrodes.

A problem encountered was the limited amounts of data collected; 16 electrodes can only produce 104 measurements. This was then reviewed by Mr McArdle.

He went on to describe what EIT has been used for. One application is to look at the impedance changes in the stomach, using food as a contrast medium. Another is to image changes in lung resistivity this time using air as the contrast medium. A set of slides illustrated the uses. Mr McArdle also commented that the impedance correlations were very close to those obtained using *Gamma camera* techniques - the standard. Other applications were:
- abnormal lung ventilation
- blood volume changes
- lung blood perfusion
- monitoring local temperature changes
- measuring blood flow

These were also illustrated with the use of slides. Possible applications include the measurement of cardiac output and diagnosis of brain death. Mr McArdle stated that the monitoring of brain output is possible but there is a need for advances in spatial resolution. Although the resolution does not have to be as good in the diagnosis of brain death a greater sensitivity is required.

Ending his presentation, he said he wanted future technological advances to include a more portable, real-time, multi-frequency system with improved spatial resolution.

The first question aimed at Mr McArdle was from Prof Hammer (University of Bergen, Norway) who wanted to know *"What is the dynamic response of your impedance imaging system? How long do you need to obtain an image?"*

The answer was *"We can collect 24 frames per second, but tend to average 40-50. The signal-to-noise ratio for real time imaging is 70dB"*.

This prompted a further question from Prof Hammer *"So can you measure muscle blood perfusion?"*

The reply - *"At present, no"*.

The next question from Dr R Williams (UMIST, United Kingdom) was *"Has anyone tried multiple sensor belts?"*

The response was *"Yes, but no positive results have been obtained at present"*.

Mr Tallantire proceeded to introduce the next speaker, Prof Beck (UMIST, United Kingdom) and his presentation entitled "Current State of Process Tomography".

Current State of Process Tomography

Prof Beck began by talking about the information available from the group status report, discussing deliverables from the concerted action and the procedures to obtain these deliverables. He went on to say that partnerships concerning research, development and users of the system are required to make *Process Tomography* successful. He then examined the number of groups and the peoples involved, in *Process Tomography*.

He went on to describe the necessary requirements for success which were:
  - task coordination. The methods of bringing new people into the activity.
  - cooperation. The need for research teams of instrument designers and process experts to get together.
  - suitability for purpose. To make something which will be used; to avoid extravagant claims and unfulfilled expectations.

He gave an example of an unfulfilled expectation; a "Sinclair C5".
This was innovative and oversold, but reliability, safety and suitability for purpose were questionable.

Prof Beck then introduced Dr L Stott (UMIST) to talk about "Standards in Process Tomography".

Dr Stott first discussed standards concerned with manufacturing standards to enable the buyer to be sure equipment is suitable for its purpose and to ensure compatibility. He went on to say that Process Tomography was not at the stage of discussing manufacturing standards, but it is useful to have standards to enable performance of different systems to be quantitatively assessed and to enable a comparison of equipment. He talked about possible items for standards. These included performance criteria for measuring systems, reconstruction systems and the total system in order to define tests to assess equipment against each other. Another possible criteria is fidelity. Looking at many different standards for techniques and applications, things which need to be considered include, cross-sectional accuracy and discrimination, position, density and reconstruction time. He suggested the use of some standard tests for simulated flow patterns (core, annulus and stratified) and the use of standard phantoms.

He proceeded to look at the possible problems. The standards required need to cover a number of different techniques and applications.

Dr Stott then asked if it is possible to devise standards, if it was desirable and if we are at the stage where we can define standards. If the answers are yes then how do we proceed to establish the standards.

This ended his contribution and he returned the session to Prof Beck who continued to talk about the necessary requirements to make tomography successful. This meant that the users (industry) and the researchers had to get along with the instrument manufacturers so that each group knows what is required from the other. This has been achieved by the ECAPT meeting.

Mr F McArdle (IBEES) commented on standards on the medical side and the Cardiff "standard" phantom, which is a 16 electrode impedance array with plug in parts so equipment and algorithms can be compared.

Prof Beck spoke about the ability to test electrical and computational integrity of systems, which is the primary requirement, leading to standards concerning electrodes and other parts of the system. He closed the session by saying that it was easier to split up the system rather than define standards for the whole system.

Dr R Green (Sheffield Polytechnic) asked Prof Beck "Is it time that some thought was given to producing standardised two component flow rigs with a calibrated sensor section which can be used to standardise other instruments to determine accuracy?"

The reply was "Yes. We should seek funding and find good ways to hold and use the standard plants".

A discussion on the session "Tomography in Perspective" followed with the chairman saying "It is difficult to envisage an all singing and all dancing standard which serves for all applications. It may be possible to derive something at this stage which could later on produce marriages resulting in more flexible arrangements. Even now there is a need for standards to allow people to decide how far they've got and whether they're going in the right direction".

Dr R Waterfall went on to comment on the time to introduce standards and produced a graph containing two "humps" and called it the "Apocalypse of the Two Elephants". Describing the curves he went on to say that *"there is an initial upsurge in research activity, followed by industrial production of the successful ideas. The optimum time for the formulation and introduction of standards is after the first hump and before the second."*

Referring to the humps Prof Beck predicted that there could be a fall in the number of people in *Process Tomography* after the research phase with a consequent lack in continuity.

Mr Tallantire then suggested that there may be a way of coalescing the humps.

Industrial visit to ICI (Chemicals and Polymers) Friday 27th March
Organised by Dr John Middleton of ICI

As part of the conference programme a visit was arranged for two parties of up to twenty persons to visit the following sites in the Runcorn area:

    i)   KLEA-134a at Rocksavage
    ii)   Fluid Dynamics Research laboratory at Widnes
    iii)   Chlorine plant at Castner-Kellner

The Cheshire chemical industry was founded in the 19th century using the local deposits of rock salt. Chlorine is produced by the well-established technique of electrolysing brine (pumped from their saltworks at Northwich) using a flowing mercury cathode. Although the plant is fully equipped with process-monitoring instrumentation, virtually all of the process-control, such as adjusting the cathode-anode spacing, is carried out manually.

At the Fluid Dynamics Research laboratory a selection of mixing vessels ranging from 500mm to 1500mm in diameter are installed in experimental rigs that can be instrumented for various research activities. In the next months, one of these vessels will be fitted with transducers for Electrical Impedance Tomography (EIT) experiments.

The KLEA-134a plant is a pilot production plant which produces small commercial quantities of an ozone-friendly chloro-fluorocarbon (CFC) replacement. The process uses hydrofluoric acid (HF). The extremely corrosive nature of hot HF means that all the pipework is manufactured from a copper-nickel alloy, Inconel, and the HF must not be allowed to cool from the vapour phase because even this alloy is not resistant to attack from wet HF. However, too high a temperature can result in fragmentation of the catalyst and this highlights the importance of accurate temperature monitoring and control in this plant.

The visits were of particular interest to the young research staff and students as it provided an opportunity to see the scale of industrial plants and experience the international dimension of the chemical industry. They also showed delegates the scope for applying tomographic techniques to pipes, mixers and reactor vessels and illustrated the relationship between laboratory-scale equipment, pilot plants and full-scale production facilities.

The importance of accurate process monitoring and control was very apparent on these visits, not only to maximise plant output but also to prevent the occurrence of an environmental incident. The ECAPT programme has an important contribution to make in developing process tomography to a point where it can be applied to plant-scale applications, such as the ones at ICI, and will assist the European effort to lead the world in this area.

CONCLUSIONS AND STRATEGY FOR INDUSTRIAL EXPLOITATION

The papers presented and discussed at this first Workshop provide an overall view of the current situation of *process* tomography. Most of the work described has started in universities during the previous 4 or 5 years. Process tomography is an enabling technology, in that the methods are frequently of general applicability to a wide range of industrial applications. However, it is noteworthy that a significant amount of the work reported was 'user demand led'.

Of the 34 papers in this book, a total of 24 include industrially sponsored work. Nine refer to work supported by the oil industry and 15 to work supported by process industries. The extent of oil industry support is not surprising because of the worldwide need to exploit new and marginal oil resources. The process industry presents a more diverse range of applications, each representing a lower capital resource and turnover than that of oilfield installations. However, as the process industry emerges from the present European recession, there is evidence that the need for increased efficiency will lead to a greater need to develop and implement appropriate tomographic instrumentation. Most critically, innovation in the area of modelling and simulation of a wide variety of existing and new process technologies is required, and optimisation of plant-scale equipment.

An emerging requirement, highlighted during the Workshop, is the need to develop tomographic methods for environmental monitoring and control. Such applications range from monitoring airborne gas and groundborne liquid emissions, through to using on-line tomographic instrumentation to provide better control for efficient combustion in power station boilers and in automobile engines.

Table 1 illustrates the balance of activity across the EC and specially invited non-EC organisations attending ECAPT. It shows that there is a workforce of 80 fulltime-equivalent scientists and engineers developing process tomography, spread over 20 institutions in 8 countries. The geographical spread is dominated by the large amount of work started in the UK in the early 1990's; there is a need to extend the subject to more EC countries. In particular, these statistics do not include a number of other workers who are active in nucleonic-based tomographic sensing methods, some of which are pertinent to the process applications.

We have been pleased with the synergy developed in association with medical tomography, particularly in electrical impedance tomography (EIT) which can be used for both medical and industrial applications. The medical EIT activity is the subject of a Brite-Euram Concerted Action on Electrical Impedance Tomography (CAIT). Similarly to process tomography, medical EIT started in research centres, and applications to clinical medicine are now emerging. To illustrate this, the coverage of a medical EIT applications conference, held in April 1992, is given in Appendix 3 and a critical paper describing a future medical application is included in Chapter 5.

TABLE 1 - ECAPT 1992 STATUS REPORT SUMMARY

GROUP	No. of people	GOALS
Aviero	3	Computer architectures for reconstruction
Barcelona	5	Multifrequency E.I.T. moisture measurement
Bergen	7 + 8 Masters students	Three phase tomography based on capacitance & gamma techniques
Birmingham	10	P.E.T. process fundamentals & on-line operation
Bolton	5	Optical tomography for laboratory & industrial use
Chr. Michelsens Institute	5	Multiphase flow. On-line chemometric & tomographic measurement
City University	3	2D/3D FEM for optimal sensor design. CAD of tomographic instruments
Delft	3	Dispersion of tagged particles. EIT for process use (including velocity measurement)
Hannover	4	Temperature, concentration & velocity fields in process equipment
Karlsruhe	4	Improving algorithms to reduce number of views. Tomographic measurements of temperature fields
Leeds	5	Real time ultrasonic tomography. Parallel reconstruction processing. Reducing field interaction errors.
Lund	7	Non-invasive temperature measurement. Multifrequency E.I.T.
Manchester	3	Image reconstruction & analysis. E.I.T. for stirred vessels
Micromath, Poland	3	E.C.T. for gas/solids flows. Optical tomography for laboratory & industrial use. E.I.T.
Schlumberger	2	Tomography for 2-phase flow investigations. Determine feasibility of oilfield applications. Tomographic measurements in multi-phase hydrocarbon flows
Sheffield Poly	6	Electrodynamic tomography. Multi-component flow in open channels. Optical fibre system for pneumatic conveyors
Surrey	6	Models for granular flows. Design & control of fluidised & spouted beds. X-ray scatter tomography for industrial-scale plants
UMIST Chemical Engineering	6	E.I.T. of process plant. E.C.T. for pneumatic conveying. 3D tomography
UMIST Electrical Engineering	16	3-component flow. Specificity & dual-mode imaging. Reconstruction with unusual geometry & missing projections. Process control using tomography.
Warsaw University	4	Solids mass flow measurement. Investigating stratified & slug flow regimes

TOTAL 20 GROUPS   108 PEOPLE   (say 80 full-time equivalent)

The formation of subgroups concerned with specific sub-systems of an overall process tomography system, was suggested by some attendees. Whilst acknowledging that the ECAPT should meet the need of developing process tomography on a basis of 'fitness for purpose' which requires an overall systems approach at the present stage, we believe that some job-specific subgroups may be needed; a report on an embryo subgroup concerned with sensors is given in Appendix 2.

Specific recommendations

1.   Strategic development of tomographic technology

The present volume represents a statement of the status of tomographic techniques applied to process engineering within Europe and the European Community. It is evident that future implementation of the technology will depend upon the successful integration of the component disciplines, which embrace specialist skills in physics, digital electronics, optics, computation, image analysis, process engineering and process control.

These skills are spread throughout the Community and need to be harnessed through continued, but closer, collaboration. In this context the present Coordinated Activity has a vital role to play but, alone, it will be insufficient to allow development of instruments for transfer into the industrial environment. ECAPT provides a forum to enable partnerships to be developed which can identify strategic technological problems, which can then be tackled via funded research. Some of the partners are already active and have the necessary resources for research, whilst others (most) do not. The following needs are evident:-

    i)   Expansion of *new* collaborative research activities with industrial (user) partners, resourced by EC and national means.

    ii)   More industrial-scale testing of emerging instrumentation at early stages in the development of a technique.

    iii)   Continued definition of, and interaction between the common technologies involved in tomographic technology, particularly in image reconstruction techniques and computational methods.

    iv)   More effective publicity and interaction with the process engineering community. For example, via presentation at existing engineering conferences rather than solely at specialised sub-discipline meetings; production of appropriate circulars, articles in professional and trade journals within all the countries participating in the ECAPT activity.

    v)   More specific targeting of industrial needs, for instance, in the areas of process and environmental control. This may involve integration of different types of tomographic sensor within the same instrument.

2.   Technological developments

To date the different tomographic techniques have been classified on the basis of 'sensor' type, with individual research groups tending to specialise in *one* type of sensor. It is recognised that often this is not the best scenario to meet industrial needs which are driven by measurement problems that may not be met by a single technique. Hence, the need for terms to define user needs (imaging speed, spatial resolution, sensitivity etc) and matching these to appropriate tomographic methods is essential. This can be achieved by invoking an integrated design strategy, supported by a database.   At present this is impeded by the lack of appropriate technical terminology and definitions of performance. This is by no means a trivial task since the various types of sensor have different attributes. However, it is an essential task in enabling industrial needs to drive the development of tomographic technology in the appropriate direction, and so identify technological bottle-necks within the instruments. The following needs are evident:-

i)   Targeting of specific technical limitations common to tomographic techniques. Key areas include:
        a)   selection and design of computer architecture for given tasks
        b)   development of image interpretation software coupled with process modelling
        c)   attention to the specific needs reported in the technical session reports in Part I.

ii)   Development of standard nomenclature and testing procedures embracing all the common sensor transducers to enable comparison of methods, and for use in i).

iii)   To evaluate the feasibility of establishing an integrated computer design package for specifying tomographic requirements for given industrial needs.

3.   Future development of ECAPT

ECAPT seeks to encourage the outworking of the strategic development of tomographic technology, as listed in 1 above. Having identified the general status of the technology, the focus of attention will now shift to the promotion of interaction between appropriate researchers and industrial users to tackle the key stages, which are governing the speed of transfer of tomographic technology into industrial practice. In future annual meetings this will be achieved by several small specialist workshop meetings covering technological developments listed in 2 above), coupled with two or three strategic overview presentations and poster presentation sessions.

PART II

WORKSHOP PROCEEDINGS

Chapter 1

Sensors

Optical Sensors For Process Tomography

P. Dugdale, R.G. Green*, A.J. Hartley, R.G. Jackson, J. Landauro

School of Engineering, Bolton Institute of Higher Education, Bolton BL3 5AB, U.K.
*Dept. of Engineering I.T., Sheffield City Polytechnic, Sheffield, S1 1WB, U.K.

ABSTRACT: This paper describes the further development of optical sensor hardware for a process tomography system in which infra-red emitters and detectors are used to exploit the optical characteristics of multiphase flow regimes. The system allows sufficient data to be captured, within the restricted time period of typical industrial processes, to produce a reconstructed tomographic image. The relation of the image to the transducer positions is discussed, and a comparison of resolution is made for different arrangements using the same reconstruction.

1.   INTRODUCTION

The work on optical sensors follows on from that done previously, enabling the necessary tomographic image reconstruction information to be obtained from a cross-section of 2 phase flow, (Dugdale et al 1991). By collimating radiation from a light source and passing it through a flow regime, the intensity of radiation detected on the opposite side is related to the distribution of the different phases and their absorption coefficients in the path of the beam. Data from an array of beams covering a cross-section of flow forms the basis for image reconstruction.

It is intended to show how the problems of data capture, in particular speed and optical management, have been overcome. Another factor affecting the resolution is the arrangement of transducers around a cross-section. This is a compromise between physical limitations and the requirements of particular reconstruction algorithms. Two such arrangements, orthogonal 8 x 8 and 16 x 16 will be discussed later and comparisons of resolution made using phantoms in a Perspex pipe of 12cm diameter cross-section with a phantom. The algorithms with which they are used are described fully in (Landauro et al 1992).

2.   DATA CAPTURE

Data capture circuitry has been developed to handle information from up to 64 pairs of optical transducers, arranged in groups or arrays of 8. The transducers of each array are numbered 1 to 8. An eight channel analog multiplexer pulses the corresponding emitters of each array simultaneously for approximately $25\mu s$ with a current of 2A. Thus the total time to pulse all the emitters in one array is $200\mu s$.

Since transducers in additional arrays are pulsed simultaneously this time is independent of the number of arrays. The pulse of current gives rise to a high intensity beam of IR radiation which in turn produces a voltage at the corresponding photodiode (Fig. 1).

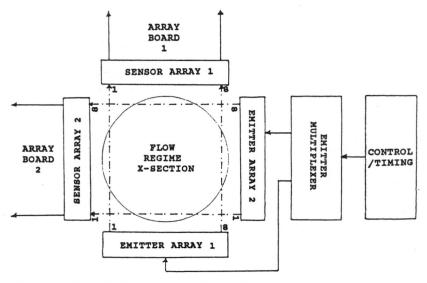

Fig. 1 : Schematic diagram of system using only two transducer arrays

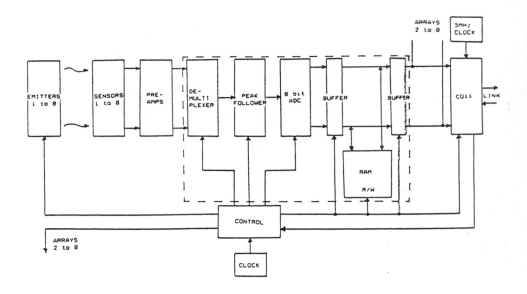

Fig. 2 : Transducer array pcb

Each array of detectors is controlled by its own array board, (Fig. 2). On this the analog voltage from each sensor is passed, after pre-amplification, to a sample and hold, converted into an 8 bit digital number and stored in a RAM. Sampling and A to D conversion occur simultaneously on adjacent boards. These boards plug into the same back plane which connects the output buses of all the boards via buffers to a C011 transputer interface chip. The C011 is multiplexed in turn to the RAMs, accepting the data from each array in turn, and passing it via its linkline into a transputer network.

Since the transputer accepts data at the rate of $\approx 0.8\mu s$ per bit an 8 bit word takes $\approx 1\mu s$ to send. However, the necessary handshaking involved adds a further $1\mu s$. The total time to send 8 such words is then approximately $16\mu s$. Since the emitters are pulsed for $25\mu s$, it is possible to access data from the RAM of an array between passing data to it from the sensors. The multiplexing of eight transducer pairs per array up to eight such RAMs, i.e. eight arrays. In this way the data capture time, for one cross-section remains at $200\mu s$, independent of the number of arrays. This is important since at maximum industrial flow rates of $10ms^{-1}$ a cross-section of flow will have moved 2mm in $200\mu s$. A slower data capture time would result in the cross-section changing as it is being investigated.

3.   OPTICAL MANAGEMENT

One of the major advantages of using infra-red radiation over other methods of obtaining tomographical data is its directional nature once configured into a beam. In order to obtain such a beam from an SFH 401 LED, a small planoconvex glass lens was used, 5mm diameter, 8.7mm back focal length. Initially, the LED was placed at the focal length of the lens. The resulting beam was approximately collimated, with the highest intensity of radiation being within a 5mm diameter. However, over the width of the pipe ($\approx 12cm$) the beam diverged enough to cover a region of 20mm diameter with radiation greater than background. Obviously since the LED had a diameter of 4.6cm it did not appear as a point source to the lens. However, such a set up was used for the orthogonal 8 x 8 transducer system (see Section 4), to accommodate 16 x 16 arrangements around a pipe of diameter 12cm a narrower beam was required. For this a small cylindrical disc was placed between the lens and the LED, in the centre of which was a pin hole. The lens was placed 8.7mm in front of the disc (see Fig. 3) which acted more like a point source. The resulting beam was better collimated, for only a small loss in intensity.

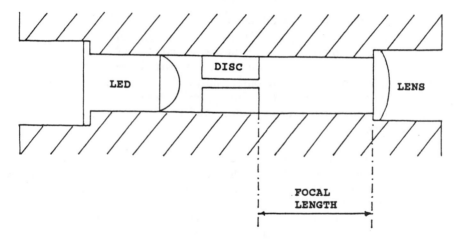

Fig. 3 : Collimation of IR radiation from an LED

For non-diametrically opposed transducer pairs the curved glass surface of the pipe affects the path of the beam. From Fig. 4 it can be seen that refraction at the walls of the pipe causes beams spaced evenly outside the pipe to move closer together inside the pipe. To get evenly distributed beams inside the pipe, the transducers need to be spaced irregularly outside. The effect is heightened the further from the diameter one moves. In practice this effect is only significant for the 2 outermost beams on both sides of the array.

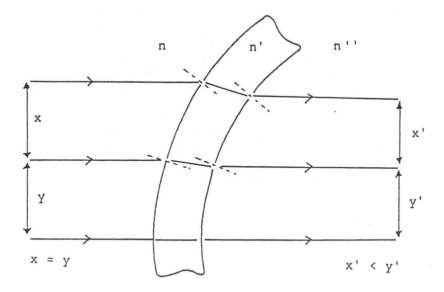

Fig. 4 : Refraction effect of perspex pipe wall on beams

4. TRANSDUCER ARRANGEMENTS

Having developed a data capture system that can accommodate any number of transducer arrays, from one to eight, initial work was carried out using the simplest arrangement possible. This consisted of two arrays of eight transducers each, placed along orthogonal projections to one another. The arrangement was built around a cross-section of Perspex pipe. Fig. 5 shows the beam width and spacing inside the pipe for one array. Although the beam diameter is approximately 5mm, the width of detectable beam is only 2mm. This is because the active area of the pin photodiode detector is only 4mm². The resulting gap between beams is then effectively 13mm. These two distances, beam width and gap between beams are critical factors in the resolution of the system. It cannot be guaranteed that regions of the minor phase with diameter less than 13mm will be detected.

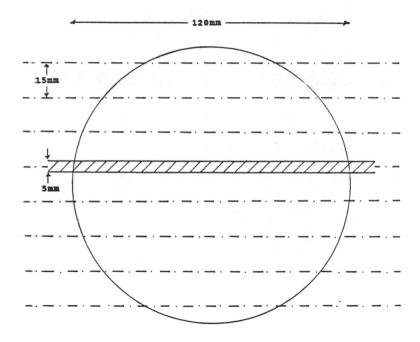

Fig. 5 : Dimensions of 8 transducer projection

The transducers were connected via the data capture system to the transputer network. This used a simple back-projection algorithm to reconstruct an image of the pipe cross-section and output it to VDU. Various rods of decreasing diameter were moved vertically around the pipe as phantom models. Below a certain diameter the image of the rod intermittently disappeared from the screen as it became lost in the gaps between the beams. The image of the smallest continually displayed rod is shown in Fig. 6.

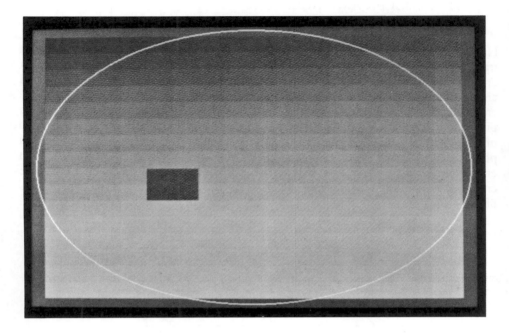

Fig. 6 : Image from 8x8 orthogonal arrangement

To increase this resolution the sensor arrangement was changed, with two arrays of 8 now along each projection resulting in an orthogonal 16 x 16 arrangement. It was only possible to place the detectors so close, without interference from adjacent beams, due to the optical management described in Section 3. Fig. 7 shows the new beam layout for one projection. Again various diameter rods were imaged and the resolution improved, as shown in Fig. 8. Minor phase regions of diameter 5.5mm and above are guaranteed to be detected. Smaller regions will suffer a finite probability of going undetected and this will increase as their size is reduced.

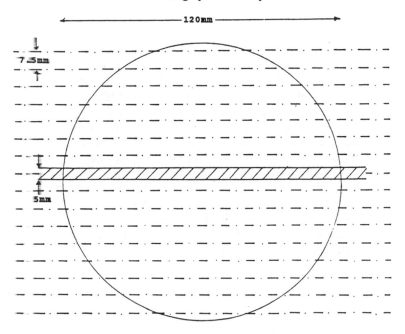

Fig. 7 : Dimensions of 16 transducer projection

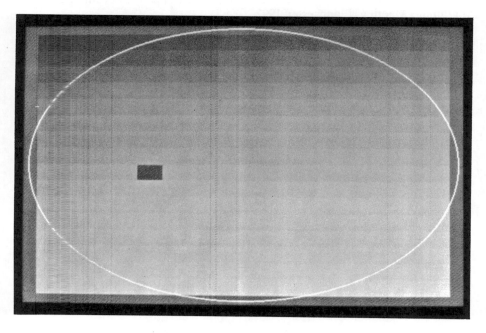

Fig. 8 : Image from 16x16 orthogonal arrangement

5.   CONCLUSIONS

From the previous section it is possible to see the relative ease with which the resolution of an optical tomography system can be increased. Further improvements can be made by increasing the number of transducer pairs along a projection. In addition, increasing the area of beam that the pin photodiode can detect by using a lens to focus the whole of the beam onto its sensitive area. Both these methods result in the gap between beams being reduced, but would require a high degree of precision in the alignment of the optics. It is felt that 16 transducers per projection is the optimum hardware design for the present. Any further improvements in resolution will have to come with the addition of more projections to the system, requiring a change in algorithm. The data capture system can accommodate data from a further two projections of 16 transducer pairs. An extra orthogonal arrangements at 45° to the present will lead to a reduction in the proportion of the pipe that is not interrogated by IR beams. The method is capable of delivering resolution of at least 2mm over the whole pipe cross-section.

REFERENCES

Dugdale P., Green R.G., Hartley A.J., Jackson R.J. and Landauro J. 1991. *"Optical tomographic imaging in industrial process equipment"*, pp227-232 in "Sensors : Technology, Systems and Applications ed K.V. Grattan, Adam Hilger 1991. (Proc 5th IOP Conference on Sensors and their Applications, Edinburgh 1991).

Landauro J., Dugdale P., Green R.G., Hartley A.J. and Jackson J. 1992. *"Algorithm for optical process tomography"*, in Proceedings of European Co-ordinated Action Programme Meeting, Manchester 1992.

MULTIFREQUENCY ELECTRICAL IMPEDANCE TOMOGRAPHY AS AN ALTERNATIVE TO ABSOLUTE IMAGING

P Riu, J Rosell and R Pallás-Areny

Departament d'Enginyeria Electrònica, U.P.C., P.O. Box 30002, 08080 Barcelona, Spain

ABSTRACT: Absolute imaging in Electrical Impedance Tomography (EIT) aims to display the distribution of conductivity (or permittivity) across a section of an object. Mathematically, it relies on solving an inverse problem by iteration methods, whose convergence and residual error depend on an initial "guess" for the unknown distribution.

Difference imaging solves this uncertainty by taking a reference measurement and using it as an initial "guess". It can image only variations in conductivity distribution with respect to the reference, and is therefore restricted to dynamic phenomena.

Multifrequency imaging uses as a reference a set of data taken at a given frequency, and then takes readings at a different frequency, making it possible to image slow-varying or static phenomena. We analyze the requirements for an object to produce an image by multifrequency tomography and determine the design specifications for an imaging instrument.

We present some *in vivo* images of a human subject obtained using a broadband system designed for research purposes.

1. INTRODUCTION

Electrical impedance tomography aims to image a cross-section of an object according to the distribution of electrical impedance in the section. This is called absolute imaging. Mathematically, it relies on solving a nonlinear inverse problem by iterative methods, whose convergence and residual error depend on an initial "guess" for the unknown distribution, the shape of the object and the position of the electrodes. Hua and Woo (1990) describe and compare several of the available reconstruction algorithms. Woo (1990) has studied their computational complexity.

A different approach to absolute imaging is the so-called adaptive or optimal current method proposed by Isaacson (1986). It also consists of making an initial guess for the unknown distribution and then taking a measurement when some given boundary conditions around the measured object are forced. Next, an error parameter is calculated that leads to a modified guess and to different boundary conditions to apply around the body. The procedure is iterated until the current lines through the object are straight, which renders the reconstruction problem linear. The advantage of this method is that the iteration is based on successive measurements instead of relying on a single measurement. However, it needs an instrument capable of modifying the boundary conditions as required, and a considerable computing capability. Also, its dependence on object's shape and electrode position is similar to that of absolute imaging. By using the adaptative method, Isaacson (1990) has obtained absolute images from a dynamic phenomenon: breathing from a human subject.

The uncertainty in image reconstruction found in absolute methods has led to the development of relative imaging methods. The most usual one is difference imaging which consists in taking a reference measurement and using it as an initial "guess". Difference imaging can image only variations in conductivity distribution with respect to the reference, and therefore is restricted to dynamic (as opposed to static) phenomena.

For static or slowly varying phenomena, multifrequency imaging has been proposed (Griffiths and Ahmed 1987). It uses as a reference a set of data taken at a given frequency, and then takes readings at a different frequency. No dynamic process needs to be involved. Therefore, structural and composition information can be derived from the images.

In this paper we analyze the requirements for an object to produce an image by multifrequency tomography and determine the design specifications for an imaging instrument. We present some images obtained from a human subject, using a broadband system designed for research purposes.

2 FUNDAMENTALS OF MULTIFREQUENCY IMPEDANCE TOMOGRAPHY

In order for a non-homogeneous object to produce a multifrequency impedance image, we need at least one of its electrical parameters (EP) to change with frequency. Usual electrical parameters considered are: electrical conductivity, permittivity, real part of the complex impedance, real part of the complex admittance, imaginary part of the complex impedance, imaginary part of the complex admittance, complex impedance modulus and complex impedance phase.

For region a in figure 1 (and for region b), and two measurement frequencies f_1 and $f_2 = f_1 + \Delta f$, we define the relative variation (RV) of a given EP with frequency as

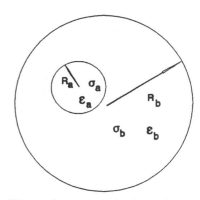

Figure 1 Small conductive region (a) embedded in a large region (b).

$$RV_a(EP) - \frac{EP_a(f_1 + \Delta f) \ - \ EP_a(f_1)}{EP_a(f_1)} \quad [1]$$

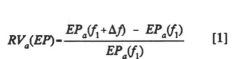

Assuming small changes with frequency, the contrast α for that object and the variation of that contrast $d\alpha/\alpha$, called conductivity resolution (Seagar *et al* 1987), are:

$$\alpha = \frac{EP_a(f_1)}{EP_b(f_1)} \qquad\qquad [2]$$

$$\frac{d\alpha}{\alpha} = \frac{d\left(\dfrac{EP_a}{EP_b}\right)}{\dfrac{EP_a}{EP_b}} = \frac{d\ EP_a}{EP_a} - \frac{d\ EP_b}{EP_b} \qquad\qquad [3]$$

If we assume small frequency increments, we can write [3] as:

$$\frac{d\alpha}{\alpha} = RV_a(EP) - RV_b(EP) \qquad\qquad [4]$$

We call this expression multifrequency contrast $MC(EP)$. Then, with these definitions, all the results from Seagar *et al* (1987) can be used in multifrequency imaging.

In principle, we can use any of the above mentioned electrical parameters for multifrequency imaging. However, measurement restrictions reduce the number of EP suitable for imaging. For some materials and frequencies, only the real part of the impedance or the admittance can be easily measured.

A simple example can help us to understand the meaning of $RV(EP)$ and $MC(EP)$. Let us consider a bidimensional object consisting of two different regions, each characterized by its own electric conductivity σ and permittivity ε, (figure 1). In the simplest case, neither σ or ε change with frequency, i.e. they are constant. Then the real part of the admittance for each region is constant with frequency and $RV_a(Re(Y)) = RV_b(Re(Y)) = 0$. The imaginary part of the admittance changes with frequency according to $Im(Y) = \omega\varepsilon$. Therefore we have for $Im(Y)$ $RV_a(Im(Y)) = RV_b(Im(Y)) = (\Delta\omega)/\omega$ and $MC(Im(Y)) = 0$. No admitance images can be obtained.

For the real part of the impedance, $Re(Z)$, the relative variation for region a (and similarly for region b) is

$$RV_a(Re(Z)) = \frac{1-d^2}{d^2+\dfrac{\sigma_a^2}{\omega_1^2\varepsilon_a^2}} \qquad\qquad [5]$$

where

$$d = \frac{\omega_2}{\omega_1} \quad ; \quad \omega_2 = \omega_1 + \Delta\omega \qquad \text{[6]}$$

The multifrequency contrast between the two regions is now

$$MC(Re(Z)) = (1-d^2)\left[1 - \frac{\omega_2^2 + \left(\dfrac{\sigma_a}{e_a}\right)^2}{\omega_2^2 + \left(\dfrac{\sigma_b}{e_b}\right)^2}\right] \qquad \text{[7]}$$

This contrast will be different from zero whenever

$$\frac{\sigma_a}{e_a} \neq \frac{\sigma_b}{e_b} \qquad \text{[8]}$$

An equation similar to [7] can be obtained for $MC(Im(Z))$.

Therefore, when we consider the complex impedance, the simple existence of conductivity and permittivity may result in an image. It is not necessary for the conductivity or permittivity to change with frequency.

The multifrequency contrast is frequency dependant. In order to obtain an image we must select both the frequency ratio d and the absolute values for the two frequencies.

If the parameters for the two regions defined previously were

$\sigma_a = 0.1$ S/m
$\varepsilon_a = 100$ (relative)
$\sigma_b = 0.2$ S/m
$\varepsilon_b = 100$

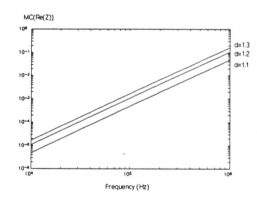

Figure 2 Multifrequency contrast as a function of frequency, and frequency ratio as a parameter, for $\sigma(a)=0.1$, $\varepsilon(a)=100$; $\sigma(b)=0.2$, $\varepsilon(b)=100$.

then the MC obtained, in the frequency range from 10 kHz to 1 MHz, when using frequency ratios of d=1.1, d=1.2 and d=1.3 is that displayed in figure 2.

We can see that the *MC* increases as frequency increases. For a radius ratio $R_a/R_b=1/10$, when region *a* is in the center of region *b* and the applied current density distribution is in the form:

$$J(\theta) - I_1\sin(\theta) + J_1\cos(\theta)$$

the expected sesitivity in the voltage change for a given *MC*

$$S - \frac{dV/V}{d\alpha/\alpha} \qquad\qquad [10]$$

can be calculated from Seagar *et al* (1987).

For example, if f=500 kHz and d=1.1 we obtain a *MC* of 10^{-2} (figure 2). The sensitivity associated is $S=10^{-2}$, thus the voltage variation dV/V will be 10^{-4}. This result means that the measurement system needs a dynamic range greater than 80 dB.

If the electrical conductivity and permittivity display a non-constant behavior with frequency, as happens for example in biological tissues, then the corresponding equations for multifrequency contrast are cumbersome and the analytical description is more involved.

The meaning of a reconstructed multifrequency image is highly dependant on the reconstruction algorithm used. For low contrasts, we have found that either the Newton-Raphson, the double constraint and the iterative backprojection methods (Hua and Woo 1990) converge to a solution that shows the difference in RV between different regions inside the object. The distribution of relative variation imaged is related only to the composition of each specific region (assumed to be homogeneous). For biological tissues, a low contrast between different regions can be obtained for example by selecting two very close measurement frequencies. Also, different materials can display the same RV for two given frequencies. In these cases, the only way to uniquely identify the EP of each region is by using a frequency sweep.

For high contrast values, some iterative reconstruction methods may become ill-conditioned. In these cases we can use non-iterative methods, such as some backprojection algorithms. But then the reconstructed image is non-linearly related to the frequency dependence of the EP measured and it is more difficult to differentiate regions.

3 DESIGN SPECIFICATIONS FOR A MULTIFREQUENCY IMAGING INSTRUMENT

In order to measure the chosen EP, we can apply a voltage or current and measure both the voltage or current being applied and, respectively, the current or voltage appearing on the object boundary. The design of the measuring instrument is simplified if the voltage or current being applied were constant and independent from the application site on the object. This, in practice, is easiest to achieve with a current generator, thus using a voltage detector. For biomedical applications we limit the current to 1 mA_{eff}.

The number of measurement points on the boundary will contribute to limiting the spatial resolution for the images. Nevertheless, the number of electrodes cannot be increased indefinitely because for a large number of electrodes the S/N ratio decreases whereas the actual image resolution does not improve (Seagar *et al* 1987). For measurements on the human torso we use 16 electrodes which requires a reasonable complex hardware and yields an acceptable resolution.

A very important parameter for a measuring instrument is its frequency range. Here we must decide the range for the "low" measurement frequency and the range for the "high" measurement frequency. The selection of each range depends on the application. For a research instrument intended to consider different applications, we propose a wide-band measurement system. Our system, initially developed for biomedical applications, can currently measure at any two frequencies between 8 kHz and 1 MHz. If we want to apply both frequencies simultaneously, it can measure at any frequency pair whose lower frequency is between 8 kHz and 64 kHz and whose higher frequency is between 125 kHz and 1 MHz.

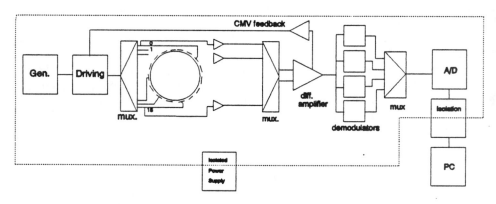

Figure 3 Block diagram of the multifrequency electrical impedance system (TIE-2sys).

Ideally, such an instrument should have a very flat frequency characteristic in both the signal generation and the signal detection parts. Alternatively, both parts must have a well known frequency characteristic. For an instrument working at a single frequency pair it is possible to use narrow-band techniques which ease its design.

Figure 3 shows the block diagram of our system (TIE-2sys). The two frequency signals are digitally synthesized and applied to a V/I converter based on an op amp supply current mirror. Current is applied to the body through two 8-channel FET-based multiplexers (MUX 08). This arrangement reduces common mode capacitance from current source to ground (< 12 pF).

Input signals are buffered using a large bandwidth op amp (AD 843) in a voltage follower configuration. The buffers' output is also used to drive the shield of the cables connecting the intrument to the body. Shielding is used to reduce crosstalk between channels and external interferences. A careful layout is also required in the two previous parts in order to keep stray capacitances between injection and detection circuits as low as possible.

Common mode voltage feedback is used in order to reduce common mode voltage in the body. This is important because of the non-ideal bipolar current source that produces a difference current to ground through the input impedance of the buffers. The measurement strategy used (driving current through adjacent electrodes and measuring voltage between adjacent electrodes) also contributes to the common mode voltage.

Voltage signals are demodulated using four switching op amps (OPA 675). We thus obtain the in-phase and quadrature components for the two frequencies used. Demodulation is performed with a phase angle of about 45° and later corrected by software. There is a variable gain amplifier prior to the demodulator. The gain in the detection channel ranges from 400 to 3200.

The demodulated signals are amplified and acquired using a 16 bit (providing 96 dB dynamic range) A/D converter (ADC 76) and transmitted via a serial/parallel interface to a personal computer which reconstructs and displays the images.

The whole system is isolated from ground, by a shielded transformer for the power supply and by optical isolators for the digital signal lines (control and data). Isolation protects the system from overvoltages on the object (and conversely) and helps in reducing interferences. Further details about the design may be found on Riu (1991).

The overall accuracy and S/N ratio has been tested using a well known resistive phantom. The index used for accuracy (static errors) is the SER (Static Error Ratio) that shows the mean relative error between each voltage measurement and the theoretical voltage calculated for the phantom. The index for S/N ratio is the NER (Noise Error Ratio) that shows the standard deviation for the overall voltages in a series of frames. Both indexes have been defined in the CAIT (Concerted Action on Impedance Tomography). A third index, the RER (Reciprocity Error Ratio) is used. This index shows the difference found in voltage measurements that must give the same value. It is useful for in vivo measurements, when no known reference is available. Some of the results from our system are given in table 1.

Static error noticeably increases for frequencies above 250 kHz. The frequency response of the shield driving circuit is mostly responsible for that fact. This circuit must have a cut-off frequency under 1 MHz in order to avoid oscillations due to cable capacitances, thus decreasing the shield efficiency. Stray capacitances also contribute to static errors at high frequencies.

Frequency	NER	SER	RER
16 kHz	0.04%	1.58%	0.9%
62 kHz	0.08%	2.7%	1.1%
250 kHz	0.4%	4.1%	7.5%
1 MHz	0.58%	17.3%	30%

Table 1 Static errors an noise for different frequencies, obtained with TIE-2sys.

4 EXPERIMENTAL RESULTS

Figure 4 shows the images obtained from saline phantom measurements using frequencies of 32 and 125 kHz. The selected electrical parameter is the real part of the impedance.

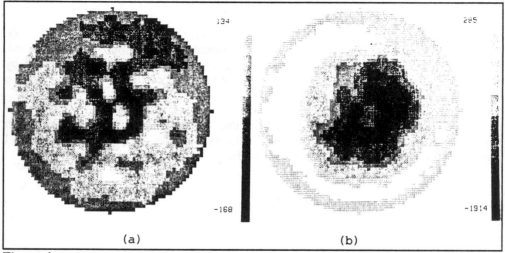

(a)   (b)

Figure 4 (a) Image from a uniform saline phantom. (b) Image from a human arm immersed inside the phantom.

Figure 4(a) shows the noise level obtained when there is only saline solution in the tank, consequently no frequency variation is expected. Figure 4(b) shows the image for a human arm placed inside the tank. Values for the reconstructed image are almost ten times greater than the noise values. The image is dark because the body impedance decreases with frequency and the water impedance is almost constant in the measurement frequency range.

The noise level for a uniform image in multifrequency mode is ten times greater than the noise level obtained with the same system, working at a single frequency, and taking dynamic measurements. The difference in noise level is due to different static errors at each measurement frequency. There are several factors to contribute to these errors: stray capacitances, shield driving frequency response and also the common mode feedback circuit, wich has a first order low pass frequency response in order to avoid oscillations.

Figure 5 is a cross section of a human abdomen, without any image averaging, using the real part of the impedance and frequencies of 16 kHz and 125 kHz. In the lower part (back), in dark color, it is possible to see the dorsal muscles (*erector spinae*). Muscle tissue displays a high negative relative variation. In the center, in light color, is the backbone. Bone tissue, in this frequency range, displays an almost constant impedance variation. In the upper part (front), it is possible to see a region with a lower frequencial change, wich corresponds to the bowels. The dark area on the right corresponds to the lower part of the liver, which displays a high negative variation in thit frequency range. Other areas in the image correspond to levels that are similar to those obtained with the saline phantom, thus no guesses may be done.

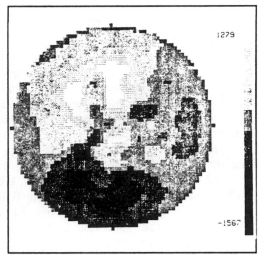

Figure 5 Cross section of a human abdomen obtained by E.I.T.

5 CONCLUSIONS

We have shown that multifrequency images can yield structural information from an object, even if the basic electrical parameters of this object (conductivity and permittivity) do not change with frequency. Nevertheless, the frequency range for the measurements must be selected according to the object's characteristics and in some cases high frequencies (> 1 MHz) may be needed.

The instrument capable of making such measurements must be designed according to the application. A general purpose broadband instrument, like the system presented in this paper, has important design restrictions, most of them derived from the fact that a flat frequency response is needed. A simpler instrument, using two fixed frequencies, can be more easily designed, because some of the design parameters can be adjusted for the particular frequencies used.

ACKNOWLEDGMENT

This work was funded by the DGICYT under project PB89-0505.

REFERENCES

Griffiths H and Ahmed A 1987, *A dual-frequency applied potential tomography technique: Computer simulations*, Clin. Phys. Physiol. Meas. **8** suppl. A 103-7.

Hua P and Woo E L 1990, *Reconstruction algorithms*, in: Webster J. G. (ed), Electrical impedance tomography (Bristol: Adam Hilger).

Isaacson D 1986, *Distinguishability of conductivities by electric current computed tomography*, IEEE Tans. Med. Imag., **5** 91-5.

Isaacson D 1990, *Thoracic impedance images during ventilation*, Annual Intl. Conference of the IEEE EMB Society, **12** No. 1 106-107.

Riu P J, Rosell J, Lozano A, Pallàs-Areny R 1991, *A Broadband system for multifrequency static imaging in EIT*, Clin. Phys, Physiol. Meas. **12** suppl. B 1-5.

Seagar A D, Barber D C and Brown B H 1987, *Theoretical limits to sensitivity and resolution in impedance imaging*, Clin. Phys. Physiol. Meas. **8** suppl. A 13-31.

Woo E J 1990, *Computational complexity*, in: Webster J. G. (ed), Electrical impedance tomography (Bristol: Adam Hilger).

Validation of Finite Element Modelling of Multielectrode Capacitive System
for Process Tomography Flow Imaging

S H Khan   F Abdullah

Measurement and Instrumentation Centre, Department of EE and Information
Engineering, City University, Northampton Square, London EC1V 0HB, UK

ABSTRACT: Finite element modelling of process tomography sensor
systems is necessary for their CAD both for performance evaluation and
design optimization. This paper involves the validation of finite
element models of a 12-electrode capacitive sensor system for multiphase
flow imaging. Various results of modelling have been compared in the
form of standing mode capacitances and sensor sensitivity distribution
with experimental data obtained from UMIST. There is good agreement
between simulation results and experiments especially for high
sensitivity regions inside the pipe.

1.   INTRODUCTION

The area of process tomography flow imaging using capacitive electrode
systems is growing rapidly with some promising results obtained already
from full scale industrial prototype. The basic principle of flow component
detection with capacitive electrodes lies in changes of capacitance values
between electrode pairs due to changes in permittivities of flow
components. Beck et al (1986) proposed to exploit this principle for
imaging multiphase flows and the practical implementation of the idea was
first made at UMIST by Huang et al (1989) who showed the feasibility of an
8-electrode sensor system for imaging two component flows. In such a
multielectrode system capacitive electrodes are mounted symmetrically
around the flow pipe and all possible independent capacitance measurements
are carried out between various electrode pairs by successive electronic
interrogation. Comparing to other existing tomography systems, capacitive
sensor systems are inexpensive, fast, noninvasive and simple in
construction; today various designs of such systems are being explored to
be used in diversified industrial applications (Dickin et al 1991,
Plaskowski et al 1991, Hammer et al 1991).

Although some of the geometric and physical parameters of capacitive
electrode systems are predetermined there is still a number of geometric
parameters which are variable and determine the overall performance of the
system during exploitation. This obviously necessitates the CAD approach
towards understanding, performance evaluation and design optimization of
these systems (Khan et al 1991). One of the main tasks of CAD of electrode
system is the solution of the so called forward problem which involves
simulation of electric field distribution inside the flow pipe. This is
done by numerical solution of the appropriate Laplace's equation by finite
element method (FEM). The data obtained from field simulations and
subsequent capacitance calculations, are then used to evaluate system

performance parameters and fed into the solution of the inverse problem of
image reconstruction the quality of which reflects the overall system
performance. It is, therefore vitally important to ensure the reliability
and accuracy of finite element (FE) modelling for CAD and design
optimization of such PT sensor systems. The obvious way to do that is to
establish confidence on modelling results by comparing them with available
experimental data. In the following sections this is done by comparing
simulation results with corresponding experimental data obtained at UMIST
from various designs of two 12-electrode capacitive systems.

2.   FINITE ELEMENT MODEL OF A 12-ELECTRODE CAPACITIVE SYSTEM

The cross section of a 12-electrode capacitive system is shown in Figure 1
which is self explanatory (see also Table 1). Radial screens in between
electrodes serve as shields to reduce high capacitance between adjacent
electrodes and increase measurement accuracy. The outer screen which is
always earthed makes the whole system stray immune. The inner radius R1 is
fixed but the rest of the parameters θ, δ_1, δ_2, scgp, scth and the number
of electrodes N are variables which determine system performance.
Capacitances between electrode pairs are measured by using special
capacitance measuring circuitry developed at UMIST (Huang et al 1991). In
this one of the electrodes (the 'active electrode') is given a constant
potential and the capacitances between this and the rest of the electrodes
('detecting electrodes' kept at virtual earth) are measured. In this way a
total of $n=N(N-1)/2$ independent capacitance measurements can be made by
choosing each of the electrodes in turn as active electrodes. The data thus
obtained are used to solve the inverse problem of determining flow
component distributions in the pipeline cross section and with a suitable
image reconstruction algorithm these are visualized on the screen in real
time (Xie et al 1991). All these could be simulated as a part of CAD before
committing to build real systems to predict their performance and optimize
geometric parameters.

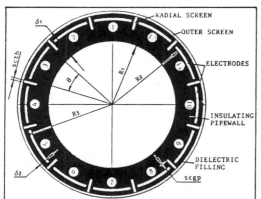

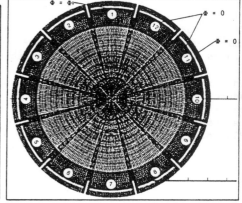

Fig. 1. Cross section of a
12-electrode capacitive system
(not in scale)

Fig. 2. Finite element model of
the 12-electrode capacitive system

By neglecting the fringing field due to finite lengths of electrodes and
assuming that flow component distribution remains the same along the length
of pipeline within electrode lengths the electric processes in the
electrode system shown in Figure 1 can be simulated by the 2D FE model
shown in Figure 2. Under appropriate boundary conditions (for example shown
in Figure 2), the electrostatic field in the electrode system is calculated

by solving the corresponding Laplace's equation

$$\nabla \ (\varepsilon(x,y) \ \nabla\Phi(x,y)) \ = \ 0 \tag{1}$$

in terms of the electrostatic potential $\Phi=\Phi(x,y)$ for space-varying permittivities of flow component distributions $\varepsilon=\varepsilon(x,y)$. The solution of this equation under proper boundary conditions by FEM gives potential values at nodal points from which field vectors $\mathbf{E}$, $\mathbf{D}$ and subsequently capacitance between any pair of electrodes are calculated.

3.   EXPERIMENTAL MODELS OF 12-ELECTRODE CAPACITIVE SYSTEM

Experiments were carried out at UMIST with two different designs of electrode system which have different inner radius R_1 and pipe wall thickness δ_1. All experiments were carried out with and without the presence of interelectrode radial screens to show their effects, quantitatively on various system performance parameters. Figure 3 shows the cross section of one of the two designs of the experimental electrode system without radial screens. In all experimental models the space between the pipe wall outer surface and the outer screen is filled with air and not with dielectric filling material. In course of experiments capacitances were measured between electrode pairs 1-7 and 1-12 when the pipe is empty; these are standing mode capacitances which we represent as C_{017} and C_{0112}

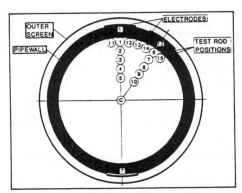

Fig. 3. Cross section of experimental model of the 12 electrode capacitive system showing test rod · positions (only three electrodes are shown)

respectively. To explore the sensitivities of various sensor designs a perspex rod of circular cross section is placed axially at different positions inside the pipeline and capacitances between 1-7 and 1-12, C_{17}, C_{112} are measured. These rod positions are represented by numbered circles inside the pipe in Figure 3. The sensitivity (relative) of the system for various test rod positions is expressed as

$$S_{ij} \ = \ \Delta C_{ij}/C_{0ij} \tag{2}$$

where, $\Delta C_{ij} = C_{ij} - C_{0ij}$, C_{ij} - capacitance between electrode pair i-j for a given rod position inside the flow pipe; C_{0ij} - standing mode capacitance between i-j. These data for different test rod positions in various electrode designs are compared with identical data obtained from simulated electrode systems. The following table shows physical and geometric parameters of electrode designs used for experimental and modelling purposes.

Table 1. List of geometric and physical parameters used in experimental and finite element models of 12-electrode capacitive systems

Parameters	Thin pipe wall model		Thick pipe wall model	
	Without radial screen	With radial screen	Without radial screen	With radial screen
1. Pipe inner radius R1, mm	68	68	78	78
2. Pipe wall thickness δ_1, mm	7	7	12.5	12.5
3. Distance between pipe wall outer surface and outer screen δ_2, mm	6	6	6	6
4. Electrode angle θ, deg.	24	24	25	25
5. Radial screen thickness scth, mm	1.6	1.6	1.6	1.6
6. Electrode thickness elt, mm	0.3	0.3	0.3	0.3
7. Radial screen penetration depth, mm	—	2	—	2
8. Electrode length 1, mm	100	100	100	100
9. Relative permittivity of pipewall material ε_{pw}	3	3	3	3
10. Test rod radius Rrod, mm	4.5	4.5	4.5	4.5
11. Permittivity of test rod material ε_{rod}	3	3	3	3

4.   FINITE ELEMENT REALIZATION OF EXPERIMENTAL MODELS

For all finite element modelling of above electrode systems a powerful 2D electromagnetic software package PE2D (Vector Fields Limited, UK) has been used on Sun Sparcstation 1. Figures 4a (thin pipe wall model without radial screens) and 4b (thick pipe wall model with radial screen) show typical FE models of experimental electrode systems set up by PE2D pre-processor. After discretisation, FE mesh for the model in Figure 4b looks like the one shown in Figure 5. Circular regions inside the pipe in all these models which are marked 1 to 10 and 'C' represent test rod positions corresponding to those shown in Figure 3. Only those regions which are marked are used to simulate test rods during modelling. The rest of the circular regions (unmarked) serve to ensure consistency and symmetry in discretisation pattern. Maximum number of triangular elements used in all models is around 10000 which is the upper limit for the version of PE2D (version 8.1) used for modelling purposes.

As can be seen from Figure 1 the geometry of the electrode system with curved electrodes, radial screens, etc. is fairly complicated to set up FE models like those shown in Figure 4 quickly and accurately. With the addition of circular regions for test rods setting up of models gets even more complicated. To tackle this a systematic approach is taken at the pre-processing stage in which all models are built up from basic 'building blocks' like the one shown in Figure 6. This group of regions is then copied to other quadrants by successive mirror reflections to get the full model (shown, for example in Figure 4b). To build this basic block all regions outside the inside of the pipe are first drawn in which the presence or the absence of radial screens is incorporated (Figure 7). The next stage is to draw holes at rod positions inside the pipe by using

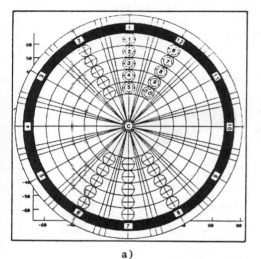
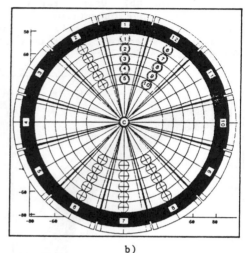

a) b)

Fig. 4. Finite element models of experimental electrode systems a) thin pipe wall model without radial screen b) thick pipe wall model with radial screen

suitably placed curvilinear quadrilateral regions shown in Figure 8. Circular regions for test rods are then drawn in local coordinate systems at rod positions by replicating respective annular regions (Figure 6). All

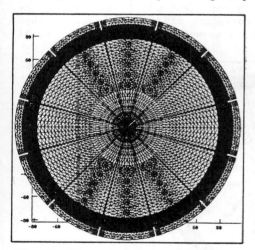
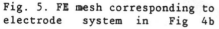
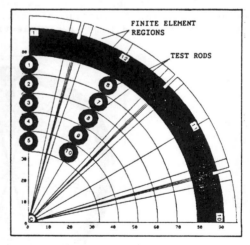

Fig. 5. FE mesh corresponding to electrode system in Fig 4b

Fig. 6. The basic 'building block' used to set up FE models

these regions are initially assigned the relative permittivity of vacuum ($\varepsilon=1$) which enables the modelling of electrode systems with empty pipes. To

simulate the electrode system with the test rod placed at one of the
positions the permittivity of the corresponding circular region in the
model is modified to that of the test rod as shown in Figure 9 where the
test rod is placed at rod position 2 between electrodes 1 and 7. In this
way the experimental designs of the 12-electrode system are simulated for
different positions of test rod placements (positions 1 to 10 and 'C' in
Figures 4a and 4b). Using PE2D's pre-processing facilities all necessary
commands for above operations are written once and stored in files which
can be easily and quickly modified and called upon to have them
automatically executed to set up models, solve equations and do necessary
post-processing for output data.

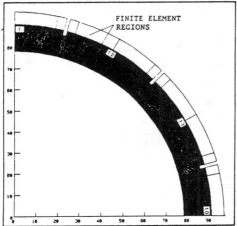

Fig. 7. First stage in building up
of the basic 'building block'

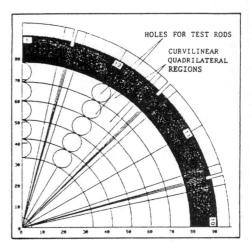

Fig. 8. Final stage in building up
of the basic 'building block'

For all FE models equation (1) is solved for electrode 1 selected as the
active electrode. A constant electric potential of 1 V is given to this
active electrode and rest of the electrodes as well as outer and radial

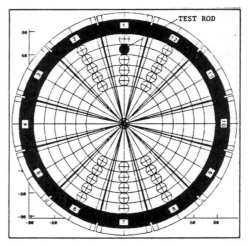

Fig. 9. Positioning of the simulated test rod in FE models

screens are kept at zero potential. Capacitances C_{17} and C_{112} are calculated between electrode pairs 1-7 and 1-12 by determining the total charge Q distributed on electrodes 7 and 12 using $Q=\varepsilon \int_s E.ds$ (Gauss's Law).

5. MODELLING RESULTS - COMPARISON WITH EXPERIMENTAL DATA AND DISCUSSIONS

Table 2 below shows standing mode capacitances C_{017} and C_{0112} obtained from simulations and experiments. These results confirm quantitatively the effects of interelectrode radial screens and pipe wall thickness on standing mode capacitances between electrode pairs. Since sensitivity requirements of capacitance measuring circuitry depend largely on minimum values of standing mode capacitances for a given sensor geometry it is important to be able to predict these values beforehand by simulations. It is equally useful to predict and determine the pattern of these capacitance changes for a possible variation of key sensor geometric parameters like R_1, δ_1 and scgp. As can be seen from Table 2 increases in δ_1 and R_1 lead to increases in values of both C_{017} and C_{0112}. For C_{017} it is due to

Table 2. Comparison between standing mode capacitances obtained from experimental and simulation models

Capacitances		Thin pipe wall model ($R_1 = 68$ mm, $\delta_1 = 7$ mm)		Thick pipe wall model ($R_1 = 78$ mm, $\delta_1 = 12.5$ mm)	
		No radial screen scgp=0	With radial screen scgp=2	No radial screen scgp=0	With radial screen scgp=2
C_{017} (pF)	Experimental	0.0124	0.011	0.013	0.0115
	Simulated	0.0172	0.0118	0.0176	0.0127
	Deviation (%)	38.70	7.27	35.38	10.43
C_{0112} (pF)	Experimental	1.217	0.424	1.493	0.618
	Simulated	1.306	0.489	1.568	0.726
	Deviation (%)	7.31	15.33	5.02	17.47

combined effects of increased electrode widths (defined by θ) and the distance between them; for C_{0112} increases in higher permittivity material between electrode pair 1-12 and electrode widths lead to increase in capacitances between them. As said earlier, radial screens are meant for reducing high capacitances between adjacent electrodes and this can be seen quantitatively from C_{0112} values obtained by simulations and experiments for electrode models with and without radial screens. At the same time presence of radial screens reduces slightly the standing mode capacitances between distant electrodes, say C_{017} which can be explained by the deviation of field lines away from those electrodes towards closer radial screens which have the same zero potential as distant electrodes.

Comparison between capacitance values shown in Table 2 shows that maximum deviation (38.7%) of simulation results from experimental ones is obtained for capacitances C_{017} the values of which far exceed corresponding values

of capacitances C0112 for which a minimum deviation of around 5% is
obtained. These differences between simulated and experimental results
could be explained by combined effects of possible experimental and
modelling errors discussed later in this section.

Variations of sensitivities (determined by equation (2)) of various sensor
models for different test rod positions are shown in Figures 10 and 11 in
which numbers 1 to 10 and 'C' along x-axis represent test rod positions
corresponding to those in Figure 4. Both simulation and experimental
results in Figures 10 and 11 clearly reflect the effects of pipe wall
thickness δ1 and radial screens (radial screen penetration depth scgp) on
sensor sensitivity distributions inside the pipe. For various rod positions
in between electrodes 1 and 7 presence of radial screens increases (15-25%)
sensitivities S17 when δ1=const. Pipe wall thickness δ1 shows to have
higher effects on sensitivity distributions S17 than radial screens. Figure
10 shows that for an about 80% increase in δ1 sensitivities S17 decrease
upto 100% (scgp=const.). All these patterns of sensitivity variations could
also be seen in Figure 11 in respect of sensitivities S112 between

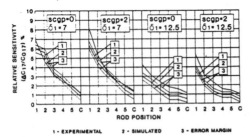

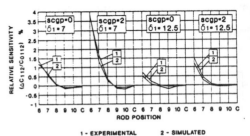

Fig. 10. Variation of relative
sensitivity S17 with test rod
position

Fig. 11. Variation of relative
sensitivity S112 with test rod
position

electrodes 1-12. For test rod positions 6 and 7 high increase in
sensitivity is observed in presence of radial screens which is most
probably due to diversions of field lines, going towards electrode 12
through high permittivity test rod at positions 6 and 7. On the other hand
the presence of test rods at positions 8-10 and at the centre 'C' diverts
field lines away from electrode 12 resulting in very small or negative
sensitivities S112 between electrodes 1 and 12. As. in the case of S17
increase in pipe wall thickness δ1 also reduces sensitivities S112 for a
given scgp=const. This is because more and more field lines tend to go
through increased pipe wall material towards electrode 12 without
penetrating into the pipeline. An extreme case for this would be the
sensitivity S112=0 for the test rod placed at position 6 in an electrode
system with extremely high δ1.

By comparing experimental and simulated sensitivity variation curves in
Figures 10 and 11 it can be concluded that deviations of simulation results
from experimental ones vary differently for different sensitivities and
electrode designs. Although there is no apparent consistent pattern of this
variation what is evident from these figures is the occurrence of maximum
deviations for low sensitivity regions between electrodes 1-7 and 1-12.
While simulation results for sensitivities S17 (Figure 10) are showing
reasonable agreement (considering, especially experimental error margins
(3)) with experimental ones some high disagreements are observed for
negative sensitivities S112 (Figure 11). This is particularly true for test
rod at positions 9-10 and 'C' for which very low values of capacitance

change ΔC_{112} are obtained.

The above disagreements between experimental and simulation results could be explained by analyzing various errors associated with both modelling and experiments. The main sources of experimental errors could be: baseline drift of sensor electronic circuit, noise voltage generated in it, geometry of electrode designs used, inaccurate positioning of test rods, etc. Discretisation errors and errors in capacitance calculations could be considered as two main sources of errors during numerical modelling.

The baseline drift of sensor electronic circuit which is caused mainly by its temperature dependency could lead to errors in capacitance measurements, especially when the circuit is switched on for a long time during experiments and temperature changes take place in between capacitance measurements for various test rod positions. For a temperature change of 10^0 C the effect of baseline drift could be comparable to an input capacitance change of 5 fF (Huang et al 1991) which is significantly higher than most capacitance changes ΔC_{ij} caused by various test rod positions during experiments. This obviously could lead to uncertainties in sensitivity values calculated from measured capacitances, especially for low sensitivity areas in between electrodes 1-7 and 1-12 inside the pipeline. The sensor electronics used at the time of above experimental studies was not baseline drift corrected and all measures were taken to reduce its effects below 0.1fF. At present, the sensor electronics provided with 12-electrode sensor systems are self-baseline drift corrected which eliminates above measurement errors (Huang et al 1991).

The capacitance measuring circuit used for sensor electrodes measures capacitances as dc voltage signals from detecting electrodes which are proportional to unknown capacitances. That is why it is important to know the level of noise voltage generated in the circuit as it contributes to errors in capacitance measurements. By taking different preventive measures to eliminate various sources of noise voltages a rms noise level of 0.07 fF could be achieved (Huang et al 1991) which is quite low comparing to measurement resolution of the circuit (0.3 fF) but comparable to some of the ΔC_{ij} obtained in experiments.

Variations in geometric features of electrode systems could be considered as potential sources of errors in measured capacitance values obtained during experiments. As can be seen from Table 1 experiments are carried out in two different models of sensor electrodes - thin pipe wall model and thick pipe wall model. It can be assumed that there are technological errors in making those models which contribute to uncertainties in their precise geometric specifications, for example precise positioning of capacitive electrodes and radial screens, concentricity of outer screen, etc. All these give inaccuracies in experimental results and lead to uncertainties in comparability of results from various models and methods of studies of sensor electrodes - experimental and numerical. For example, simulation results show that both capacitances C_{17} and C_{112} change with the variation of outer screen distance δ_2 from electrodes (Khan et al 1991). For a 12-electrode system standing mode capacitances C_{017} and C_{0112} could increase upto 0.4 fF and 0.05-0.09 pF respectively for each mm increase in δ_2 which are comparable and sometimes significantly higher (in case of C_{0112}) than most of the values of ΔC_{ij} obtained from experiments.

Inaccurate positioning of test rod at given positions inside the pipeline

during experiments could be considered as one of the main causes of
disagreements between experimental and simulation results, especially for
test rod positions in regions of high sensitivity. While in numerical
modelling simulated test rods could be placed almost exactly at positions
(1-10 and 'C') shown in Figures 3 and 4 it is far more difficult to do that
in experimental models. For experimental results shown in Figures 10 and 11
inaccuracies in the positioning of the test rod at various positions are
considered to be ±3 mm. The effects of these 'positioning errors' on
sensitivity variation curves could be roughly estimated from gradient of
these experimental curves shown in Figures 10 and 11. For example +3 mm
positioning error at test rod position 2 (model with $\delta_1 = 7$ mm and scgp=0 in
Figure 10) would give an error of 13% in sensitivity (S_{17}) calculations;
for position 6 (model with $\delta_1 = 12.5$ mm and scgp=2 mm) in Figure 11 this
would reach upto 25% for sensitivity S_{112}. Higher gradients of sensitivity
variation curves for test rods at high sensitivity regions inside the pipe
show that positioning errors are higher in those regions.

Errors associated with numerical modelling are usually inherent to the
particular modelling method and package used and with correct modelling
strategy they could be minimized to get required accuracy. As said earlier,
two main sources of modelling errors in the simulation of sensor electrodes
by FEM are finite element discretisation and capacitance calculations from
field solutions. Discretisation errors are minimized by proper and adequate
refining of FE mesh. Any discretisation error which cannot be corrected by
further mesh refinement is maintained consistent for various models to
ensure comparability of simulation results. For results shown in Figures 10
and 11 FE meshes for all models have been adequately refined to minimize
discretisation errors. To show this adequacy simulation results from full
models (Figures 4a and 4b) have been compared with those from half models
(with twice finer mesh for the same number of FE triangles as in full
models) which shows, for example that for the thick pipe wall model
($\delta_1 = 12.5$ mm, scgp=0) the difference in calculated capacitances C_{017}
obtained from full and half models is only 1.3%. In terms of sensitivity
this gives a deviation of less than 1% for test rod at position 1.

Errors in capacitance calculations from field solutions are usually
associated with numerical integration by which total charge distributed on
detecting electrodes is calculated (section 4). Using PE2D's
post-processing features these errors could be reduced to an insignificant
value by selecting suitable tolerance factor in line integration.

6. CONCLUSIONS

In light of above discussions, simulation and experimental results produced
in Table 2 and Figures 10 and 11 it can be concluded that numerical
simulation of capacitive electrode systems by FEM could be used confidently
to design these systems, predict and evaluate performances at various
stages of their CAD.

7. ACKNOWLEDGEMENTS

The authors would like to thank SERC for financial support and professor M.
S. Beck and his Group at UMIST, especially Dr. S. M. Huang (now with
Schlumberger Cambridge Research Limited, UK) for providing us with
experimental data and Dr. C. G. Xie for valuable suggestions and
discussions at various stages of the work.

9. REFERENCES

Beck M S, Plaskowski A and Green R G 1986 *Proceedings of the 4th International Symposium on Flow Visualization, 26 - 28 August 1986* (Hemisphere Publishing Corporation) pp 585 - 588

Dickin F G, Hoyle B S, Hunt A, Huang S M, Illyas O, Lenn C, Waterfall R, Williams R A, Xie C G and Beck M S 1991 *Sensors: Technology, Systems and Applications* ed K T V Grattan (Bristol: Adam Hilger) pp 191-196

Hammer E A and Nordtvedt J E 1991 *Sensors: Technology, Systems and Applications* ed K T V Grattan (Bristol: Adam Hilger) pp 233-238

Huang S M, Plaskowski A B, Xie C G and Beck M S 1989 *J. Phys. E, Sci. Instrum.* 22 pp 173 - 177

Huang S M, Xie C G, Thorn R, Snowden D and Beck M S 1991 *Sensors: Technology, Systems and Applications* ed K T V Grattan (Bristol: Adam Hilger) pp 197-202

Khan S H and Abdullah F 1991 *Sensors: Technology, Systems and Applications* ed K T V Grattan (Bristol: Adam Hilger) pp 209-214

Plaskowski A, Bukalski P, Habdas T and Skolimowski J 1991 *Sensors: Technology, Systems and Applications* ed K T V Grattan (Bristol: Adam Hilger) pp 221-226

Xie C G, Plaskowski A and Beck M S 1989 *IEE Proc.* 136 (4) pp 173 - 183

Xie C G, Stott A L, Plaskowski A and Beck M S 1990 *Meas. Sci. Technol.* 1 pp 65 - 78

Xie C G, Huang S M, Hoyle B S and Beck M S 1991 *Sensors: Technology, Systems and Applications* ed K T V Grattan (Bristol: Adam Hilger) pp 203-208

Improved electrical impedance tomography data collection system and measurement protocols

Mi Wang[1], Fraser J. Dickin, and Maurice S. Beck

Process Tomography Unit, UMIST,
Department of Electrical Engineering & Electronics,
P.O. Box 88, Manchester. M60 1QD.
([1]Visiting from the Chinese Academy of Sciences)

Abstract

An improved electrical impedance tomography (EIT) data collection system with the following programmable specifications is described; alternating current injection range - 0 to 30 mA (in 256 steps), frequency range - 75 Hz to 153.6 kHz (in 12 steps), phase shift of phase-sensitive demodulator - 0.7° to 180°, number of electrodes - 32, current sources - separately mounted on each electrode, current source output impedance - 2.5 MΩ at 76.8 kHz, common mode rejection ratio (CMRR) of differential programmable gain amplifier - more than 75.6 dB at 76.8 kHz. The significance of each of the specifications will be emphasised and results from the improved system comparing the performance of a number of data collection protocols will be given.

1. Introduction

A number of EIT data collection systems have been built by biomedical research groups in America and Europe for use in clinical observations. Notably, the largest group, at Rennselaer Polytechnic Institute (RPI), Troy, NY, appear to have assembled the most complicated and expensive system. The group at Sheffield University, with their latest 'real-time' applied potential tomography (APT) system, have also opted for a high-speed data processing approach which utilises a number of Transputers to perform qualitative image reconstruction and several Texas Instruments digital signal processors (DSPs) to manipulate the measured voltage data. Due to the constraints imposed by the strict safety requirements of clinical instrumentation, the majority of biomedical EIT data collection systems are correspondingly restricted in the range of measurements they can make. The wide dynamic range of measurement conditions occurring in the process industry cannot therefore be easily encompassed by the limited biomedical EIT apparatus. Hence, the primary aim of the authors, in designing an EIT system to demonstrate the feasibility for tomographic visualisation of process equipment, was to make the system as 'flexible' as possible for use on a number of different process applications. Thus the following outline specification was drawn up to maintain optimal flexibility and accuracy whilst accommodating the majority of process applications encountered by the authors:

a) *injected ac. current frequency bandwidth* - 75 Hz up to 153.6 kHz
b) *injected ac. current amplitude* - 0 to 30 mA (peak-to-peak)
c) *methods of current injection* - adjacent, opposite, multireference, and multisink
d) *analogue to digital converter (ADC) resolution* - 12 bits minimum ($\approx$ 0.025%)
e) *mode of measurement* - either serial or parallel
f) *maximum number of electrode modules* - 64

The first two requirements a) and b) are the most restricted ones in biomedical systems: usually limited to currents less than 5 mA in amplitude and over 20 kHz in frequency to avoid patient discomfort. To overcome the problems associated with process vessel size it is useful to have the facility to either increase or decrease the amplitude of injected currents in order to optimise the signal-to-noise ratio (SNR) of the measured voltage signal. Also, for slowly changing processes, more accurate measurements are facilitated at lower frequencies of injected current. Hence, the motivation for the ranges given in a) and b) above.

The requirement in c) for several different methods or 'protocols' of injecting ac. current, described by Brown and Seagar (1985), is readily achievable by utilising more than one current source/sink pair. The adjacent and opposite protocols only require one current source and sink pair thereby minimising the cost the associated circuitry. Conversely, the multireference method requires that all but one of the electrodes has an identical fixed amplitude current source attached to it. The corresponding voltage measurement is taken across a grounded load connected to the free electrode. The multisink method is a compromise between the adjacent/opposite methods and the multireference method in that only a limited number of fixed amplitude current source/sink pairs are necessary to acquire voltage measurements. A further current injection method employed by the RPI group is called the 'adaptive' method since each electrode has a different current amplitude source/sink on it. The method is so-called because a set of electrode current amplitudes are iteratively generated for internal objects to optimise the SNR of the measured voltages. Thus, the applied currents are said to be 'adapted' to the object(s) inside the vessel. The adaptive method, although attractive from an image reconstruction stand-point since it optimises the accuracy of the measured voltage data, is both expensive to implement and time consuming. The RPI group have implemented an independent programmable current source on each electrode of their 32-electrode ACT3 system. Every electrode also has an associated DSP device (AD2101) which demodulates and filters the measured voltage signal. The combined cost of the hardware for *each* electrode is reputed to be around £2,800. The specification outlined in part d) will enable up to 64 fixed-amplitude current sources to be attached to the process vessel. By making the current source constant amplitude and performing the voltage measurement demodulation and filtering sequentially using analogue circuitry, the combined hardware cost per electrode is reduced to £35. Further, the option of making voltage measurements in parallel, encompassed by specification e), similar to the RPI ACT3 and Sheffield real-time systems is realisable by employing additional voltage demodulation and filtering sub-systems.

The overall accuracy of the voltage measurements is governed by the resolution of the ADC. A 12-bit ADC has a resolution of 1/4096 or approximately 0.025% of the input signal. A 16-bit ADC has a resolution of 1/65536 corresponding to 0.0015% of the input signal. Once again, cost is the limiting factor: a typical 12-bit successive approximation, sample and hold, ADC

with a conversion time of 3 μs costs around £40. A 16-bit ADC with similar conversion time specifications presently costs approximately £700. To conduct preliminary investigations, it was felt that a 16-bit ADC was unnecessary and that a 12-bit device would suffice. It must be noted however, both the RPI and Sheffield systems employ 16-bit converters since their DSP devices can handle 16-bits of data as quickly as 12-bits thereby yielding higher accuracy.

The following sections are arranged in such a way as to describe the key components of the data acquisition system (DAS) shown in Figure 1. Starting at the bottom left corner of Figure 1 and moving in a clockwise direction, Section 2 describes the operation of the voltage generator. Section 3 explains the structure of the electrode module attached to each electrode on the process vessel. Section 4 describes the voltage measurement demodulation and filtering functions. Finally, Section 5 discusses the performance-related aspects of the circuitry covered in the previous three sections and outlines the approaches adopted by the authors in maintaining the flexibility versus accuracy trade-off.

2.   Voltage generator

The voltage generator, shown in the bottom left corner of Figure 1, is an important integral part of all EIT DAS's. To minimise the number of harmonic components in the 'probe' signal, the voltage generator is required to produce a sinewave-shaped output. However, with the emergence of fast and accurate signal processing devices, both digital and analogue, researchers are now beginning to examine the use of multifrequency EIT (Record *et al* 1992) in which the material is interrogated simultaneously by a range of different frequencies. The resultant measurements are then processed by frequency-selective circuitry to yield more detailed analyses of the material.

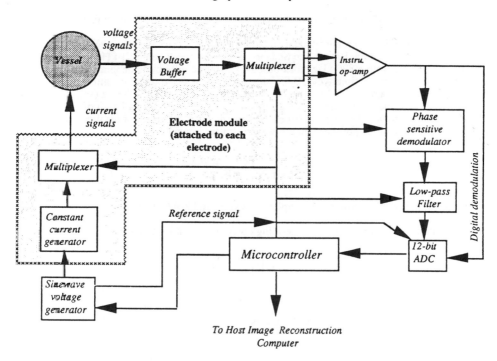

Figure 1   Structure of the UMIST process tomography data acquisition system

Two important attributes of the voltage generator for use in EIT are:

i)   good amplitude stability - for example, in a sequential measurement 16 electrode system where the applied ac. current is at 50 kHz, the amplitude must remain stable (to ±0.1%) for at least 320 ms.

ii)   low harmonic distortion - the phase sensitive demodulator (see Section 4) uses the oscillator output to synchronously rectify the measured voltage signal. The noise contribution from the harmonic coefficients (see later analysis) is also rectified by the demodulator causing an error. This error can be reduced by employing a switching demodulator (in which only odd-numbered harmonics cause errors) or a digital demodulator in combination with a digital function generator.

The Wien-bridge oscillator is a traditional sinewave generator which exhibits low output signal distortion. Van der Walt (1981) used three FET op-amps to construct a Wien-bridge circuit which had a distortion of 0.01% @ 5 kHz Some monolithic function generators such as the Exar XR-2206 (0.5% distortion), and the Datel ROJ-1K can also produce a good-quality sinewave. The main problem in using the above circuits is that it is difficult to get both a variable frequency sinewave signal *and* a synchronous (square wave) signal used for demodulation, as well as being able to adjust the phase shift (see Section 4) at different frequencies. The solution, also adopted by other groups, is to utilise an EPROM-based staircase function generator. The EPROM is programmed with a digitised sinewave signal. This signal can be stored as a variable number of samples, usually 16 or 32, depending on the required accuracy of the reconstituted signal. A counter is used to repetitively clock the stored 'staircase' wave form out of the EPROM which is then converted into a voltage by a zero-order hold digital-to-analogue converter (DAC) and subsequently filtered by an op-amp stage to remove the unwanted harmonic components. This digital approach generates both a sinewave voltage output as well as two synchronous square waves. One of the square waves is supplied to the analogue phase sensitive demodulator as a synchronous demodulation signal and the other is used to produce an ADC conversion pulse if synchronous digital demodulation is desired.

Evans and Towers (1980) produced detailed mathematical descriptions of sinewave generators from staircase wave forms. Brown and Seagar (1985) also produced a 51 kHz sinewave with 16 values per cycle from a 820 kHz clock based on a staircase function generator for their first clinical APT system. A final year B.Sc. degree student at UMIST designed and built a programmable generator with adjustable frequencies from 500 Hz to 62.5 kHz (selectable over 9 steps) with 32 values per cycle from a 2 MHz clock. The generator had a 53 dB attenuation of the second harmonic when the fundamental frequency was 30 kHz. For ideal conditions, the harmonics components C_m of the staircase wave form are given by,

$$|C_m| = \frac{1}{2} \left| sinc\left\{\frac{m\pi}{N}\right\} \right| \tag{1}$$

where: $m = kN \pm 1$, N = number of samples per cycle, and $k = 0, 1, 2, .., \infty$

From equation (1), a simple formula describing coefficients can be derived,

$$|C_m| = \frac{\frac{1}{2} \left| sinc\left\{\frac{\pi}{N}\right\} \right|}{m} = \frac{|c_1|}{m} \tag{2}$$

The total harmonic distortion (THD) is defined below,

$$THD = \sqrt{1 - (sinc(\pi/N))^2} \times 100\% \tag{3}$$

In the case of 32 samples per cycle (i.e. N=32), the coefficients are shown in Table 1. The total harmonic distortion (THD) for three different values of N are shown in Table 2.

Harmonic	Coefficient	Value
Fundamental	C1	0.4992
31	C31	0.0161
33	C33	0.0151
63	C63	0.0079
65	C65	0.0077
67	C67	0.0074

Table 1   Coefficient values for N = 32 using Equation (2)

N	THD (%)
6	13.071
32	5.6645
64	2.8336

Table 2   Total harmonic distortion values for different values of N using equation (3)

The harmonic components are easily removed by a low-pass filter for N » 1. The UMIST system uses an active second order Butterworth low-pass filter the amplitude function of which is given below from (Harry 1979),

$$B_p(\omega) = \frac{1}{(1 + \omega^{2p})} \approx \frac{1}{\omega^{2p}} \qquad (if\ \omega \gg 1) \tag{4}$$

where ω is the normalised angular signal frequency and p is the number of filter poles (2 in this case).

The attenuation A of the power function between the corner frequency (F_c) and the filtered frequency (F_b) is given by,

$$A = 10 \log_{10}\left(\frac{B_p(\omega_b)}{B_p(\omega_c)}\right) = 20\,p \log\left(\frac{F_c}{F_b}\right) \qquad (5)$$

For N=32 and p=2, the attenuation of the lower harmonic (31st) is -59.65 dB at the output of the filter. Considering the original coefficients of the first harmonic and the fundamental frequency, the total attenuation of the lower harmonic (31st) is -89.48 dB. In practice, the main distortion does not arise from the staircase wave form but from the switching of the DAC and the harmonic distortion from the op-amps. The resultant distortion contains a number of low-order harmonics. It is thus imperative to use a high speed DAC and low harmonic distortion op-amps when constructing the voltage generator. When using an AD7545 ADC coupled to a 2-pole active low-pass Butterworth filter, the attenuation of the second harmonic was found to be lower than 65 dB @ 38.4 kHz, 57.2 dB @ 76.8 kHz and 45.5 dB @ 153.6 kHz. All of the high order harmonics from the staircase wave form were lower than 70 dB (see Section 5).

Because the voltage to current converter (VCCS - Section 3.1) and filter stages produce a combined phase delay (5.6° @ 38.4 kHz by the VCCS and approximately 45° by the filter), it is necessary to maintain a synchronous reference with the measured signal at the input of the demodulator. In order to obtain a synchronous signal for input to the demodulator reference, the signal from the sinewave voltage generator is passed through a phase shift circuit, which will delay the phase of the reference signal by the same amount as that of the injected sinewave signal caused by hardware. Since a wide band of frequencies and a wide range of current amplitudes are inherent in the system, different phase delays at the output of the VCCS will be generated particularly at high frequencies. It is difficult to adjust the phase delay using the above approach for all situations. Thus the EPROM-based staircase wave generator was altered to generate square waves in phase with the original sinewave which can be used for either analogue or digital demodulation. The phase of square waves are shifted relative to the sinewave by microcontrolled switches from 0.7° to 180° and more precise adjustment can be achieved by using adjustable 5 to 500 ns delay lines. For the enhanced sinewave generator shown in Figure 2, the lower 5-bits of the EPROMs address line are connected to the output of a CMOS counter which clocks out 32 samples of the staircase wave. The high 8-bits of the EPROM are controlled by a microcontroller, which selects one of 256 staircase waves with different pre-calculated phase shifts also being stored in the EPROM. The most significant bit and bit 2 of the counter output also form the synchronous signals and are used elsewhere.

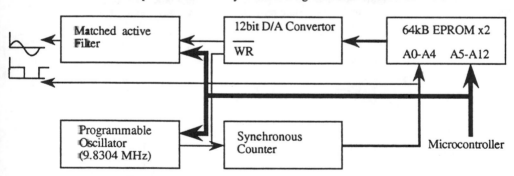

Figure 2   Enhanced digital sinewave voltage generator with programmable synchronous square wave output

3.   Electrode module

A distinct problem in clinical EIT systems is the distance of the ac. current injection source to the electrodes. Many clinical instruments suffer from the effects of stray capacitance arising from lengths of coaxial cable (typically 100 pF/m for UR95-type cable) connecting the current source to the injecting electrodes. Rigaud *et al* (1990) suggested that a module containing the necessary current injection and voltage measurement circuitry be constructed on the electrode thereby removing the problems associated with stray capacitance. Thus the authors constructed a small batch of such modules, called 'electrode modules', shown in Figure 3. Each module is mounted directly onto the vessel via male and female subminiature gold-plated SMB connectors to the electrode.

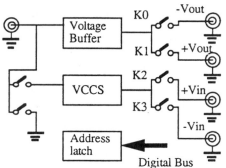

Figure 3   Electrode module showing connection of routing switches to injection point, voltage buffer and voltage controlled current source (VCCS).

Switches K0 and K1 in Figure 3 are employed to route the output voltage to one input of the differential op-amp. Switches K2 and K3 select one of the input sinewave voltages (one is inphase the other inverted) so that the VCCS can be configured as either a current source or a current sink to enable various data collection protocols (Brown and Seagar 1987) to be used.

3.1   Voltage controlled current source (VCCS)

The VCCS is probably one of the most critical aspects of a current injection EIT data collection system. The simplest form of a VCCS is an inverting amplifier (Figure 4a). The output current error produced by such a circuit is less than 0.0003% for a typical open-loop gain of 600 @ -90° (Webster 1990). However, it cannot be used for systems requiring more than one current source, or on systems with a grounded load (which are prevalent in the process industry). An extension of the above circuit is accomplished by using a transformer to isolate the output of the op-amp from Z_L (Figure 4b). Due to the limitation of inductance associated with the transformer, it still cannot be used in a system requiring high accuracy due to its inherent low output impedance.

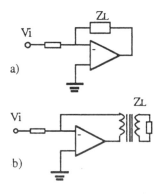

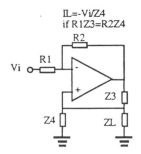

Figure 4
Fundamental negative feedback VCCS designs
a) simplest circuit,b) extension of a)
using transformer coupled load

Figure 5
Single op-amp VCCS with positive feedback
used by Nowicki and Webster (1989)

Positive feedback VCCSs are a popular alternative. Nowicki and Webster (1989) used a single op-amp with positive feedback and obtained a respectable performance at 50 kHz for a 5 mA current amplitude output (see Figure 5). Having tested the same circuit, the authors found it to be unstable when the voltage dropped across load was higher than 10 V.

Lidgey et al (1990) introduced a VCCS employing an op-amp supply current technique to obtain high performance (see Figure 6). The circuit does not use positive feedback and thus operates in a unity gain condition. Hence, it is inherently stable and has a wide bandwidth. Its performance is limited by the inherent inaccuracies in the current-mirror portions of the design. For example, it is difficult to maintain the mismatch of the required transistor pair lower than 0.1%. In fact, the best commercially available matched transistor pair costing £13 is only ±0.2% @ 10μA. Hilland (1991) built a VCCS using a similar circuit: the current mirrors were based on a CA3096E transistor array; and the second harmonic produced by the VCCS was reported to be 8 dB @ 30 kHz fundamental frequency.

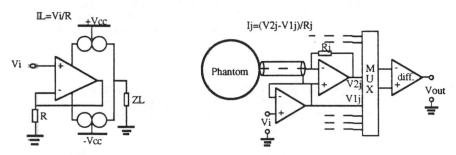

Figure 6   **Figure 7**
Op-amp supply current sensing VCCS   Dynamically adjustable VCCS by Lidgey and Zhu (1991)

Lidgey and Zhu (1991) presented a new front-end architecture shown in Figure 7. In essence, the circuit is a voltage driver, but its current can be measured easily by a differential op-amp. In operation, a voltage V_i is input and the corresponding output voltage V_{out}, measured. The input voltage V_i is altered until sufficient accuracy in I_j calculated by V_{out}/R_j was obtained. The circuit has a relatively straightforward structure and manages to produce a high accuracy injection current at a frequency of 10 kHz. However, this circuit is difficult to modify to accommodate the high speed and high frequency specifications given in Section 1.

The VCCS finally adopted by the authors is based on a positive feedback architecture the schematic circuit for which is shown in Figure 8 below,

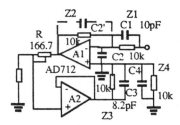

Figure 8   Two op-amp VCCS with positive feedback used in the authors' system

The transconductance term of the circuit in Figure 8 is given by,

$$G_T = -\frac{Z_2}{Z_1 R} \tag{6}$$

and its output admittance is given by,

$$G_{out} = \frac{1 - \dfrac{1 + \dfrac{Z_2}{Z_1}}{1 + \dfrac{Z_3}{Z_4}}}{R} \tag{7}$$

$$I_1 = \frac{V_i \, Z_2}{Z_1 \, R} \tag{8}$$

If the ratio of Z_2/Z_1 is equal to the ratio of Z_3/Z_4, G_{out} should tend to zero, but due to the input capacitances C_2 and C_4 of the differential op-amp, A1, two capacitances C_1 and C_2 are present between both inputs to A_1 (see Figure 8) and ground. Among them, the equivalent capacitance C_2' is used to represent C_2 from Miller's theorem. It is necessary to complement Z_1 and Z_2 with C_1 and C_2 in order to attain a higher VCCS output impedance. Also, the value of R should be chosen to be as large as possible according to equation (6). Unfortunately, due to the finite limit of the op-amp power rails, the voltage dropped across R can lower the saturation voltage V_s of the VCCS.

$$V_s = V_{pp} - I_L \, R - 5 \, v \tag{9}$$

The VCCS produces significant phase shift at high frequency (over 20 kHz). This produces errors in phase sensitive demodulated data if there is no phase compensation. As described in Section 2, the authors system employs an accurate programmable phase shift function which can adjust the matched phase error to less than $0.7°$.

Although the technique of direct connection between the vessel and electrode modules is used, the driven shield technique is necessary to cancel any stray capacitance associated with the SNB connectors. The choice of op-amp for the voltage buffer is also critical. In order to obtain a high input impedance for the voltage buffer, FET or CMOS input op-amps are used. Due to stray capacitance of the output transducer cable (about 100pF/m), instability of the VCCS will be produced with some types of CMOS op-amp, such as the AD711 and the TL081c. The LF411 JFET input op-amp was found to have a good performance for either input impedance or driving capacitance load.

Through the use of compensation techniques, the bandwidth and the amplitude of current from the VCCS extends linearly from 75 Hz up to 153.6 kHz and the current from 0 to 30 mA respectively. Also, the output impedance of the electrode module is increased to 1.74 MΩ @ 153.6 kHz, and 2.5 MΩ @ 76.8 kHz.

4. Voltage measurement, demodulation and filtering

The voltage measurement circuitry (Figure 9) extends from the voltage buffers in the electrode module to the digital data output from the ADC.

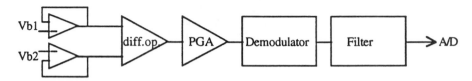

Figure 9   The voltage measurement, demodulation and filtering components of the UMIST
EIT data acquisition system

One of the most problematic measurement errors arises from common mode voltage (CMV) because of the limitations of the op-amps. To establish the bounds of such voltage measurements a four electrode simulation circuit based on a measurement model suggested by Brown and Seagar (1985) was constructed (Figure 10). The current source and sink both have an output impedance Rs to ground. The current passes through a multiplexer with an 'ON' resistance R_m, and an equivalent capacitance C_m to represent the multiplexer's 'IN' and

'COMMOM' terminal leakage capacitances. The equivalent contact resistance R_{e1} and R_{e2} is larger than R_m since they are connected serially in the injection circuit and cause the major part of the CMV. Stray capacitance C_s appears directly between the wires at the driving electrodes and those at the measuring electrodes. At each interface between the electrode and conducting region there is a stray capacitance C_v to ground. The conductive region is simplified to R_1, R_2, R_3 and R_4 ($R_4 > R_3 > R_2 > R_1$). The input impedance of the voltage buffer is mainly determined by the input capacitance C_{b1} and C_{b2} at high frequency. R_{mb1} and R_{mb2} are the sum of the output impedances of the op-amp and multiplexer. C_{c1} and C_{c2} are the sum of the stray capacitances of the transfer cable, between the output of the multiplexer and the differential op-amp.

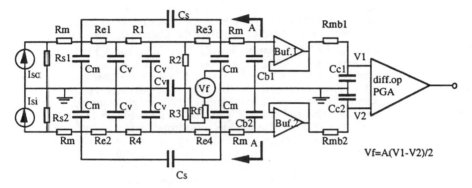

Figure 10 Four-electrode measurement model

The common mode voltage is generated due to a leakage current and is determined from a combination of the injecting current value, the electrode contact resistance, and the conductivity of the conductive region. The error caused by the CMV is formed from the difference between the output impedance, looked at from the A-A direction, and the mismatched input impedance of the op-amp, and the coupling components.

At the differential programmable gain amplifier (PGA) (PGA202): if the output impedance of the common voltage are identical to the two inputs of the PGA, the CMRR only depends on the mismatch error of integrated circuit. The CMRR will be increased, i.e. the error will be reduced, if the gain of the PGA is increased. The PGA202 has CMRR of 32db @ gain 1, 53db @ gain 10 and 73db @ gain 100 and gain 1000 all @ 100 kHz according to its specification. After the compensation values of 24.8db @ gain 1, 69.7 dB @ gain 10, 74.1 dB @ gain 100 and 71.9 dB @ gain 1000 were obtained from the authors' system when the frequency was 153.6 kHz. For an imbalance of output impedance of the CMV, the maximum realisable CMRR is as below (Garrett 1981),

$$CMRR_{max} = \frac{1}{4\pi f\, \Delta R_s\, \Delta C_s} \tag{10}$$

According to Figure 10, if $\Delta R_s = R_{mb1} - R_{mb2} = 50\ \Omega$ which is contributed to mainly by the mismatched multiplexer 'ON' resistance, $\Delta C_s = C_{c1} - C_{c2} = 20$ pF is contributed to mainly by multiplexer's output capacitance and the stray capacitance of cable, the CMRR at 76.8 kHz will be 60.3 dB. In order to increase the CMRR at this stage, a transformer can also be used, for which a higher CMRR will be attained. It is worth noting the balance of output impedance of the transformer: a differential op-amp is still necessary because a common voltage is still maintained on the output of the transformer (see Figure 4b) caused by mutual inductance and stray capacitance between the primary and secondary coils. Particularly, the error caused by CMV at the voltage buffer will become a sum of differential signal and a common voltage. According to Murphy (1988), the differential signal from the common voltage at the output of the two op-amps will be:

$$V_o = (4\pi f\ \Delta R\ \Delta C)^2 V_{cm} + j(4\pi f\ \Delta R\ \Delta C)V_{cm} \tag{11}$$

Among them: ΔR is the difference in the output impedances looked at from the A-A direction, which is mainly from contact resistance of electrodes and the impedance of the conductive region; ΔC is the difference in the output capacitance, which is mainly from the connecting cables and multiplexers. Because $\Delta R \gg \Delta R_s$, the error caused at the voltage buffer is larger than that at the differential op-amp. Besides reducing the mismatched impedance, discussed above, such as ΔR_s, ΔC_s, ΔR, ΔC, the best method is to reduce the common voltage. One method used by Brown and Seagar (1985), is the technique of common mode voltage feedback (CMFB). In clinical applications, electrical isolation of the current generator enables common mode feedback to be applied to a common reference electrode and so improve the common mode rejection ratio. Figure 11 is a simplified circuit for the adjacent injection model. If $Z_{c1} = Z_{c2} = Z_{c3}$, $Z_1 = 0.1\ Z_2$, $|Z_2| \ll |Z_{cn}|$, then V_1 is $4IZ_1$, V2 is $3IZ_1$, and V3 is $-7IZ_1$. There a feedback current is induced. If the $I_f = -9IZ_1/Z_c$ to ground it merely cancels the current through the Z_{c2}, and so the common voltage V_2 will be zero. However, the CMFB is not without limitation. Because of the phase delay of the feedback circuit, it will cause a phase error in the demodulation and possible feedback oscillation (Murphy 1988) at high frequency. Thus, due to there being no voltage being dropped across Z_{c2} an ideal CMFB in Figure 11, point 2 can be connected to ground directly (Figure 12) since electrical isolation is no longer necessary in industrial applications. The current change in the floating model is similar to the CMFB of Figure 11. The feedback path of the CMFB and GFM methods is generally through any unused electrode in contact with the conductive region. This is necessary to remove the influence of contact impedance between the electrode and the low frequency ac. signal caused by the feedback.

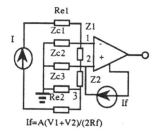

If=A(V1+V2)/(2Rf)

Figure 11
Common mode feedback (CMFB)
in the adjacent model

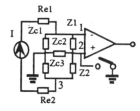

Figure 12
Grounded floating measurement (GFM)
in the adjacent model

The other method to reduce the error caused by the CMV is to use a low CMV injection method and some coefficients of the phantom. The common mode voltage in subsequent tests (see Section 5) is more than 6.6 V(p-p) for the adjacent method, larger than 5.5 V(p-p) in the multireference method, more than 4.4 V(p-p) in opposite method and lower than 0.63 V(p-p) in the multisink method. The multisink injection method was devised specifically for use on metal walled phantoms which has the advantage of a lower CMV. Increasing the surface area of the electrode in contact with the process material, increasing the conductivity of process material, and decreasing the amplitude of injection current can all act to reduce the CMV of the conductive region.

Physical models similar to the one shown in Figure 10 were also developed by the authors to represent the opposite, multireference and multisink current injection methods. Due to lack of space, these circuits will be described in the oral presentation.

4.1 Demodulation and filtering

Demodulation, in the authors' system, is achieved either by switched demodulation or digital demodulation. It is well known that the phase shift of the signal must be less than 1.266° for

12-bit accuracy in switched demodulation. Demodulation for the quadrature wave is much more sensitive than for the in-phase wave. For example, a quadrature signal deviated by only 0.015° can be located with a 12-bit ADC. The DAS is initially calibrated at the quadrature position for the injection current phase and then the correction phase is subtracted by 90° to represent the reference phase at the demodulator for in-phase demodulation. The minimum adjustable phase shift is 0.7° by microcontroller and 5 ns delay by manual delay line adjustment.

At the output of a switching demodulator an in-phase signal Y can be expressed using Fourier series by,

$$Y(\omega t, \theta) = \frac{2}{\pi} V_m \cos\theta + \frac{4}{\pi} V_m \sum_{n=1}^{\infty} \frac{1}{4n^2 - 1} (2n \sin 2n\omega t \sin\theta - \cos 2n\omega t \cos\theta) \quad (12)$$

where θ is the phase shift of the signal and $(-\pi/2 < \theta \leq 0)$

Using a 2 pole active low-pass filter the d.c. component of Y is obtained. The corner frequency F_c of such a filter is calculated from,

$$F_c = 2F_0 \sqrt[p]{\delta} \quad (13)$$

where F_0 is the fundamental frequency of the signal, p is the number of filter poles, and ∂ is the accuracy which is 1/4096 for a 12-bit ADC.

The filter settling time is given in (Webster 1990) and can be determined from,

$$\frac{V_o}{V_i} = 1 - e^{-\omega ct} \left\{ 1 + \omega_c t + \frac{\omega_c^2 t^2}{t!} + \ldots + \frac{(\omega_c t)^{n-1}}{(n-1)!} \right\} \quad (14)$$

The settling time with different poles at 76.8kHz are shown in Table 3 and at different frequencies with 2 fixed poles in Table 4.

pole	$\omega_c t$	F_c (Hz)	T (mS)
1	8.3247	37.5	35.3
2	10.799	2400	0.716
3	14.923	19200	0.123

Table 3   Low-pass filter settling times ($F_0 = 76.8$ kHz) for different numbers of poles p

F_0 (kHz)	2.4	9.6	38.4	76.8	153.6
T (mS)	22.9	5.7	1.43	0.716	0.358

Table 4   Low-pass filter settling times (p = 2) for different fundamental frequencies F_0

The matched filter can be constructed using op-amps or from a monolithic switched capacitor Butterworth low-pass filter such as the MF4. The latter is easier to implement and has a better performance. Using digital demodulation and simplified demodulation algorithms, a SNR much closer to the theoretical value can be attained since the synchronous sampling signals can all be obtained from the EIT DAS.

The data collection speed of an EIT system is mainly limited by the filter and its associated couplings. Because there are several coupling circuits from the current generator to the ADC input, the transition effects will occur as the electrode is switched to connect to the measurement circuit with the multiplexer. In a flexible data collection system, it is difficult to satisfy both the high speed and wide bandwidth. In the Mk.1b several parts of the coupling circuit and some function circuits are placed in a small module which can be exchanged easily in order to satisfy the different requirements. The fastest speed of collection for 1 frame of 104 measurements is 40 ms at 38.4kHz using the digital demodulation method.

5.   Performance of data collection system

5.1   Output impedance of current source

For the electrode module described in Section 3, the current source is accompanied by a voltage buffer and a multiplexer. Hence, the measured output impedance is influenced by both the buffer and multiplexer. A purely resistive load was attached to the output of the module. The voltage dropped across different resistive loads for the same current and frequency was measured and inserted into equation (15) to determine the impedance Z_s listed in Table 5 below,

$$Z_s = \frac{\Delta V}{\Delta I} = \frac{V_2 - V_1}{(V_2/R_2) - (V_1/R_1)} \tag{15}$$

F (kHz)	Vr1 (mV)	Vr2 (mV)	I_1 (mA)	ΔI (mA)	Impedance (MΩ)
153.6	2458.0	125.830	2.456	0.0013	1.7449
76.8	3284.2	167.970	3.282	0.0012	2.5159
38.4	3276.2	167.669	3.274	0.00088	3.5449
19.2	3294.6	168.584	3.292	0.00036	8.6628
9.6	3295.5	168.633	3.293	0.00042	7.4713
4.8	3294.5	168.489	3.292	0.0014	2.2414
2.4	3289.3	168.250	3.287	0.00087	3.6028

Table 5   Current source(module) output impedance

[Note: R_1 =1000.7Ω, R_2=51.2Ω. Sample electrode was number 15 and was measured with a Fluke 8842A meter]

The phase shift caused by the electrode module when measuring the phase shift with the quadrature measurement technique was found to be 185.6° @ 38.4 kHz.

5.2   VCCS harmonics

The harmonics were measured on a HP4195 spectrum analyser. At the output of the sinewave voltage generator, the attenuation of second harmonic is lower than 65 dB @ 38.4 kHz, 57.2 dB @ 76.8 kHz and 45.5 dB @ 153.6 kHz. All of the high order harmonics from the 31st order upwards were lower than 70 dB, which were due to the staircase wave form. The attenuation caused by the electrode module is 6 dB @ 38.4 kHz and 76.8 kHz.

5.3   Common mode rejection ratio (CMRR)

The CMRR was measured at the output of the PGA with a Fluke 8842A voltmeter. The results for different values of the PGA gain are given in Figure 13. The input common mode voltage at the differential inputs of the differential input amplifier are 12 V (p-p) sinewave from a Farnell LF1 generator. The CMRR @ 153.6kHz were as follows: 24.8 dB @ gain 1, 69.76 dB @ gain 10, 74.31 dB @ gain 100 and 71.87 dB @ gain 1000.

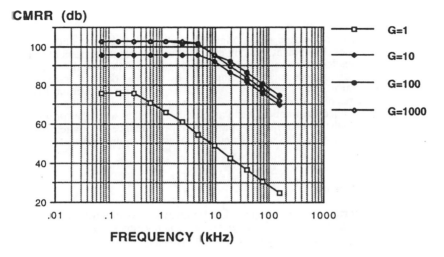

FREQUENCY (kHz)

Figure 13   CMRR of the authors' system for different values of PGA gain

5.4   Input offset voltage of the signal measurement stages

The digital output of the ADC in the authors' system in response to zero at its input is ± 1LSB when the gain of the programmable gain amplifier was changed from 1 to 1000.

5.5   Gain error of the signal measurement stages

The errors were +0.19% at gain 1, +0.12% at gain 10, +0.38% at gain 100 and +1.4% at gain 1000 all measured at a frequency of 9.6 kHz, which were acquired from the digital output of the ADC, and the input voltages were measured with the Fluke 8842A voltmeter (the accuracy of the Fluke 8842A is ±0.08%+100 digital)

5.6   Accuracy of the signal measurement stages

A voltage was placed at the input of the DAS which was also measured with the Fluke 8842A voltmeter. The digital data from the output of the ADC showed a deviation of lower than +0.5% from 0.6 kHz to 76.8 kHz.(the accuracy of the Fluke 8842A voltmeter is ±0.07% +150 digital @ 0.6 kHz to 9.6 kHz, ±0.19% +150 digital @ 38.4 kHz and ±0.5% +300 digital @ 76.8 kHz)

5.7   Load range

The load range can be determined by an approximate equation given below,

$$V_s = V_{pp} - I_L R - 5 v \tag{16}$$

where: V_s is the saturation voltage, V_{pp} is the amplitude of the supply voltage (30 V in this case), I_L is the current through the load, and R is the value of the feedback resistor in electrode module (66.7 Ω).

5.8   Accuracy for the adjacent electrode method

A resistor network was used to determine the DAS error for this form of measurement method. The majority of errors were lower than ±1%, the maximum error was 5% corresponding to two readings taken when the measurement electrode pair was diametrically opposite the current injection pair.

6. Conclusion

The specifications of a flexible data collection system built by the authors to enable investigation of process equipment utilising electrical impedance measurements were given. The structure and function of the key circuits constituting the system were also described along with a comparison of equivalent circuits employed by other workers. A trade-off between system flexibility, measurement accuracy, cost, and speed of data acquisition was achieved. The result was a data collection system with 7 programmable frequencies and 256 selectable levels of ac. current injection frequency and amplitude as well as a number of voltage signal measurement, demodulation and filtering options. The performance criteria relevant to such a data collection system were also highlighted and measured figures given for the authors' system.

7. Acknowledgements

This work is supported by the European Coal and Steel Community and UMIST under agreement number 7220/EA/829. MW also gratefully acknowledges the Chinese Academy of Sciences Scholarship and additional support from the Xinjiang Institute of Physics.

8. References

Brown, B.H., and Seagar, A.D, (1985), "Applied Potential Tomography: data collection problems", IEE Int. Conf. on Electric and Magnetic Fields in Medicine and Biology, London, 4 - 5 Dec.

Brown, B.H., and Seagar, A.D, (1987), "The Sheffield data collection system", Clin. Phys. Physiol. Meas., 8A, pp. 91-98.

Evans, W.A., Towers, M.S., (1980), "Hybrid techniques in waveform generation and synthesis", IEE Proc., 127,3.

Garrett, P.H., (1981), "Analogue I/O: acquistion, conversion, recovery", Reston Pub. Co., Virginia.

Harry, Y.F., (1979) "Analog and digital filters: Design and realization", Prentice-Hall, New Jersey.

Hilland, J., (1991), "Optimization of data acquisition and signal processing for use in process tomography", final year project report, Dept. E.E & E., UMIST.

Lidgey, J., Vere-Hunt, M., and Toumazou, C., (1990), "Development in current driver circuitry), Proc. CAIT Conf., Copenhagen, pp. 183-190.

Lidgey, J., and Zhu, Q.C., (1991), "Electrode current determination from programmable voltage sources", Proc. CAIT Conf., York.

Murphy, D., and Rolfe, P., (1988), "Aspects of instrumentation design for impedance imaging", Clin. Phys.Physiol. Meas., 9A, pp. 5-14.

Nowicki, D.J., and Webster, J.G., (1989), "A one-amp current source for electrical impedance tomography", Proc. Ann. Int Conf. IEEE Eng. in Medicine and Biol. Soc., 11, pp. 457-8.

Record, P.M., Gadd, R., and Vinther, F., (1992), "Multifrequency tomograms", Submitted to J. Clin. Phys.and Physiol. Meas.

Rigaud, B., Anah, J., Givelin, P., Graziotin, P., Morucci, J.P, (1990) "Multifunction electrode module for electrical impedance tomography, Proc. CAIT Conf., Copenhagen. pp. 217-225.

Van der Walt, E.G., (1981), "A Wien-bridge oscillator with high-amplitude stability", IEEE Trans. Instr. Meas., IM-30, pp. 292-4

Webster, J.G., (1990), Editor of "Electrical Impedance Tomography", Adam Hilger, Bristol.

A digital signal processor based architecture for EIT data acquisition

G M Lyon and J P Oakley

Signal Processing Group, Dept. Electrical Engineering, The University, Manchester, M13 9PL, UK.

Abstract

This paper describes a novel system architecture for electrical impedance tomography data acquisition, based on Motorola's DSP96000 series digital signal processor. The principle aim is to produce a system that is modular and flexible in order to address various research aspects of electrical process tomography. The architecture is able to support unusual electrode configurations with no limit placed on the number possible. The same circuitry performs both signal injection and measurement, thus eliminating the need for analogue signal multiplexing. The system will allow fast data sampling and image frame rates, and provides support for future real-time image reconstruction.

1   Introduction

Existing EIT data acquisition systems have mainly been based on analogue electronics, with all the signal processing performed in the analogue domain before digital conversion and storage. These designs have the usual problems associated with analogue circuits, such as noise, stray capacitance, bad component matching, input offsets and cable loading. The speed of operation of analogue systems is also limited by factors such as switching transients, multiplexing overhead and conversion delays. These problems all stem from the serial data acquisition method.

In order to improve both the signal fidelity and data acquisition speed a modular Digital Signal Processor (DSP) based architecture is proposed, based upon Motorola's DSP96002 device. The system is intended for use in the dynamic imaging of concentration profiles in stirred vessels, with a typical system configuration shown in figure 5. This paper forms a statement of intent rather than a report of an operational system. We hope to report and possibly demonstrate a DSP based system at a future ECAPT meeting.

2   Idealized system architecture

In order to provide a truly modular architecture it would be desirable to have one DSP for each electrode, or electrode measurement pair, as shown in figure 1. With suitable front end electronics associated with each DSP we are able to configure, with external software, each module to behave either as a measurement device or as an excitation device or as both.

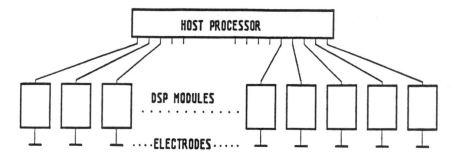

Figure 1, Idealized system architecture

In measurement mode the module samples, digitally demodulates and digitally filters the incoming signal producing real and quadrature data. In excitation mode the DSP generates the excitation waveform, either from a waveform stored in memory, or by computing the waveform from a mathematical expression. As each DSP module only caters for a single electrode, the system places no restriction on the number of electrodes used. The number of electrodes also has little effect on the speed of operation as all its actions are in parallel. The DSP modules however must be synchronized to ensure measurement concurrency. The system also requires a master process to control the operation of the DSP modules, to set up the measurement sequence, and to collate the demodulated data for each image.

3   Proposed system architecture

In order to reduce the cost of the one processor per electrode system while retaining most of the benefits we propose a pseudo-parallel architecture in which each DSP module is used to measure and excite a number of electrodes.

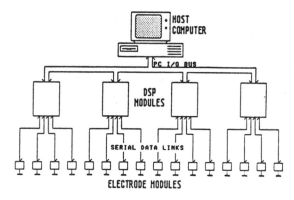

Figure 2, Proposed system configuration

We intend to build a system using 4 electrodes to each processor. The target configuration is initially 24 electrodes but this is likely to be extended to a greater number at a later stage in the research. Figure 2 shows the configuration of a 16 electrode system.

3.1   Electrode module

An analogue front end circuit is an essential part of the system providing the interface
between the analogue electrode signals and the digital processing domain. It has been
suggested by Record et al (1990) that a single ended or common mode measurement
technique would be more advantageous. However the resolution of present ADC devices
prohibits such measurement techniques. A differential amplifier is still required to obtain
a good quality signal with sufficient variation due to impedance changes. Programmable
gain is also required to take advantage of the ADC's quantization range. A conversion
device with 12 or more bits resolution and a sampling rate of several hundred kHz would
be required, for example Motorola's DSP56ADC16. Having a modular front end however
removes the need for signal and source multiplexing, and this has a beneficial effect on the
signal quality. Figure 3 shows functionally the form of the analogue front end circuitry,
or electrode module. It also shows signals coming from (n-1) and going to (n+1), the
adjacent electrode modules. The module communicates with the DSP via a serial digital
data link, allowing location of the module close to the electrode.

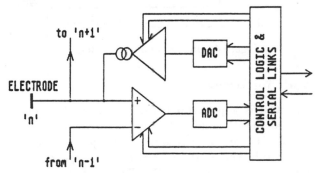

Figure 3, Electrode Module

3.2   DSP module architecture

The Motorola DSP96002. despite having internal RAM and ROM, requires external memory space for program and data storage. This area of RAM can be accessed by the host
processor, enabling the device to be directly programmed and controlled by the host.
The host will also be capable of resetting the DSP to enable concurrent execution of the
DSP program routines. The DSP must also be able to send data to the electrode modules
under its control. This is achieved using serial data links, allowing the DSP to be placed
some distance from the measurement site. Figure 4 shows the basic structure of the DSP
module. In order to reduce the physical size, circuit board complexity and cost, and
increase reliability the design will make extensive use of erasable logic arrays (ELAs) for
the DSP support logic including: interrupt control, memory control and the PC interface
control and buffering. By using erasable ASICs the hardware configuration also becomes
partially programmable. allowing quick and easy rectification of any design errors.

3.3   The host processor

The host machine is an IBM PC clone. based on the Intel i486 processor and chosen
for its good performance/price ratio. and to allow use of Motorola's 96000 development

system, providing DSP emulation and debugging facilities. The PC uses the extended EISA bus architecture; this allows a fast data transfer rate (up to 32Mbits/s) achieved by direct parallel word transfer to and from the DSP modules. The PC will also provide the user interface, non-volatile memory and a platform for image reconstruction.

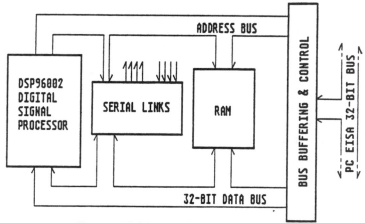

Figure 4, DSP module: block diagram

3.4   Speed and performance

The Motorola DSP96002 is a powerful IEEE floating point signal processing device, capable of performing at 20 MIPS and 60 MFLOPS. In practice however the floating point speed will be less than this figure since maximum throughput implies that a floating point multiply, addition and subtraction are performed on independent data in a dual clock cycle. A more realistic figure would be 40MFLOPS since this corresponds to the multiply add cycle of digital filters. For real time operation the complexity of the demodulation and filtering algorithm applied will be limited to the number of instructions that can be executed between each sampling of the signal, or each change in the desired excitation signal. For example if we apply a 10kHz sine wave to the vessel and wish to sample the signal at ten times this frequency then the DSP will be able to execute 400 instruction cycles between each sample. With, 4 electrodes per DSP each signal will have to be processed within 100 clock cycles. At faster sampling rates the processing time will decrease and may not allow sufficient time to apply anything but the simplest processing algorithms, e.g. sample and store to RAM.

A similar system to the one proposed is in use for real time medical EIT imaging. using parallel sampling channels and digital demodulation (Smith et al 1990). This system achieves an overall signal to noise increase of 20dB when used on a cylindrical phantom, compared with the serial analogue acquisition method. This is achieved using 6 samples per period of a 10kHz sinusoid demodulated over 20 cycles. We would wish to improve on this figure by the use of faster and more resolute sampling, a wider range of frequencies and excitation waveforms, and variable sampling periods.

3.5   Time gating

In most practical situations the frame rate (the number of images per second) will be determined by an application related event. In our case this will be the speed of impeller rotation in a mixing vessel. This data capture rate may not always be as fast as the maximum possible rate, particularly with large mixing vessels. The speed of frame capture however must still be as quick as possible to avoid image blurring due to the dynamic nature of the mixing process. In order to make good use of any idle time between frame captures the captured data is processed during this period before the next frame requires sampling. By time gating the frame sampling in this manner the data can be processed in real time, with complex algorithms, and free from interruption by sampling input and excitation output signals.

4   System Applications

We see the EIT data acquisition system described as applicable to many time-varying dynamic processes. Our particular interset is in the dynamic imaging of mixing in stirred vessels. Other possible applications are assessing flow rates in pipelines via cross-correlation, and monitoring of fluidized beds and hydro-cyclones. The scale of such processes varies greatly, with mixing vessels having diameters from 0.1 metres all the way up to 5 metres. Having the analogue front end circuitry separate from the digital processing large distances, several metres, can be placed between the two parts of the system, An optical link could be used to cover greater distances, e.g. from a control room to a plant process vessel.

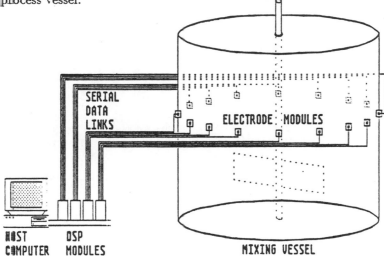

Figure 5, System application: Imaging a stirred mixing vessel

Figure 5 shows a typical configuration for monitoring a mixing vessel. This has 4 DSP modules, each controlling 4 electrode modules mounted around the outside of the vessel. Due to the flexible design of the system its use is not restricted to EIT. Other methods of data collection could be used such as capacitive or ultrasonic measurements by changing the front end's transducer elements.

Acknowledgement

This work was supported by a SERC Total Technology award in collaboration with ICI Chemicals and Polymers.

References

[1] Boniface A. 1990 *Looking into Process Plant* , The Chemical Engineer, 26 July 1990

[2] Brown B H. 1990 *Proc. EIT Workshop, Copenhagen: COMAC-BME* pp9-13

[3] Dickin et al. 1992 *IEE proceedings-G* , **139** No.1 72-82

[4] Motorola
    DSP96000 IEEE Floating-Point Dual-Port User's Manual
    DSP96000 Interface Techniques and Examples
    from: European Literature Distribution Centre, 88 Tanners Drive, Blakelands, Milton Keynes, MK14 5BP, England.

[5] Record P, Gadd R and Rolfe P. 1990 *Proc. EIT Workshop, Copenhagen; COMAC-BME* pp168-174

[6] Smith R W M, Brown B H, Freeston I L and McArdle F J. 1990 *Proc. EIT Workshop, Copenhagen; COMAC-BME* pp212-216

A prototype electrodynamic tomographic imaging system for pneumatic conveyors.

AR Bidin[1,3], RG Green[1], ME Shackleton[1] and RW Taylor[2].

1. School of Engineering Information Technology, Sheffield City Polytechnic
2. Department of Adaptive System Engineering, York University
3. Department of Electronics & Computer Engineering, Universiti Pertanian, Malaysia

Abstract: This paper describes the initial work which has been completed on a tomographic imaging system using electrodynamic sensors for application to pneumatically conveyed solids.

A mathematical model of the effect of a single charged particle on an array of sensors has been developed. A range of expected values has been predicted and used to design a simple reverse construction method.

Practical tests have been carried out. Eight sensors are equally spaced around the circumference of a 100 mm diameter plastic pipe and the system surrounded by an earthed screen. Each sensor output is buffered and uses driven guard techniques to maximise sensitivity. These outputs are amplified and conditioned for the data capture system.

A series of tests have been carried out to verify that the model is correct and to estimate the accuracies which have been attained.

1 Introduction

Electrical sensing is by far the most common technique used in process tomography. A lot of work has been done on electrical capacitance and, more recently, on electrical impedance based on earlier work in the medical field by Brown and Barber (1985). The work described in this paper is the first known attempt to investigate electrodynamic imaging.

The sensor electronics are based on earlier work by Shackleton (1981) who used a ring electrode to detect induced charges. Results from this work showed remarkable potential for such transducers to be applied in industry. Further to this, Gregory (1987) used a dual-location pin electrode system and cross-correlation to measure the velocity of shot leaving the nozzle of a shot-peening machine.

The imaging system currently developed by the authors makes use of an eight-channel electrodynamic transducer with eight sensors mounted at equal spacing around the circumference of a conveyor to pick up induced charges. A simple image reconstruction is developed using this data to produce an image of the flowing material.

2 An electrodynamic measurement system

The generation of electrical charge in pneumatic transport of materials has been known for many years. The magnitude of this charge is dependent on various factors such as the type of material, whether conducting or non-conducting, the quantity involved, moisture level, air flow rate and the physical dimensions of the conveyor.

The transducer system consists of two basic components: the pin electrode as the sensing device and the signal processing electronics. Capacitance and impedance sensors make use of an injected current into the system to produce a field. However, in electrodynamic tomography, the field is due to the conveying material and the electrodes are therefore passive.

Ring electrodes are not suitable for measuring induced potential on the sensors around the walls, because they do not provide information about spatial distribution. Pin electrodes, apart from being cheap and simple to construct, give point data along the circumference. Eight electrodes are used and the sampling has to be very fast and instantaneous for the sensors to capture the data simultaneously during the flight of the particles through the sensing volume. By having these sensors around the walls of the pipe, the difference of the strength of the measured output voltages gives a relationship with the position of the inducing charge.

The range of particle size in this work is 1-100 microns. The maximum potential that particles of this size range can attain is estimated by Shackleton (1981) to be in the range of 10^{-5} to 10^{-1} volts. The transducer was therefore designed to have a gain of 500 to give an output of up to 5 volts.

The input to each channel of the transducer is from a guarded buffer receiving the output from a sensor. In this way capacitance effects due to the leads being in the active field are eliminated and the sensitivity of the output measurement is enhanced. By introducing an input impedance input of about 5 MΩ, the effect of the potential due to the field is minimised and the measured potential is primarily due to induction. This is verified by the experiments described in the section below.

3 The Induction Model

A vertically downward flow of particles in a pipeline is considered for the modelling. On a macroscopic level, these particles flow in a turbulent manner causing changes in particle concentration.

It may be assumed that the net effect of the negative and positive charges on the various particles in the particulate cloud will result in a volume of charge travelling in the axial direction of the pipeline, but not necessarily through the central axis of the pipeline. Analogously, on a microscopic level, it is possible to assume for a low loading flow that only one particle is being viewed by the sensors in any short sampling time, as reported by Beck et al (1990).

The assumptions for the model are:

   1. The point charge is travelling in an axial direction parallel to the axis of the pipe.

   2. This particle has a constant, finite amount of charge which is not dissipated during the time it travels through the sensing volume.

   3. There is no interacting field external to the sensing volume because the dielectric pipe material is non-conducting.

   4. The charge is spherical with constant surface density.

The sensors along the pipe wall detect the passing charged particle. The potential measured on any one sensor is described by a relationship depending on the effects of induction, the field of the particle or possibly both these effects.

For a single charged particle, assumed as a point charge, the field is uniform radially over its surface,

$$E = \frac{q}{4\pi r^2 \varepsilon_o} \tag{1}$$

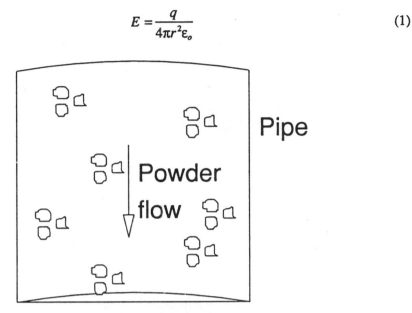

Figure 1. The Physical Model.

It is assumed in this model that this point charge induces a potential onto the surface of a pin electrode used to sense the change in potential at a point on the wall of a non-conducting or dielectric pipe.

For a given sensor, such as that shown in figure 2, the surface area is πr_e^2 which is normal to the flux. The area of the charge, assumed to be spherical, is $4\pi r^2$. So the proportion of flux for each sensor is

$$\frac{\pi r_e^2}{4\pi r_i^2} \tag{2}$$

For an unknown charge q, the induced charge for the i'th sensor will be proportional to q. Hence,

$$Q_{induced} = \frac{kr_e^2 q}{4r_i^2} = \frac{k_1 q}{r_i^2} \tag{3}$$

But $Q_{induced} = C V_{induced}$ and C, the capacitance of each sensor, is made constant by keeping the same distance between each sensor and the concentric earth shield,
Hence,

$$V_{induced} = k_2 \frac{q}{r_i^2} \tag{4}$$

From Figure 3, the distance from the charge to the sensor is given by the geometrical relationship

$$r_i = \sqrt{r^2 + R^2 - 2Rr\cos(\theta - \alpha)} \qquad (5)$$

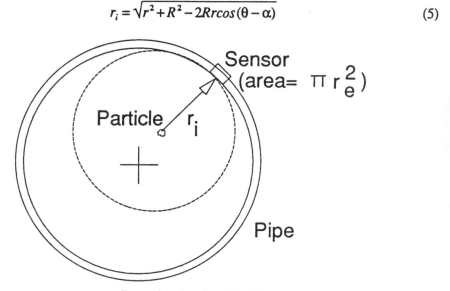

figure 2 Induction Model

The angle θ is the radial position of the charge while α is that of the sensor location from a reference diametrical axis. The distance between the i'th sensor and the charge is r_i.

Because q and k are unknowns in the above equation, the voltages for a given r are normalised over the maximum voltage to cancel out any constant terms in the model due to sensor or pipe geometry and size of charge. Hence,

$$V_{normalised} = \frac{V_i}{V_{max}} \qquad (6)$$

From this model, an estimate of the profile of the boundary voltages can be produced. It is possible to simulate different positions of the charge by changing the values of r and θ. However, changing θ will only give an angular offset to the profiles as shown by the results. Hence, only the results for $\theta = 0$ are shown.

For these calculations a charged particle is first placed at the centre of the pipe and then moved radially outwards towards the wall of the pipe. The voltage profiles produced at various radii along a chosen zero radian diametrical axis are plotted on the one graph; see Figure 4.

It is found that with the charge at the centre the voltage profile produced is uniform as expected. However as the charge is moved outwards towards the pipe wall along the reference radial axis the increase in voltage intensity is proportional to the distance or radius squared for the induction model. This voltage is proportional to distance or radius for a field model discussed elsewhere by Bidin et al (1992). Because normalised voltages are used, the unknown quantities in charge size, area of electrode surface and other geometrical correction factors are cancelled out.

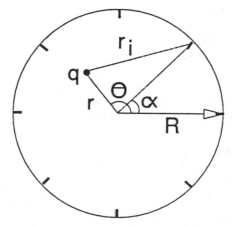

Figure 3. Geometry of the charge and sensor.

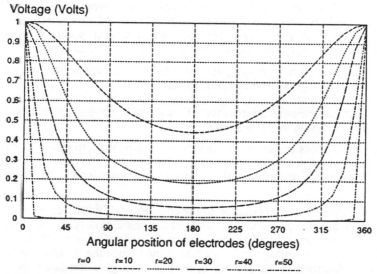

Figure 4. Variation in normalized induced voltage by a charge at various radial displacements (R=50).

The reconstruction of the radial position is obtained by a simple method of plotting the ratio of the maximum to minimum voltage obtained against the test radial positions and then interpolating the measured range to find the unknown radial position. This is discussed further in the next section.

4 Experiments for Model Verification

The experimental rig shown in figure 5 was designed to verify that the model accurately represents the phenomenon of pick-up potential on the pin electrodes.

The response from each sensor in the time domain is shown in Figure 6. Each channel response is displayed on the oscilloscope and the peak voltage is then measured. The peak-voltage is proportional to the strength of the induced charge on each sensor. The strength of the induced charge depends on the initial charge on the bead as well as the sensor-bead distance.

As the induced charge gets weaker, either due to small bead charge or the sensor being relatively far from the charged bead, the amplitude of the output sensor response diminishes and so does the signal to noise ratio. Theoretically, this can be corrected by increasing the charge on the bead. However, if too large a charge is used, the output potential on the nearer sensors will go into saturation. This difficulty is more pronounced as the bead is dropped near the pipe walls.

The data was processed statistically from a set of four tests at each of the five radial positions chosen. The mean and standard deviation values were used to plot the voltage profile of the pipe boundary. Normalised values were used as explained in section 3. This was advantageous not only from the computational point of view but also experimentally as the charge on the bead is never the same in each test.

The results were plotted on special graphs where the theoretical profiles were already plotted for several charge positions along a reference axis. The results were plotted in such a way that the sensor with maximum value is fixed as the reference sensor at $\theta = 0$ and the readings from the other sensors were then plotted on the graph in a cyclic manner. Typical results are shown in figures 7a-e.

From the voltage profiles around the boundary of the pipe wall, the position of maximum voltage suggests which sensor is closest to the charge inside the pipe. In a single charge situation, the position of minimum voltage should be diametrically opposite the location of the charge.

In order to determine the radial position of the charge, a calibration chart is used. Values of the ratio of maximum to minimum voltages are calculated for several radial charge positions. These are then plotted to show the range and radial position as demonstrated in Figure 8. Hence, the voltage ratio, as determined from the voltage profile obtained by the method described in the preceding section, will give the radial position of the charge. In reconstructing the image, the task of determining the values r and θ is therefore achieved.

The algorithm for image reconstruction is as follows :

1. Construct a theoretical voltage profile for a given geometry of sensor array based on the model described in chapter 4 and verified by experiment. Repeat this procedure for several charge positions.

2. Construct graphs from the above profile on a plot of normalised voltage versus sensor angular position as well as a calibration chart of voltage ratio versus charge radial location

3. Obtain measurement of sensors in the time domain.

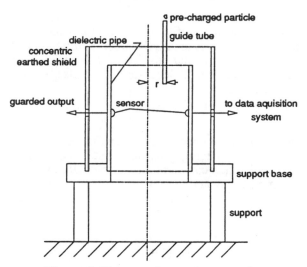

Figure 5. The experimental sensor rig.

4. Estimate the angular position of charge from the record of the sensor which has highest measured voltage.

5. Find the range of maximum-minimum voltage ratio reading and use the calibration chart obtained in step 2 to estimate the radial position of charge.

The results from the experiment showed a close agreement with the model. The results were close to the estimated profiles for all charge locations except at the centre. This is extremely good given the difficulty with regards to ascertaining the right model and geometry of rig construction throughout the work.

With the charge at the centre, it is extremely difficult to obtain results close to the theoretical because the charge has a certain amount of freeplay as it falls through the guiding tube and therefore can come out of the tube mouth at a slight angle and so become off-centre. The diameter of guide tube is 13mm, that is an error of 6.5/50 or 13% off-centre is possible.

For charges located at 15mm, 22.5mm, 30mm and 37.5mm the results were extremely close to the theoretical. This verifies that the induction model used to describe the voltage profile is correct for the setup of the instrumentation in the experiment.

Three factors were found to be critical in obtaining good results:

1. The earth shield should be concentric with the pipe. This was not obvious in the first instance because earlier work was based on metal conveyors. However, scrutiny of the results from tests made early in the project using box shield suggests a certain amount of potential due to field distribution influenced the readings.

2. To make the measurements more sensitive the correction of the field effects was minimised by controlling the input impedance of the transducer as well as the buffer.

3. The buffer was included to ensure a steady potential on the input to the transducers and to isolate the sensors from effects external to the pipe.

It is interesting to observe that in the hardware situation, it is easy to reconstruct the image of the charge through such a profile by deciding at which sensor the maximum voltage is recorded. If the charge is axially between two neighbouring sensors, then simple interpolation will give the angular position of the charge. Hence, the resolution is increased by increasing the number of electrodes. It can also be increased by reducing the distance between these electrodes.

5 Conclusions

The results from this work show encouraging possibilities of using electrodynamic measurements for tomographic imaging. The work is still at a basic research stage. The potential for industrial application can be realised especially in the powder processing industry where charge monitoring and process studies can be made.

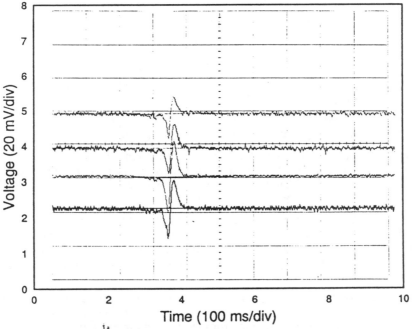

Figure 6. Typical outputs from the sensors.

r=0 mm

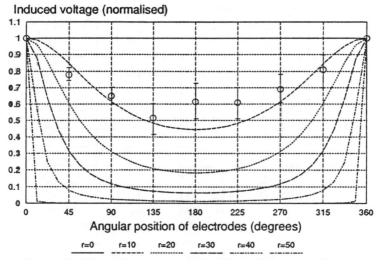

Figure 7a. Normalized voltage profile: r=0 mm, R=50 mm.

r=15 mm

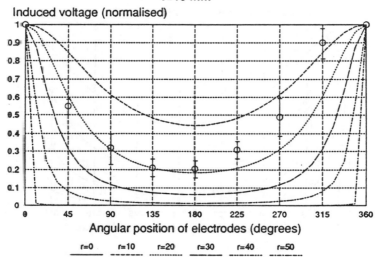

Figure 7b. Normalized voltage profile: r=15 mm, R=50 mm.

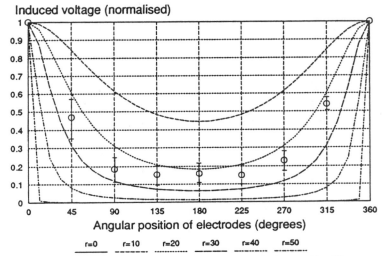

Figure 7c. Normalized voltage profile: r=22.5 mm, R=50 mm.

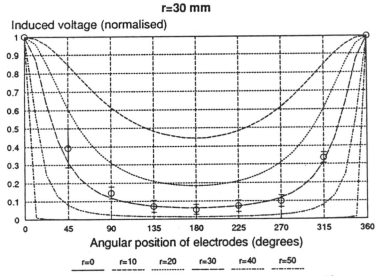

Figure 7d. Normalized voltage profile: r=30 mm, R=50 mm.

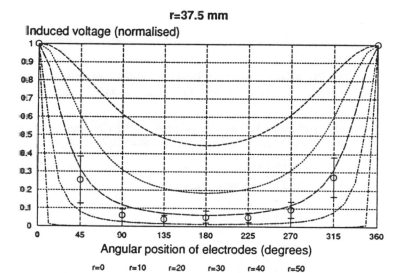

Figure 7e. Normalized voltage profile: r=37.5 mm, R=50 mm.

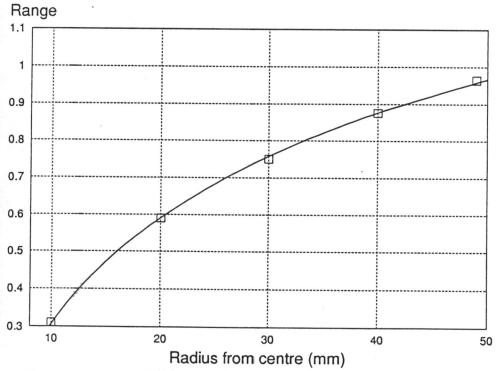

Figure 8. Relationship between charge radial position and measurement range.

6 References

Barber DC and Brown BH 1984 *Applied Potential Tomography*, J Phys E: Sci Instrum v17:723-731.

Beck MS Green RG Plaskowski AB and Stott AL 1990 *Capacitance measurement applied to a pneumatic conveyor with very low solids loading*, Meas Sci Technol 1 p561-564.

Bidin AR Green RG Shackleton ME and Taylor RW 1992 *Process tomography using electrodynamic measurements*, ICEMI 92 20-22 October 1992 Tianjin China.

Gregory I 1987 PhD Thesis, UMIST.

Shackleton ME 1981 MPhil Thesis, Bradford University.

Low Value Capacitance Measurements for Process Tomography

W.Q.Yang and A.L.Stott

Department of Electrical Engineering and Electronics, Process Tomography Group, UMIST, P.O. Box 88, Manchester M60 1QD, U.K.

ABSTRACT: The design fundamentals of stray-immune capacitance transducers based on operational amplifiers with capacitance feedback are described. A new method for measuring low value capacitance for process tomography is presented. It has the following new features: (1) stray immune a.c. bridge with feedback balance; (2) measurement of both unknown capacitance and loss conductance; (3) combination of forward signal with feedback signal and (4) communication with transputer imaging system.

1. INTRODUCTION

Although capacitance transducers have been widely used both in the laboratory and in industry for many years, new methods of measurement, particularly for low value capacitance, are still being reported. Recent developments include charge/discharge (Huang, 1988), a.c. impedance measurement based on an operational amplifier (Stott, 1990), self-balance capacitance-to-DC-voltage conversion (Hagiwara, 1987), lock-in detection (Marioli, 1991), phase measurement (Natarajam, 1990) and switched-capacitor (Cichocki, 1991).

Electrical capacitance tomography (ECT) presents a particularly difficult measurement problem. The precise requirements depend on the application and the electrode system used but typically the measurement can range from 0.1 pF to 10 pF with a desired accuracy of 1% of reading. If a capacitance transducer is required with a measuring range of 0.1-10 pF and a resolution of 0.1 fF, the linearity of the measuring circuit should be 1×10^{-5} and the signal-to-noise ratio should be nearly 100 dB, i.e. the acquired measurement data should be a binary digit with 17 bits. It is difficult to achieve such a high accuracy by the usual open loop methods.

In a practical measurement systems stray capacitances are always present, e.g. between the measurement electrode and an earthed screen. A screened cable of only 10 cm long can have a stray capacitance of 10 pF, which is often much larger than the measured capacitance. Additionally stray capacitances may vary as the external or internal electric field changes or with slight mechanical movements. Therefore, the capacitance transducers used in process tomography must be stray-immune, i.e. stray capacitance must have no effect on the capacitance measurement.

Another factor which influences the measurement of low value capacitance is the drift of the measuring circuit. Since the unknown capacitance is very small, the measurement system should have a high sensitivity, i.e. the gain of measuring circuit must be sufficiently large. Circuit drift due to ambient temperature changes, component variation etc. has considerable effect on the accuracy of the measurement system. Therefore, ideally, the capacitance transducer used in process tomography should be drift free.

In addition, there is usually a loss conductance in parallel with the unknown capacitance. So the capacitance transducer should be able to measure both the capacitance and the conductance.

A further consideration is that to obtain data from a non-stationary object, e.g. a flow system, the measurement system must operate as fast as possible, say, 1 ms for individual capacitance measurements.

Summarising, a capacitance transducer for process tomography should have the following characteristics:

(1) immunity to stray capacitance;
(2) low drift;
(3) high sensitivity, 0.1 fF;
(4) good linearity, 1×10^{-5};
(5) large signal-to-noise ratio, 100 dB;
(6) be unaffected by loss conductance;
(7) adequate range, 0.1-10 pF;
(8) short measurement time, 1 ms.

Currently the UMIST Process Tomography Group has found the most satisfactory capacitance transducer for ECT to be the differential charge/discharge type reported by Huang. This has a sensitivity of 0.3 fF and has operated satisfactorily with a 12-electrode sensor system. To achieve better image resolution, however, it is necessary to increase the number of electrodes and consequently an improved transducer is required.

On the basis of the above considerations, the authors present a new scheme for low value capacitance measurement. Firstly, the measurement system which is based on a.c. bridge with feedback is described. Then the hardware and software for realizing the measurement method are given. Finally the present state of developing the measurement system and the intended applications of the system are discussed.

2. GENERAL DESCRIPTION OF SYSTEM

The basic measuring circuit based on an operational amplifier is shown in Fig.1.

C_x is the unknown capacitance, C_{s1} and C_{s2} are stray capacitances to earth and V_s is a sinusoidal excitation voltage source. C_{s1} is driven directly by the voltage source and so has no effect on the measurement of C_x. Since the feedback point is kept at virtual earth by the operational amplifier there is zero potential difference across C_{s2}. So C_{s2} also has no effect on the measurement of C_x. Therefore, the capacitance measuring circuit

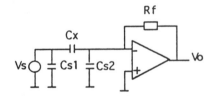

Fig.1 Basic Capacitance Measuring Circuit

based on an operational amplifier is stray-immune. The output voltage of the circuit is given by

$$V_o = -j\omega C_x R_f V_s \qquad (1)$$

where, ω and V_s are the anglular frequency and r.m.s. amplitude of the excitation voltage respectively and R_f is the feedback impedance. Clearly, to achieve high sensitivity, large values of ω, V_s and R_f should be used.

When measuring small capacitance changes to an accuracy of, say, 0.1 fF with a large standing capacitance present, say, 10 pF, it is difficult to achieve the required accuracy by conventional open loop measurement techniques. The solution proposed in this paper is to use a self balancing a.c. bridge. A schematic diagram of this measurement system is given in Fig.2.

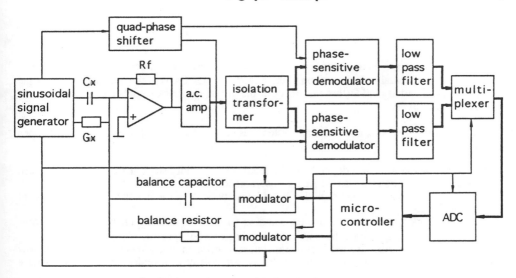

Fig.2 Capacitance Measurement System with Feedback

The signal generator provides a 500 KHz sine-wave voltage. This excitation voltage is applied to both the unknown capacitance C_x and the parallel loss conductance G_x. The output voltage of the operational amplifier is then composed of two orthogonal components:

$$V_{out} = -R_f G_x V_s - j\omega C_x R_f V_s \tag{2}$$

The amplified AC signal passes through an isolation transformer to the phase sensitive demodulators. To demodulate the two orthogonal components of the a.c. signal, four reference signals at 90° phase intervals are required. The 90° and 270° reference signals are used to obtain the information related to C_x and the 0° and 180° for G_x. The demodulated signal comprises a d.c. component and a 1 MHz a.c. component plus harmonics. The low pass filter rejects the a.c. signals and the two d.c. signals representing the unknown capacitance and conductance pass, via the multiplexer, to a single ADC in which the analog voltages are converted into digital signals and input to the micro-controller. On the basis of these input signals the micro-controller produces the digital feedback signals needed to null the forward loop capacitance and conductance signals. These digital feedback signals are used via two multiplying DACs, to set the amplitudes of two 500 KHz sinusoidal signals derived from the excitation voltage. The two voltages are fed back to the input operational amplifier through the balance capacitance and balance resistor respectively. In the ideal situation, the feedback signals will balance the signal from C_x and G_x.

The principle is similar to that of the balanced a.c. bridge. However, in the conventional balanced a.c. bridge, balance is obtained by adjusting the balance impedance, while in this system balance is obtained by varying the amplitudes of the voltages applied to fixed balance impedances.

When balance is obtained the values of C_x and G_x are related to the digital feedback signal thus

$$C_x = \frac{C_b V_b}{V_s 2^N} D_c \tag{3}$$

$$G_x = \frac{V_b}{R_b V_s 2^N} D_g \tag{4}$$

where, C_b and R_b are the balance capacitance and balance resistor respectively, V_b is the r.m.s. amplitude of the sinusoidal voltage applied to the multiplying DACs, N is the feedback range of the multiplying DACs and D_c and D_g are the values of the digital feedback signals for capacitance and conductance respectively.

It is evident that the feedback measurement system has several advantages over conventional open loop measurement:

(1) The measuring accuracy depends on the feedback loop only since the changes of forward loop gains have no effect on the final measurement;
(2) The feedback measurement provides better linearity because the linearity is only dependent on the DACs;
(3) The feedback signals can balance the standing value of C_x and G_x, enabling an excitation signal of large amplitude to be applied and giving a better signal-to-noise ratio;
(4) Using a balance capacitor with zero temperature coefficient and a balance resistor with low temperature coefficient, the measurement system will have low drift due to temperature change;
(5) The measurement is not affected by variation of the excitation voltage.

In practice, it is impossible to obtain a perfect balance because of the limited resolution of the digital feedback signal. However, the resolution of the measurement can be improved by combining the digital feedback signal with the resultant forward signal (the error signal). A possible method is illustrated by Fig.3.

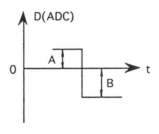

As the digital feedback signal is increased the resultant forward loop signal will decrease towards zero until one additional feedback bit will change the polarity of the forward signal

Fig.3 Combination of ADC and DAC

from "+**A**" to "-**B**". Assuming adequate gain in the forward loop "**A**" and "**B**" will be measured by the ADC with high resolution and can be combined with the feedback measurement thus

$$C_x = \frac{C_b V_b}{V_s 2^N} \left(D_c + \frac{A}{A+B} \right) \tag{5}$$

$$G_x = \frac{V_b}{R_b V_s 2^N} \left(D_g + \frac{A'}{A'+B'} \right) \tag{6}$$

3. HARDWARE AND SOFTWARE

This section describes in detail two important circuit blocks shown in Fig.2 and gives the flow diagram of the micro-controller.

3.1 Sinusoidal Signal Generator and Quad Phase Shifter

The digital synthesiser shown in Fig.4 produces the excitation signals with small distortion and precise phase shifts.

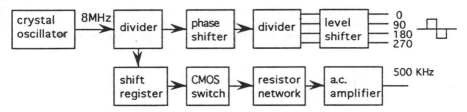

Fig.4 Sinusoidal Signal Generator and Quad Phase Shifter

. The sinusoidal signal is produced by a precise resistor network with 16 steps. This digital synthesiser has the following features:

(1) high frequency stability, 1×10^{-4};
(2) stable sinusoidal amplitude;
(3) four reference square-wave signal with 90° phase intervals;
(4) adjustable reference phases with respect to the sine-wave exciting signal in the range of 360°.

3.2 Phase-Sensitive Demodulator

The demodulators in Fig.2 utilize CMOS switches as shown in Fig.5.

A transformer is used to isolate the demodulator ground from the ground of the preceding circuits. The phase relation between the input sinusoidal signal and the reference square waves is dependent on the ratio of C_x to G_x. Assume a situation where the input signal and the reference signal are in phase. In the first half of the reference square wave circle, switches "1" and "3" are closed while switches "2" and "4" are open. Hence the output terminal "D" of the isolation transformer is kept a ground potential and the output voltage V is applied to the load resistor R_1. In the second half, switches "2" and "4" are closed while switches "1" and "3" are open. Now the output terminal "C" is held at ground and the signal -V is applied to the load resistor. The action of the

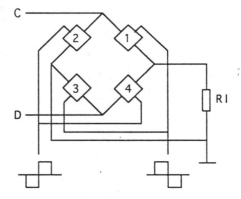

Fig. 5 Phase-Sensitive Demodulator

switches is equivalent to multiplying the input signal by a square wave with magnitude of ± 1 at the same frequency and phase as the reference signal, thus producing phase-sensitive demodulation.

The advantages of the demodulator are:

(1) wide frequency range up to 500 KHz;
(2) small signal loss due to the CMOS switch with low "ON" resistor;

(3) high signal-to-noise ratio due to full-wave output;

3.3 Control and Measurement Software

The measurement system is controlled by a micro-controller type MCS-51. The units controlled include the multiplexer for selecting the capacitance or conductance signal, the ADC, the multiplying DACs and the SPST switch for electrode connection (explained in the following section). The flow diagram for obtaining capacitance and conductance measurements is shown in Fig.6.

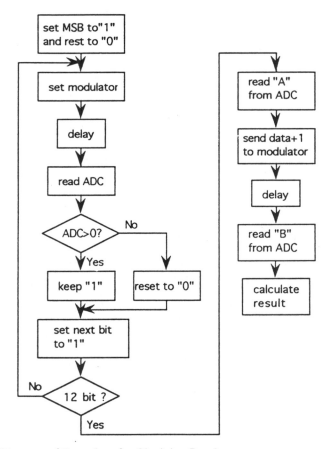

Fig.6 Flow Diagram of Procedure for Obtaining Result

The routine to obtain the measurement is divided into two stages. During the first stage, "1" is set from MSB to LSB successively for each of the multiplying DACs. If the resultant forward signal remains positive the "1" is kept, but if the forward signal becomes negative the bit is reset to "0". The measurement system acts as a 12-bit successive-approximation analog-to-digital converter and after processing the full 12 bits the system is balanced to within 1 bit.

In the second stage, a more accurate result is obtained by combining the digital feedback signal to the multiplying DAC with the forward signal "A" and "B" as measured by the ADC using the method discussed in Section 2.

This subroutine program is used for both capacitance and conductance measurements which are carried out alternately.

4. PRESENT STATE AND PENDING APPLICATIONS

This capacitance measurement system has been designed for use in process tomography. The proposed ECT system is shown in Fig.7.

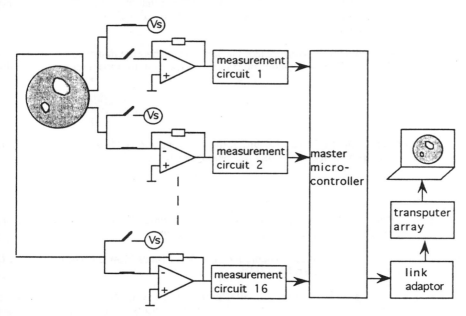

Fig.7 Electrical Capacitance Tomography System

This is a 16-electrode imaging system with each electrode assigned to one complete measurement circuit. Every electrode is used in turn as the excitation electrode while the other electrodes are used as detection electrodes. Thus fifteen measurements are processed concurrently. The selection of excitation and detection electrodes is carried out by a MASTER micro-controller.

This is effectively a master-slave micro-computer network, comprising one MASTER micro-controller and sixteen CHANNEL micro-controllers. The MASTER micro-controller sends commands to each CHANNEL micro-controller and collects the resultant channel measurements. The MASTER micro-controller is connected to the image reconstruction computer system (the transputer array) by means of a link adaptor which acts as serial-to parallel or parallel-to-serial device. The transputer array both sends instructions to the MASTER micro-controller and receives the measurement data via this link adaptor.

To date, the design of the ECT system has been completed and all circuit units have been "bread boarded" and tested. Currently the system PCBs are being made, including one signal generator, sixteen measurement channels and one MASTER and link adaptor boards.

The capacitance measurement system will be used initially for multi-interface level measurement.

5. SUMMARY

A stray-immune capacitance transducer based on an operational amplifier is being developed. Two digital feedback signals are applied via two multiplying DACs to null the unknown capacitance and loss conductance signals so that the transducer behaves essentially as a balanced a.c. bridge. The measurement is determined by the amount of feedback applied, consequently the stability, accuracy, linearity and signal-to-noise ratio should be better than that of a conventional open loop measurement system. The measurement resolution is improved by combining the digital feedback measurement with the residual forward (error) signal.

A 16-electrode ECT system is being constructed. The sixteen channels are managed by a MASTER micro-controller. The MASTER micro-controller communicates with transputer through a link adaptor.

ACKNOWLEDGEMENT

The authors appreciate Prof. M.S.Beck for providing the opportunity to work in UMIST. Dr. C.G.Xie is thanked for his help in constructing the measurement system.

REFERENCES

S.M.Huang, A.L.Stott, R.G.Green and M.S.Beck, Electronic Transducer for Industrial Measurement of Low Value Capacitances, *J.Phy. E: Sci. Instrum.* **21**, 1988, 242-250

A.L.Stott, Correlation and Capacitance Techniques for Solid Mass Flow Measurement, *Ph.D. Thesis, The University of Manchester*, May 1991

N.Hagiwara, M.Yanase and T.Saegusa, A Self-Balance-Type Capacitance-to-DC-Voltage Converter for Measuring Small Capacitance, *IEEE Transactions on Instrumentation and Measurement,* **IM-36 (2)**, June 1987, 385-389

D.Marioli, E.Sardini and A.Taroni, Measurement of Small Capacitance Variations, *IEEE Transactions on Instrumentation and Measurement*, **40 (2)**, April 1991, 426-428

S.Najarajan and B.K.Herman, Measurement of Small Capacitances Using Phase Measurement, *IEEE Comput. Soc., 22nd Southeast. Symp. on System Theory*, Cookville, TN., 11-13 March 1990, 46-50

A.Cichocki and R.Unbehauen, Switched-Capacitor Transducers with Digital or Duty-Cycle Output Based on Pulse-Width Modulation Technique, *Int. J. Electronics*, 1991, **71 (2)**, 265-278

Comparison of Excitation Methods for Electrical Capacitance Tomography

M. S. Bair and J. P. Oakley
Dept. Electrical Engineering, University of Manchester

ABSTRACT: In this paper we report the results from a comparative study of imaging performance for a fixed sensor configuration with two different excitation schemes. The first scheme is to excite a single electrode, as in the UMIST system. In the second scheme, opposing pairs of electrodes are excited with opposite potentials of equal magnitude. The images are reconstructed using a simple back projection algorithm.

The imaging performance of the dual excitation system is remarkably similar to that of the single excitation system, in spite of the fact that the sensitivity distributions for the measurements are quite different. We conclude that the limiting factor is the reconstruction algorithm used.

1. INTRODUCTION

Electrical Capacitance tomography is now established as a viable means for imaging industrial processes in which the components have different permittivities. Various configurations of active and sensing electrodes have been reported. For example, the UMIST system for flow tomography [Huang et al 1989] uses twelve electrodes of which, at any one time, only one electrode is active and other eleven electrodes are sensing. Another system used by the Department of Energy in Morgantown USA [Fasching et al 1988 and 1990] has a quite different configuration in which potentials are simultaneously applied to several electrodes at once. The geometrical configuration of the electrodes affects the electrical field distribution inside the pipe and so does the excitation method. It has been reported [Oakley et al 1991] that the sensitivity distribution, which is used in reconstruction algorithm, is proportional to the electrical field strength and can be calculated directly from field simulations. The dual excitation method, which is described in section 5, generates a higher electrical field strength than that of the single excitation method in the centre of pipe and so potentially provides more information above the centre area of the pipe. Images reconstructed by single, dual, and a combination of single and dual excitation, have been obtained and compared in this study.

2. SYSTEM DESCRIPTION

Our capacitance tomography simulation system is designed to image the distribution of two different permittivity materials (relative permittivity 1 and 3). The configurations are the same for both the single excitation and the dual excitation methods. Twelve capacitance sensors are used and the inside area of the pipe is divided into 1080 regions. The system screen and isolation guards are always connected to ground 0V. The geometry of the pipe is shown in Figure 1. The whole simulation is divided into two stages, the forward problem and the inverse problem shown in Figure 2. In the forward problem, it is assumed that the system is electrostatic and no space charge in the pipe. The electrical field can be solved by solving Laplace's equation and associated boundary conditions (Dirichlet boundary conditions are applied.)

$$\nabla \cdot [\epsilon(x , y) \nabla \phi(x , y)] = 0 \tag{1}$$

A standard finite element electromagnetic field simulation package, PE2D [Vector Field Limited 1991], has been used to solved the forward problem. The capacitances between all possible independent combinations of electrode pairs and the electrical field strength at each region inside pipe are measured. A permittivity value is assigned to each of the 1080 regions (or picture elements). A-*priori* knowledge about the sensitivity distribution of the capacitance measurements is used in the reconstruction algorithm which is based on simple back projection. The sensitivity distribution is calculated from the electrical field strength distribution in the pipe. Then the measured capacitances are weighted by sensitivity and back projected to form images on a computer screen.

3. SENSITIVITY DISTRIBUTIONS

A mathematical model for multi-electrode capacitance sensor has been designed to calculate the sensitivity distributions inside the pipe [Oakley et al 1991]. The capacitance change, caused by the disturbance of a small non-homogeneous material at region A, should be proportional to the sensitivity at that region. It can be expressed as

$$\Delta C_{ij} = \lim_{A \to 0} S_{ij} (x , y) \cdot \epsilon \cdot A \tag{2}$$

Then the sensitivity at that small region can be written as

$$S_{ij} (x , y) = \frac{\Delta C_{ij}}{\epsilon \cdot A} \tag{3}$$

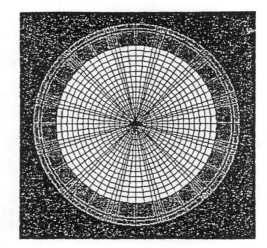

Angle of electrode   : 24°
Radius of inner pipe : 0.0762M
Radius of outer piper : 0.0982M
Radius of electrode   : 0.0912M
Length of guard   : 0.008M
Thickness of electrode: 0.001M

Figure 1. The geometry for 12 electrodes capacitance tomography

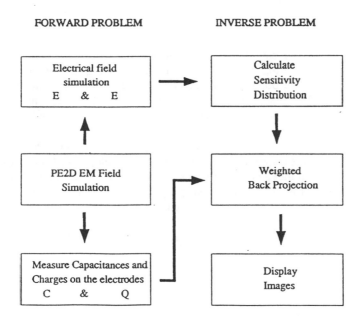

Figure 2. Capacitance tomography simulation system diagram

It is shown in [Bair 1991] that

$$\Delta C = \frac{\epsilon_0 \chi_e E \cdot E_d V}{\phi^2} \tag{4}$$

where E is the excitation field intensity,
E_d is the detecting field generated by unit charge on the sensing electrode.

so that the sensitivity is given by:

$$S_j (x, y) = \frac{\Delta C_j}{\epsilon A} = \frac{\chi_e E \cdot E_j}{\phi^2_j} \tag{5}$$

where E_j is detecting field strength generated by the total charge on the sensing electrode.

4. SINGLE EXCITATION METHOD

Forward Problem

In this method, only one electrode is active and eleven electrodes are sensing at any one time. The capacitance measuring is carried out in the following manner. Firstly, electrode 1 is connected to a positive potential 1V and the other electrodes (electrode 2 through 12) are grounded to 0V. Then the capacitance between electrode 1 and 2, 1 and 3, ..., 1 and 12 are measured. Eleven independent capacitances measurements are obtained in this way. Secondly, electrode 2 is connected to a positive potential, 1V, as an active electrode and others kept in the ground 0V as sensing electrodes. Then the capacitance between electrodes 2 and 3, 2 and 4 , ..., 2 and 12 are measured. (the capacitance between electrode 1 and 2 has been measured in the first step). Ten independent capacitance measurements are then obtained. This process continues until electrode 11 is connected to a positive potential 1V as an active electrode and electrode 12 connected to ground 0V as a sensing electrode and one independent capacitance measurements is obtained. A total of 66 independent capacitance measurements are obtained and stored. In the same time, the electrical field strength at all regions inside the pipe is measured and stored.

Inverse Problem

The dielectric permittivity distribution will be reconstructed by 66 capacitance measurements. However, the number of unknown variables (pixel grey levels) is much greater than the numbers of known data items. The sensitivity distributions are calculated according to the equation (5). Figures 3a to 3f show the sensitivity distribution between electrode pairs 1-2, 1-3, ..., 1-7 respectively. The other 60 sensitivity distributions for all possible independent combinations of electrode pairs can be achieved by appropriate rotation of those 6 sensitivity distributions.

The capacitance changes on the electrode j, while electrode i is active, are calculated as

$$\Delta C_{ij} = C_{ij}^R - C_{ij}^E \qquad (6)$$

where ΔC_{ij} : measured capacitance change,
  C_{ij}^R : capacitance due to a non-homogeneous material in the pipe,
  C_{ij}^E : capacitance when pipe empty,

These capacitance changes are weighted by sensitivity and back projected by using simple back projection method to form the an image of permittivity distribution, using the formula:

$$G(x, y) = \sum_{i=1}^{i=11} \sum_{j=i+1}^{j=12} \Delta C_{ij} \cdot S_{ij}(x, y) \qquad (7)$$

where $S_{ij}(x,y)$: the sensitivity of pixel (x,y) respect to electrodes i and j.

Three kinds of phantom, shown in Figure 5a to 7a, have been used in simulations and images of permittivity distribution obtained in this way are shown in Figure 5b to 7b. The capacitance data was obtained using PE2D.

5. DUAL EXCITATION SYSTEM

Forward Problem

In this method, the system screen and the isolated guards are still keep at ground. One pair of the opposing electrodes (1 and 7, 2 and 8, ..., or 6 and 12) are excited with opposite potentials of equal magnitude, (+1V and -1V), as an active electrodes and other ten electrodes are sensing electrodes. The charges are measured in the following way. Firstly, electrodes 1 and 7 are excited with a positive potential, +1V, and a negative potential, -1V, respectively and other electrodes are kept at ground. The charges on all electrodes except electrodes 1 and 7 are then measured. Ten charge measurements are collected in this step. Then active electrode pair is changed to 2 and 8, 3 and 9, and so on up to 6 and 12. A total of 60 independent charge measurements are measured and stored.

Inverse Problem

The analysis of the dual excitation system is similar to that of the single excitation method. The sensitivity distributions can be calculated from (5). The sensitivity distributions between electrode 1 and 2, ..., 1 and 6, 1 and 8, ..., 1 and 12 are shown in Figures 4a to 4j respectively. The other 50 sensitivity distributions for all possible independent combination of electrode pairs can be obtained by appropriate rotation of those ten distributions.

The charge change on electrode j, while electrodes i and i+6 are excited by a positive and a negative potential respectively, is calculated

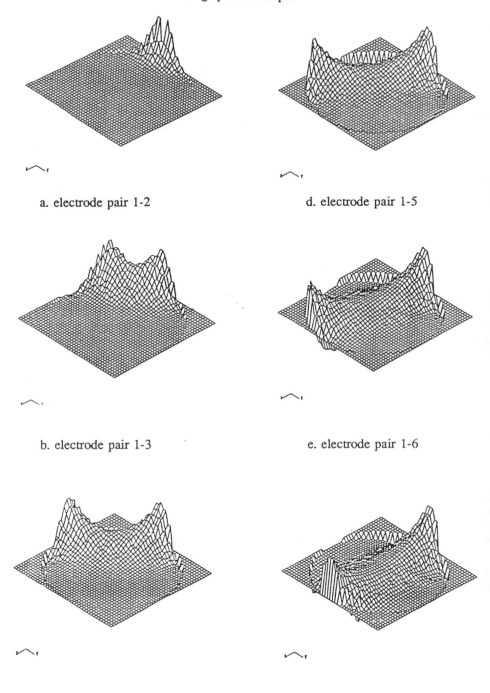

a. electrode pair 1-2

d. electrode pair 1-5

b. electrode pair 1-3

e. electrode pair 1-6

c. electrode pair 1-4

f. electrode pair 1-7

Figure 3. Sensitivity distributions for single excitation system

$$\Delta Q_{i,j} = Q_{i,j}^R - Q_{i,j}^E \qquad (8)$$

where $\Delta Q_{i,j}$: measured charge change,
$\quad Q_{i,j}^R$: charge due to a non-homogeneous material in the pipe,
$\quad Q_{i,j}^E$: charge when pipe empty,

These charge changes are weighted by sensitivity and back projected by using simple back projection method to form a image of the permittivity distribution, which is represented as grey level.

$$G(x , y) = \sum_{i=1}^{i=5} \sum_{j=1}^{j=12} \Delta Q_{i,j} \cdot S_{i,j}(x , y) \qquad\qquad i \neq j , \; i \neq j \pm 6 \qquad (9)$$

where $S_{i,j}(x,y)$ is the sensitivity at pixel (x,y) respect to electrode j, when a positive and a negative potential are applied to electrodes i and i+6.

The images reconstructed by using simple back projection method are shown in Figures 5c to 7c.

6. COMBINATION SYSTEM

The single and the dual excitation methods are combined together. The forward problem is completed in two steps. The first step is using single excitation method to measure 66 capacitance measurements and the second step is using dual excitation method to measure 60 charge measurements. Then the permittivity distribution represented in grey level is

$$G(x , y) = \sum_{i=1}^{i=11} \sum_{j=i+1}^{j=12} \Delta C_{i,j} \cdot S_{i,j}^s(x , y) + \sum_{\substack{i=1 \\ i \neq j, \; i \neq j \pm 6}}^{i=6} \sum_{j=1}^{j=12} \Delta Q_{i,j} \cdot S_{i,j}^d(x , y) \qquad (10)$$

The images reconstructed by using simple back projection method are shown in the Figures 5d to 7d.

7. CONCLUSION

Images reconstructed by simple weighted back projection method from single, dual and combination excitation methods have been obtained. It was expected that the reconstructed images would be difference for the different excitation systems, because the weighting factors, sensitivity distributions, are dramatically different for the different excitation systems, shown in Figures 3 and 4, and the back projection is simply a weighted sum of the sensitivity

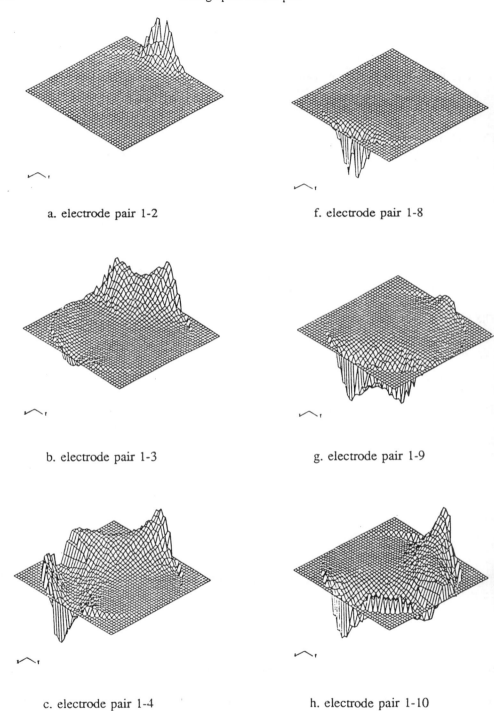

Figure 4. Sensitivity distributions for dual excitation system

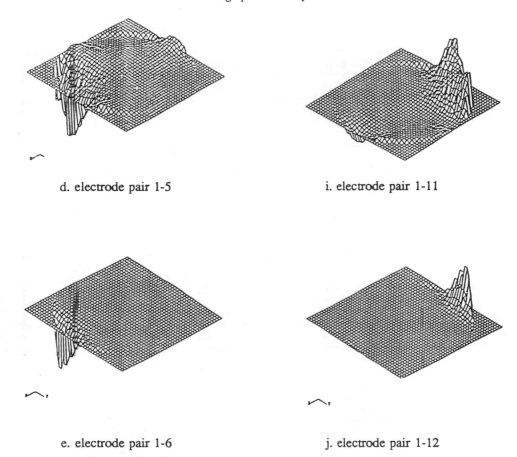

d. electrode pair 1-5   i. electrode pair 1-11

e. electrode pair 1-6   j. electrode pair 1-12

Figure 4. Sensitivity distributions for dual excitation system (continue)

functions. However, all of the reconstructed images are blurred in a similar way and seem almost identical. This shows that the sensitivity distribution is not the significant factor which determines image quality. The limiting factor for image resolution from back projection seems to be the high degree of overlap between the sensitivity distributions for different excitation electrode (or electrodes pair). The comparisons for the area which the grey level is higher then 90% and 80% of the maximum grey level is shown in Table 1 and Table 2. All of the methods produce quite similar images for the centre phantom (phantom 3) and the boundary areas (object near boundary). However, for the phantom 2, the single excitation method shows better resolution.

The areas of the phantom which applied in this study are about 10% of the whole pipe. In the future we will make the same comparison for larger phantom objects where the soft field effect is important in order to see whether dual excitation method gives any advantage. We will also be investigating the use of more sophisticated reconstruction algorithms in these systems.

Table 1. The areas which grey level is higher then 90% of the maximum grey level.

Area(M^2*10^{-4})	Phantom 1	Phantom 2	Phantom 3
Phantom	11.6745	10.93392	12.9717
Single	0.78372	11.5867	81.0732
Dual	0.78372	13.78248	81.0732
Combine	0.78372	12.161	81.0732

Area of whole pipe is 1.82415E-2 M^2

Table 2. The areas which grey level is higher then 80% of the maximum grey level.

Area(M^2*10^{-4})	Phantom 1	Phantom 2	Phantom 3
Single	1.56744	27.9728	98.098
Dual	1.56744	56.1057	98.098
Combine	1.56744	38.5208	98.098

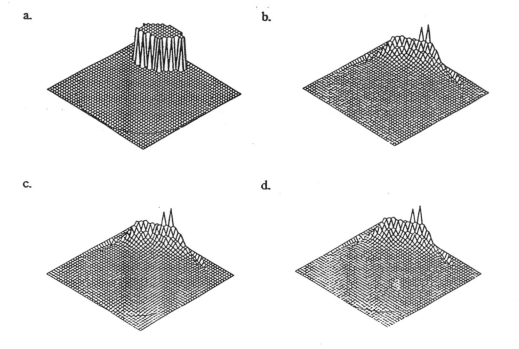

a. phantom b. single excitation c. dual excitation d. combination
Figure 5 Test phantom 1. and reconstructed images

a.

b.

c.

d.

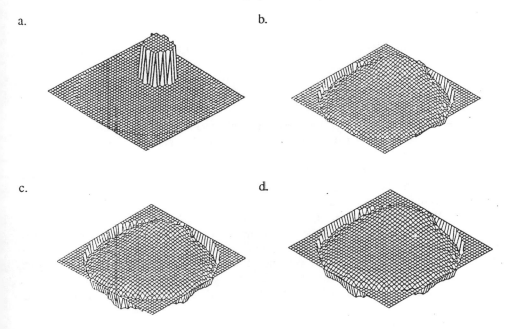

a. phantom b. single excitation c. dual excitation d. combination
Figure 6 Test phantom 2. and reconstructed images

a.

b.

c.

d.

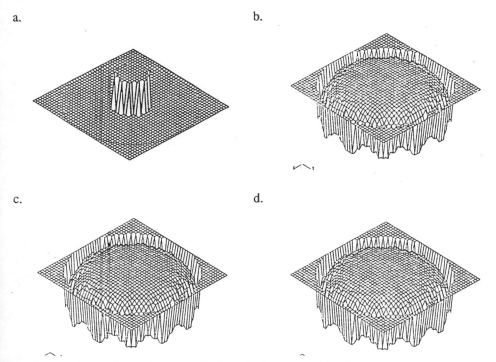

a. phantom b. single excitation c. dual excitation d. combination
Figure 7 Test phantom 3. and reconstructed images

ACKNOWLEDGMENTS

The first author would like to thank the National Defence Department of the Republic of China for financial support.

REFERENCE

Fasching G.E., Smith N.S. 1988 'High resolution capacitance imaging system', Technical note, U.S. Department of Energy, Office of Fossil Energy, Morgantown Energy Technology Centre, Morgantown, West Virginia, U.S.A.

Fasching G.E. Smith N.S 1990 ' Three-Dimensional Capacitance Imaging System', Technical note, U.S. Department of Energy, Office of Fossil Energy, Morgantown Energy Technology Centre, Morgantown, West Virginia, U.S.A.

M. S. Bair 1991 PT group internal report (27 November 1991)

Oakley J.P And Bair M.S.   'A mathematical model for the Multi-electrode capacitance sensor' (to be published)

S. M. Huang, A. B. Plaskowski, C. G. Xie, and M. S. Beck 1989 'Tomographic imaging of two phase flow using capacitance sensors', L. Phys. E. Sci. Instrum 22 173-177

Vector Field Limited 1991 ' The PE2D Reference Manual', 24 Bnakside, Kidlington, Oxford OX5 1JE, U.K.

Investigation of electrode geometries for use in cyclonic separators

MZ Abdullah[1,] WF Conway[1,] T Dyakowski[2] and RC Waterfall[1]

[1]Dept. of EE&E, UMIST

[2]Dept. of Chem. Eng,UMIST

Abstract

In electrical impedance tomography (EIT), the electrodes are normally fabricated from a conductive material in order to reduce the inherent effects caused by the electrode-electrolyte interface. The size and geometrical shape of these electrodes are normally chosen so as to increase the accuracy of the measured data. However, the number of electrodes which can be employed in any given application is limited by the size of the vessel. Because of the complex electro-chemical behaviour of the metal electrodes, there seems to be a lack of information in the literature on the relationship between the electrode parameters and other measurable quantities obtainable from the electrodes. In EIT, one of the parameter which is still not well understood is the dependency of the differential voltage measurements on the size and type of materials used for the electrodes and vessel. We show experimentally that, as the size of the vessel is reduced (to that of a 2 inch hydrocyclone),the effect of the electrode size, shape and material on the accuracy of the measured voltages becomes more pronounced. By measuring the impedance of a variety of electrode materials, we have found that the impedance of a rectangular (20 x 12mm) nickel plated brass electrode is more stable compared to that of smaller sized electrodes. We calculated the response for each types of electrodes using a finite element model and compared the results with measured values. For two different saline solutions studied, an agreement between calculated and measured values is better than 1% for rectangular electrodes. Larger discrepancies have been found for other types of electrodes. For these reasons, we conclude that the rectangular electrode is the most suitable for use in the hydrocyclone imaging system.

1. Introduction

In EIT, a set of electric currents are applied to an object and the resulting external voltage distributions are measured through an array of electrodes attached to the object boundary. These voltages together with a suitable reconstruction algorithm can be used to reconstruct an approximation to the internal electrical resistivity distribution of an object. In the case of the iterative reconstruction algorithm, such as the modified Newton-Raphson(MNR) method described elsewhere (Yorkey *et al* 1987), an accurate and reliable reconstruction of the object resistivity distribution requires precise measurements of the boundary voltages. It has been reported by several EIT workers (Isaacson *et al* 1990 & Owen *et al* 1992) that an iterative reconstruction can only yield meaningful results if the accuracy of the measured voltages is less than 20%. Beside the measuring circuitry and the mathematical modelling used for image reconstruction, the design of the electrodes to obtain optimum accuracy is very critical.

The EIT technique has received much attention for clinical use (Barber *et al* 1984) and the electrodes used for process applications have to be modified somewhat from their medical counterparts. Unfortunately, these two areas of application are completely different in many respects namely: the object size and its internal structure; magnitude of applied currents; image resolution; and safety considerations. Furthermore, it is important to know in advance the kind of application the electrodes are used for and other important criteria such as corrosive and abrasive properties in order to fabricate the correct electrode geometry. In the case of hydrocyclone imaging, one constraint is that the reconstructed image must accurately reflect a wide resistivity band width of the object. For example, the resistivity(the inverse of conductivity) of the air core at the centre of the hydrocyclone can be considered as an insulator whilst the background resistivity is in the range of a few milli-Siemens/cm representing an extreme range to quantify. Quantification of the reconstructed images is possible with the use of the MNR algorithm but the accuracy of the images produced depends, in-turn, on the accuracy that the voltages can be measured to. Since these voltages are measured through an electrode, this necessitates their optimal design to a better signal to noise ratio. However, for a 2 inch diameter hydrocyclone, the design of such electrodes is non-trivial largely due to the small sized of the hydrocyclone which consequently demands accurate geometrical placement, size and electrode material.

In this paper, the properties of 5 different sets of electrodes are discussed having measured their impedances using a multi-bridge meter. All tests were carried out at 50 kHz, a typical frequency used in process applications (Dickin *et al* 1992). For each type of electrode, we investigated their electrical response by measuring voltages between adjacent electrodes when excited with a known a.c current. Using the finite element method, we predicted the voltages and compared these with their measured counterparts. From this, we were able to choose the most suitable electrode for our 2 inch hydrocyclone.

2. Impedance measurement

The conduction of currents in the system comprising the electrode-electrolyte interface differs greatly to the electronic conduction occurring in metal. Electrolytes conduct current by transportation of ions which travel in opposite directions toward the electrodes. This phenomenem has enabled many investigators to model the equivalent circuits of the electrode immersed in an electrolyte by discrete resistive and capacitive elements (Geddes 1972, Pollak 1973 & Weinman *et al* 1964). To reduce the d.c electrode potential at the electrode/metal interface an a.c current is used. This gives rise to frequency dependent effects which have to be included in the electrode equivalent circuit. In EIT, we normally limit the frequency to less than 100 kHz. In this range, the high frequency effects are reduced and the electrode equivalent circuit can be simplified as shown in Fig 1 (Geddes 1972).

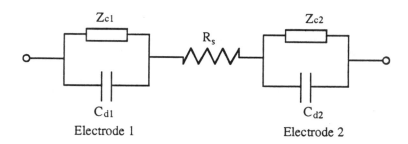

Fig 1 Low Frequency equivalent circuit for electrode
Z_C = Warburg (or contact) impedance
C_d= Double layer capacitance
R_s= Bulk resistance of saline solution

From Fig 1, the component that to be measured is the total impedance between two the electrodes. This may include either the real or the reactive component of the equivalent circuit shown above. At low frequency, the capacitive effect is negligible and the total impedance is dominated by the real part (the resistance) between two electrodes. Assuming the electrodes are identical($Z_{c1}=Z_{c2}=Z_o$), the total impedance $|Z_T|_{real}$ between the two electrodes can be written as,

$$|Z_T|_{real} = R_s + 2|Z_c|_{real} \qquad (1)$$

Z_C in (1) has no simple representation in terms of frequency independent resistances and capacitances. It is simply for this reason that others (Barber *et al* 1984 & Ider *et at* 1990) have avoided making measurements on the current driving electrodes. An earlier attempt to circumvent this difficulty was tried by Cheng *et al* (1989) who included Z_C in their model. However, both R_s and Z_C are very complicated elements which are not only functions of frequency but also on the geometrical shape of the electrodes. In his calculation, Cheng introduced some correcting factors to reduce the artefact caused by electrode geometry. The interested readers are referred to his paper for further explanation.

In our investigation, to make impedance measurements, 16 electrodes of 5 different types were attached to the model of a hydrocyclone body. The spacing between electrodes was dependent on their size. Since we used the 4-electrode measurement method in our reconstruction algorithm (Abdullah *et al* 1992), the impedances between all adjacent electrodes are measured. This gives a total of 16 readings for each type of electrode. We used the Wayne-Kerr multibridge meter with an accuracy of 0.05 mΩ @100kHz. The schematic diagram of the measurement circuitry is shown in Fig 2 and the results are presented in Fig 3(a).

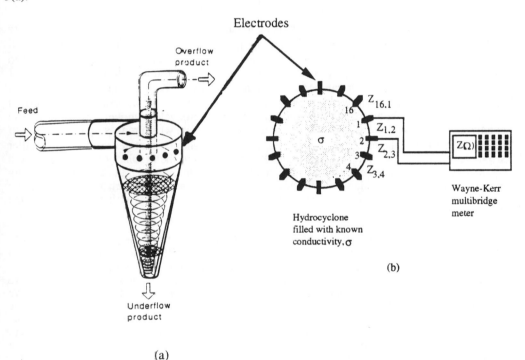

Fig 2 (a) Front view of the 2 inch hydrocyclone
  (b) Arrangement for measuring $|Z_T|_{real}$ with
     multi-bridge meter. Electrodes evaluated are
     Type 1 : 20 x 12 mm nickel plated brass(rectangular)
     Type 2 : 8mm diameter silver palladium(circular)
     Type 3 : 3mm diameter silver(circular)
     Type 4 : 3mm diameter brass(circular)
     Type 5 : 1.5mm diameter gold plated(circular)

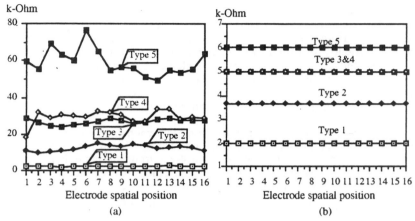

Fig 3 Measured (a) and calculated (b) electrode
impedances for all spatial positions

All measurements were performed using a homogeneous saline solution of conductivity
$225\mu S/cm$. Since our model is made-up of a circular vessel, the measured $|Z_T|$real values will
theoretically be constant and independent of the electrode spatial position. Referring again to
the graph in Fig 3(a), $|Z_T|$real for type 1 electrode appears to be much more stable compared
to the others. Furthermore, it can be seen that the stability of $|Z_T|$real degrades as the size of
electrode is reduced.   Unlike the vessel with larger diameter,   we find that the current
streamlines flowing between two electrodes inside the hydrocyclone model tend to propagate
evenly toward the boundary. This will cause the effective area which makes up the $|Z_T|$real to
be very sensitive to the electrode position especially at higher current densities or for smaller
sized electrodes. In addition, Yorkey et al (1985) has reported the problem of shunting caused
by the internodal resistance lowered by the electrode size. In our case, the electrode shunting
effect will lead to an imbalance in the flow of currents between two electrodes. The solution
to this problem is to increase the resistance between two electrodes either by reducing the
currents or increasing the inter-electrode gap.

It is sometimes more instructive to compare the measured $|Z_T|$real with the values
obtained by calculation. However, an accurate calculation is difficult to achieve because Z_c in
equation (1) cannot be easily modelled. It is also noted that the effective length between any
two neighbouring electrodes varies quite markedly, i.e., the equipotential lines between these
electrodes can be formed in many different paths. Obviously, the choice of a single effective
length will lead to an error. In addition, the geometrical factors describing the electrode
position cannot easily be determined using a direct mathematical method rather, these factors
can only be obtained through an iterative technique (Pollak 1973). The author's have found that,
unless a number of asumptions concerning the geometry and process conditions inside the
vessel are made, the iterative mathematical technique is prone to adverse errors. One of the
main assumptions to satisfy the requirements of the mathematical technique is that no
interface product are formed on the surface of the electrodes. Consequently, it is almost
impossible to calculate $|Z_T|$real with a sufficiently high degree of accuracy. For these reasons,
no attempt has been made to calculate the actual $|Z_T|$real but instead to estimate them from
existing circuit theory.   In order to do this, the theory proposed by Gisser et al (1988) was
used:

$$|Z_T|_{ij}\,\text{real} = \frac{V_{ij}}{J_{ij}} \text{ for } i = 1,2...,16 \text{ and } j=i+1 \text{ for } i{\leq}15, j=1 \text{ for } i=16 \qquad (2)$$

where V is the voltage appearing on the electrode and J is the applied current density. Using the Fourier expansion technique (Ider et al 1990), it is possible to calculate V for given J and is given by:

$$V_{ij} = \frac{2J_{ij}}{\sigma} \Lambda_c \tag{3}$$

where $\Lambda_c = \frac{1}{\beta\pi} \sum \frac{1}{n^2} (\frac{r}{R})^n \sin\frac{n\beta}{2} [\cos(n(\alpha_1-\theta)) - \cos(n(\alpha_2-\theta))]$

Substituting (3) into (2) gives

$$|Z_T|_{,real} = \frac{2}{\sigma} \Lambda_c \tag{4}$$

Employing equation (4) we estimated $|Z_T|_{real}$ for all types of electrode and the results are summarised in Fig 3(b). Except for type 1 electrodes, the measured $|Z_T|_{real}$ for all other electrodes is lower than those estimated using equation (4). The disagreement is expected and the reasons are given above.

In EIT, $|Z_T|_{real}$ is not measured directly but its distribution is estimated from a set of voltages measured on the electrodes. This can be performed in many ways and we have chosen the MNR algorithm because its convergence properties are superior to other iterative techniques (Yorkey et al 1987). However as discussed in section 1, the accuracy of the estimated resistivity distribution cannot be guaranteed if the voltages measured for the homogeneous bath cannot be accurately determined. In the following section, we used the finite element method to predict the boundary voltages for all types of electrode and compared these results with measured values.

3. Boundary voltage calculation using the finite element method

3.1   The forward solver

The mathematical model which describes the potential distribution ϕ defined over a space domain Γ filled with conductivities σ can be derived from Maxwell's equation and is given by:

$$\nabla \cdot (\sigma\nabla\phi) = 0 \text{ in } \Gamma \tag{5}$$

Equation (5) represents the most fundamental equation which is found in almost any EIT literature. Equation (5) describes the potential distribution ϕ in an in homogeneous isotropic medium Γ resulting from a.c current excitation wherein the variation of σ must be known. The applied currents in-turn produce vector character current density $\mathbf{J}$ whose direction υ is always normal to $\partial\Gamma$. The problem of solving ϕ for a given $\mathbf{J}$ and σ can thus be designated as the boundary value problem of the second kind (Weber 1950). Mathematically, the boundary condition can be written as

$$\sigma\frac{\partial\phi}{\partial\upsilon} = \mathbf{J} \text{ on } \partial\Gamma, \tag{6}$$

Applying Kirchoff's current law, the total currents that flow into the domain Γ bounded by $\partial\Gamma$ must correspond exactly to the total of currents flowing out of Γ. Thus, the electric current density is solenoidal. Hence,

$$\oint_{\partial\Gamma} \sigma\frac{\partial\phi}{\partial\upsilon} = 0 \tag{7}$$

Similarly, the resulting boundary voltages **V** can be written as

$$\oint_{\partial\Gamma} V = 0 \tag{8}$$

Since we do not make any measurement on current driving electrodes, the best electrode model which can be used to solve equation (5) is the shunt model (Isaacson *et al* 1990). We used this model in our forward solver to give the following boundary conditions

$$\int_{+ve} \sigma\frac{\partial\phi}{\partial\upsilon} = I \text{ on positive current electrode} \tag{9a}$$

$$\int_{-ve} \sigma\frac{\partial\phi}{\partial\upsilon} = -I \text{ on negative current electrode} \tag{9b}$$

In practice, a set of K electrodes are attached to the domain boundary $\partial\Gamma$ and currents are applied at $\partial\Gamma$ while voltages at other electrodes are measured. Equation (7) and (8) can be modified to give

$$\sim \sum_{l=1}^{k} I_l = 0 \tag{10a}$$

and
$$\sum_{l=1}^{k} V_l = 0 \tag{10b}$$

Thus, equation (5) together with a conditions in (9) and (10) can be solved yielding a unique set of solution. We used the finite element method (FEM) to solve equation (5) even though, for a simple model such as for the circular geometry, an analytical technique is also possible. We prefer the FEM because for its flexibility in handling the inverse problem described elsewhere (Abdullah *et al* 1992). The solution of equation (5) using the FEM is based on minimisation of total energy density function ζ and for a two dimensional case can be expressed in integral form as a

$$\zeta = \frac{1}{2}\iint \nabla.(\sigma\nabla\phi)dxdy \tag{11}$$

We divided the domain Γ into a set of N first order triangular elements each having their own assigned σ. Thus, we can reduce (11) to discrete form,

$$\zeta = \frac{1}{2}\sum_{\sigma=1}^{N} \nabla.(\sigma\nabla\phi)dxdy \tag{12}$$

From equation (12), the unknown quantity that we are trying to solve is the potential vector characterised as a finite number of M nodes placed at vertices of each element in the FEM. To enable integration to be carried out in each element, we represent each element by a linear interpolation function connecting ϕ. This is

$$\frac{1}{2}\sum_{\sigma=1}^{\nu}\nabla.(\sigma\nabla\phi)dxdy = \zeta(\phi_1,\phi_2,\phi_3,.....,\phi_m) \tag{13}$$

Solving equation (5) is now identical to finding the minimum of function ζ for variables $\phi_1,\phi_2,\phi_3, . . . ,\phi_M$. Taking the partial derivatives with respect to each variable in (13) and equating them to zero leads to the following

$$\frac{\partial\zeta}{\partial\phi_i} = 0 \text{ for } i=1,2,3,....,m \tag{14}$$

Equation (14) gives set of M linear algebraic equations in M unknowns written as

$$[A]x = b \tag{15}$$

Here $[A]$ is a square positive definite matrix of order M while the unknowns x are the voltages that we are interested in. For M=69, K=16 and N=104, this gives 13 unique independent voltages for each projection (Barber *et al* 1984) which are solved using Cholesky's decomposition algorithm. The results comparing the measured and calculated voltages for all types of electrode are given in Fig 4.

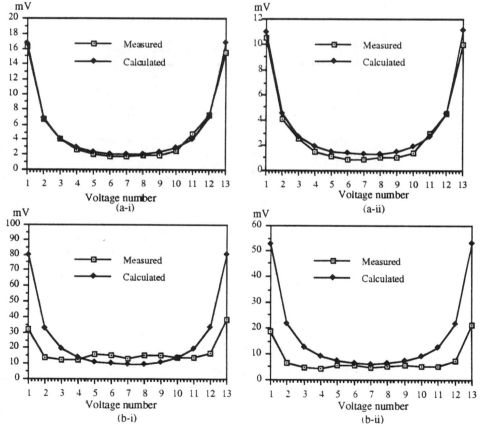

Fig 4 (continue overleaf)

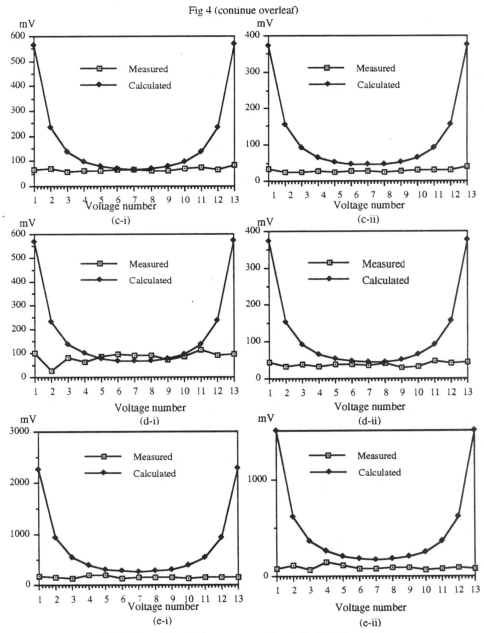

Fig 4 (continue overleaf)

Fig 4 Comparisons between measured and calculated boundary
voltages for (i) 2.63 mS-cm and (ii)4 mS-cm conductivity bath.
(a) Type 1 electrode
(b) Type 2 electrode
(c) Type 3 electrode
(d) Type 4 electrode
(e) Type 5 electrode

From Fig 4, it can be seen that the agreement between the measured and calculated boundary voltages for type 1 electrodes is close for the two different conductivities studied. For other types of electrodes, the agreement is less satisfactory, especially for voltages measured near the current driving electrodes, i.e., voltage numbers 1,2,3,11,12 and 13 shown in Fig 4. The disagreement was due to the fact that, for smaller sized electrodes, the induced voltage will be higher thus requiring a voltmeter with higher input impedance to measure the voltage to a more accurate signal-to-noise ratio. Another factor affecting the measurement accuracy is the electrode geometry error explained in section 2 which is difficult to remedy unless accurate placement of electrode (to within ± 1%) is made. Consequently, we feel that the type 1 electrode is the most suitable for used in the 2 inch hydrocyclone.The prototype quantitative EIT system for use on hydrocyclones producing images at the frame rate of approximately 30sec/frame is shown in the photograph in Fig 5. The reconstructed image shown in Fig 5 depicts a simulated air core developed at the centre of the hydrocyclone.

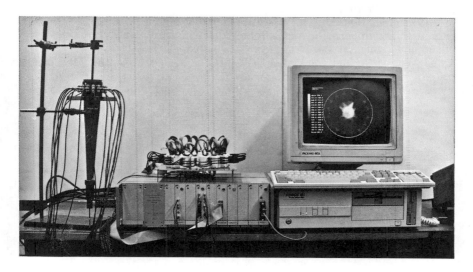

Fig 5 Hydrocyclone imaging system using EIT technique.
The image simulates the air core at the centre
of the hydrocyclone using a 6mm diameter plastic rod.

4. Conclusion

It is desirable in EIT to model the calculated voltages to the same precision as those measured. In practice, this is difficult to achieve since numerous factors must be accounted for. One of these is the design of the electrode. We show experimentally that, as the vessel diameter becomes small, the highest possible reconstruction accuracy of the conductivity cannot be accomplished with arbitrary electrode geometries. Results from experiments on the 2 inch hydrocyclone have indicated that, for the two dimensional case compared to small point-sized circular electrode of 8mm diameter, the larger rectangular shaped electrodes can be modelled quite easily in the forward solver. This modification enables the voltage on the electrodes to be accurately predicted. This finding has enabled us to build the first prototype of the pseudo real-time quantitative imaging system using the EIT measurement technique. Further experimental work is necessary to investigate this relatively new imaging technique for process applications

5. Acknowledgements

This work has been supported by the European coal and steel community (ECSC) under agreement number 7220/EA/829. The authors are grateful to Dr FJ Dickin, Dr CG Xie and Mr XJ Zhao for useful discussions and suggestions. MZ Abdullah acknowledges financial support from the Malaysian government.

6. References

MZ, Abdullah, SV Quick and FJ Dickin 1992: *ECAPT Conf.*,March 1992.
Barber DC and Brown BH 1984:*J.Phys. E: Sci. Instrum*, 723-733.
Cheng KS, Isaacson D, Newell JC and Gisser DG 1989: *IEEE Trans. Biomed. Eng*, 918-923
Dickin FJ, Williams RA and Beck MS 1992: *IEE Proc G*, 72-82(in press).
Geddes LA 1972: *IEEE Spectrum*, 41-48.
Gisser D, Isaacson D and Newel JC 1988: *Clin. Phys. Physio. Meas*, 35-41.
Ider YZ, Gencer NG, Atalar E and Tosun H 1990: *IEEE Trans. Biomed. Eng*, 918-923.
Isaacson D and Cheney M 1990: *Inverse Problems in PDE*, ed Cotten D, Ewing R and Rendell W.
Owen E and Daily W 1992:*Submitted*.
Pollak V 1973:*Medi. Biol. Eng*, 461-464.
Weber E 1950: *Electromagnetic Fields*, John Wiley & Sons.
Weinman J and Mahler J 1964; *Med. Electron. Biol. Eng*, 299-309.
Yorkey TJ, Webster JG and Tomkins WJ 1985; *IEEE 7th Ann. Conf. Eng. Med. and Bio. Soc*, 632-637.
Yorkey TJ, Webster JG and Tompkins WJ 1987: *IEEE Trans. Biomed. Eng*, 843-852.

A simulation study of sensitivity in stirred vessel electrical impedance tomography

G. M. Lyon and J. P. Oakley

Signal Processing Group, Dept. Electrical Engineering, The University, Manchester, M13 9PL, UK.

Abstract

There is current demand in the process industry for high resolution tomographic imaging. One major application area is the imaging of concentration profiles within stirred mixing vessels. This paper reports on a study of the spatial distributions of sensitivity for various possible measurements in such vessels. The following three cases are addressed: [1] an non-intrusive case, with no stirrer present; [2] stirrers of known geometry, conductivity and potential; [3] stirrers with attached electrodes. The results of the study show that the sensitivity, and also spatial resolution can be improved by taking advantage of the stirrer's presence.

1   Introduction

One current area of research at Manchester University is the development of an EIT system specifically for obtaining tomographic images from stirred vessels. The main application area of this EIT system is for the validation of fluid flow (CFD) models to aid in the design of mixing vessels. For this purpose the highest possible resolution is required, particularly in the centre of the vessel where circulation of material is greatest. Present EIT systems give a non-uniform distribution of spatial resolution with the resolution lowest in the central area of the vessel. One possible improvement would be to increase the number of electrodes surrounding the vessel; for example going from 16 to 32. This would effectively double the spatial resolution near the vessel wall, but would have significantly less impact on the resolution at the vessels centre. Continuing this argument to its limit, by repeated doubling of electrode numbers, results in a negligible increase in central resolution (Seagar 1987). A comparison of existing 16 and 32 electrode EIT systems showed little difference in their spatial resolutions of 10%-20% (Webster 1990). Much of the initial work in EIT was for medical applications, where electrodes could only be located on the outside of the patient for in-vitro imaging. With a stirred mixing vessel we have the opportunity to place electrodes in the centre of the vessel, by attachment to the stirring rod or impeller. This study was performed in order to determine whether the presence of the stirrer and use of central electrodes can increase the quality of the images obtained.

2   Simulation procedure

The sensitivity studies were all performed by modeling the vessel using Poisson's Equation in Two Dimensions, PE2D, a finite element electro-magnetic simulation package supplied by Vector Fields Limited. Electrostatic field simulations were performed to determine the potential distributions within the vessel for various electrode configurations. The resulting data was post-processed by software to determine the sensitivity distributions, and allow comparative analyses of the cases studied.

2.1   Definition of Sensitivity

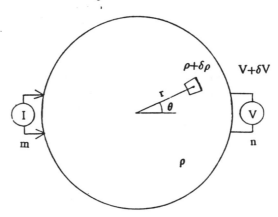

Figure 1; Sensitivity diagram

The use of sensitivity coefficients for image reconstruction was defined by Brekon and Pidcock (1987), and can be stated as eqn(1).

$$S_{(m,n,r,\theta)} = \frac{\delta V(m,n)}{\delta \rho(r,\theta)} = \int_e \underline{E}_m \cdot \underline{E}_n \, dS \tag{1}$$

δV is the change in the measured signal across an electrode pair 'n' when the conductivity in element $e(r,\theta)$ is changed by a small amount $\delta \rho$, while the region is excited by a unit current source across a second electrode pair 'm'. This is shown in figure 1. Brekon and Pidcock also showed that this result is equivalent to the dot product of the electric fields produced by a unit current source at 'm' and 'n', integrated over the elements area, e. Reconstruction of images by this method was first reported by Kotre (1989).

2.2   Finite Element Modeling

The vessel is modeled as a cylinder with the finite element simulations performed in a plane perpendicular to the vessel's axis. As shown in figure 2(i) the elemental mesh is circular in shape, with the stirrer located at the centre of the mesh. The model assumes no external interaction and an insulative vessel wall. The vessel modeled has a radius of 30cm. this being the smallest size of interest for many vessel design prototypes. However, this dimension is not critical to the outcome of the results. The stirrer was modeled outside the plane of the impeller and as such is rotationally symmetrical and small in size with a radius of 1cm. this being considered realistic if electrodes are to be mounted onto the stirrer as in case [3].

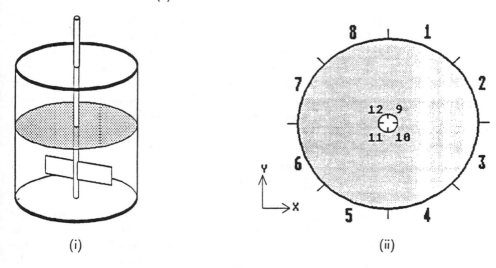

(i)   (ii)

Figure 2; (i) Vessel model, (ii) Electrode pair labels

The modeling of current sources (Neumann boundary conditions) using PE2D is not possible in practice. Applying Thevenin's theorem, an equivalent voltage source can be modeled, yielding a Dirichlet bounded problem. The vessel model uses a single source, multi-reference or adaptive vessel excitation has not been considered by this study. The simulations all use near to the maximal number of possible mesh nodes, 10000 (Vector Fields 1991). This reduced the overall RMS error to less than 5% in all the simulations. Figure 3(i) shows a typical equi-potential distribution for a vessel containing an insulative rod.

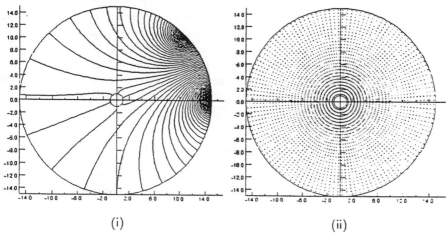

(i)   (ii)

Figure 3; (i) Equi-potential distribution, (ii) Sample points within vessel

2.3   Sensitivity Calculations

In order to calculate the sensitivity distributions the potential gradient within the vessel
must be obtained. The PE2D simulation results were sampled using a cylindrical-polar
frame of reference, with 30 samples radially repeated through 128 angles of rotation,
yielding a total of 3840 sample points, as shown in figure 3(ii). The field at each sample
point was resolved into orthogonal x-y components $(\vec{E_x}, \vec{E_y})$. To reduce the number
of required simulations the simulation data was rotated through multiples of the angle
between adjacent electrodes. Equation (2) was used to obtain field values $(\vec{E_x'}, \vec{E_y'})$ for
$(\vec{E_x}, \vec{E_y})$ rotated through an angle θ.

$$\vec{E_x'} = \vec{E_x}\,cos(\theta) - \vec{E_y}\,sin(\theta) \tag{2}$$
$$\vec{E_y'} = \vec{E_x}\,cos(\theta) + \vec{E_y}\,sin(\theta)$$

The rotated data was also inverted if necessary to ensure the correct polarity of the
sensitivity calculations. The sensitivity calculations were performed in a discrete form,
with the assumption that the area of integration, e, is infinitesimally small, and the
potential gradient in this area constant. The area integral was thus removed from the
sensitivity equation and the calculations form a discrete map of relative sensitivity at the
sampled points throughout the vessel, using equation (3).

$$S_{[m,n,r,\theta]} = \underline{E}_{m[r,\theta]} \cdot \underline{E}_{n[r,\theta]} \tag{3}$$

To show the results graphically the sensitivity data is transformed to a Cartesian frame
of reference.

3   Cases studied

Three main cases have been considered in this study and are described in the following
sub-sections with sample graphical results of the sensitivity distribution calculations. In
all cases the material inside the vessel modeled is homogeneous. A total of eight equally
spaced electrodes have been located around the edge of the vessel. This may seem low
compared to that used in practice, but was considered sufficient to validate the suitability
of the various cases considered. In all cases the source was connected to two adjacent
electrodes. Figure 2(ii) shows the electrode pair labels used in the following sub-sections.
Electrode pairs 9 to 12 are only used in case[3].

3.1   Case[1]: Non-intrusive model

In this case the vessel was modeled without the presence of a stirrer to provide a comparative reference for cases [2] and [3]. Models and physical phantoms of this kind have
been used in the development of many existing EIT systems.
Figure 4(i) shows the sensitivity distribution plot for electrode pairs 1 and 4, where
the X-Y axes correspond to those shown in figure 2(ii). This shows that the region of
positive sensitivity follows approximately the shape of the equi-potential lines used in
simple backprojection (Barber et al 1984). Of note are the areas of negative sensitivity
close to the electrode pairs. This is caused by the increase in conductivity concentrating

the field in these regions causing the field gradients to decrease in other areas of the vessel, including that across the measurement electrode pair.

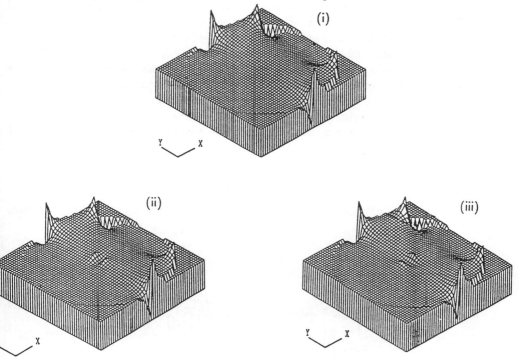

Figure 4; (i)non-intrusive, (ii)insulative stirrer, (iii)metallic stirrer

3.2 Case[2]: Addition of a stirrer

This case studies the addition of a stirrer within the vessel. Firstly an insulative stirrer is modeled, followed a metallic stirrer.

3.2.1 Insulative Stirrer

In order to model the insulative stirrer a 'hole' was placed in the centre of the mesh. thus representing a infinitely insulative region.

Visual inspection of the the simulated field's equi-potential line distribution showed no noticeable change from those in the non-obtrusive case, except for a small area surrounding the stirrer. This would suggest very little change in the sensitivity distribution when compared to the non-intrusive case (sect 3.1). Figure 4(ii) shows the sensitivity between electrode pairs 1 and 4, hence showing the only marked changes are in close proximity to the stirrer. This change is quantified in section 4.

3.2.2 Metallic earthed stirrer

In most practical mixing vessels the metallic stirrer is connected to earth for safety and mechanical reasons. If the simulation was performed without a stirrer in homogeneous conditions then the voltage at the vessels centre would be half the excitation voltage due to the vessels symmetry. In order to minimize the stirrer's distortion on the field the excitation electrodes were set to equal voltages with opposing polarity, with respect to the stirrer voltage. The graph in figure 4(iii) shows the sensitivity distribution for electrode pairs 1 and 4. It can be seen that the only area of noticeable change, when compared to case 1, is in close proximity to the stirrer. This shows that by appropriate vessel excitation, the presence of the metallic stirrer can be accounted for to allow sensible EIT measurements to be made.

3.3   Case[3]: Centrally mounted electrodes

This model places an extra 4 electrodes to an insulative stirrer at the centre of the vessel.

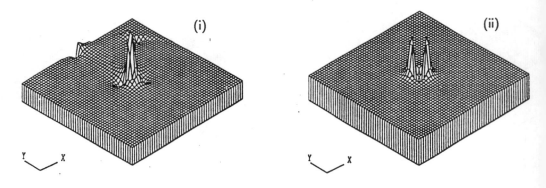

Figure 5; (i)Sensitivity between central and outer electrode pairs,
(ii)Sensitivity between two central electrode pairs

The sensitivity distributions of electrodes 1 to 8 were identical to those modeled with the insulative stirrer (section 3.2.1), assuming high electrode impedances. The graphs in figure 5 show sensitivity distributions for electrode pairs 1 and 9 and for 1 and 11. The graph for pairs 1 and 9 shows the sensitivity between central and surrounding electrode pairs. This shows an increase in sensitivity in the central area of the vessel, focused in a sector of the central area, allowing this area to be spatially decomposed. The graph for electrode pairs 9 and 11 shows the sensitivity between opposing electrode pairs attached to the stirrer. The sensitivity graph clearly shows that the highest sensitivity values are located in the central region of the vessel, therefore giving the best opportunity to increase the spatial resolution at the centre of the vessel. Due to adding only 4 extra electrodes the spatial decomposition at the vessels centre could not be determined with great accuracy. A larger number of electrodes might be desired for this reason.

4   Simulation Analysis

4.1   Overall image sensitivity and resolution

Figure 6 shows the sensitivity distribution over a complete image for cases [1] and [3]. The plots show that the increase in central sensitivity is limited to the central region of the vessel; the mid region of the vessel has not shown an average increase. The graph in figure 7 shows the percentage change in average sensitivity as a function of the vessel's radius for cases [2] and [3], with respect to the non-intrusive case, [1].

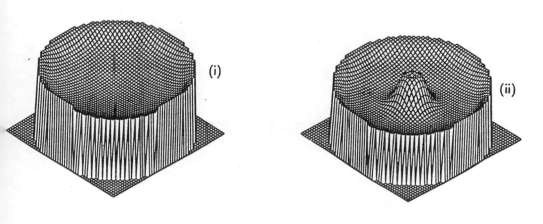

Figure 6; (i)Non-intrusive image sensitivity,
(ii)Central measurement image sensitivity

The graph shows that for the insulative and metallic stirrers. the change is limited to the central region of the vessel and the change in sensitivity is less than 1% except in the inner 5cm of the vessel's radius. The change in sensitivity for case [3] is 450% at the vessels centre, but is up to 20% less in the mid region of the vessel.

The increase in sensitivity shown by case[3] will help image reconstruction achieve a much greater central resolution. Seagar (1987) suggested a simple method to determine the spatial resolution throughout a circular region based on the electrode spacing. For a 16 electrode system Seagar predicted effective resolutions of 0.20 and 0.55 at the regions surface and centre respectively. These values being fractions of the vessel's diameter. Applying the same argument to our vessel model with the addition of 8 central electrodes, and scaling due to the small distances between central electrodes. gives a central effective resolution of 0.025. This equates to an improvement in central resolution of 700%. The change in resolution along the vessel's radius will not be linear and the increase in spatial resolution will be limited to mainly the inner third of the vessel radius.

In single source EIT systems two main types of excitation are used, adjacent as used in this study, or opposing were the excitation electrodes are placed on opposite sides of the region. Opposing excitation achieves a greater overall sensitivity, but with reduced resolution. In order to improve the sensitivity in the mid-region of the vessel excitation between a central and outer electrode could be applied.

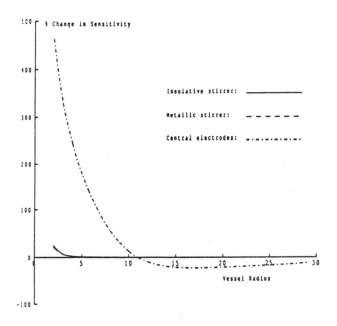

Figure 7; Relative changes in sensitivity as a function of vessel radius

4.2   Simulation validation

The data presented by this study is based on the mathematical relationship stated by Brekon and Pidcock (eqn.(1)) and its subsequent interpretation to allow sensitivity calculation. One possible verification method would be to model a non-homogeneous vessel and simulate the conditions arising from changing conductivity values at various points, such as that shown in figure 1, where the conductivity, ρ, of the small area, e, centred at (r,θ), is increased to $\rho+\delta\rho$. Instead of this approach practical measurements were made using a cylindrical phantom and the conductivity at particular points, (r,θ), altered by probing the phantom with a small metallic rod.

Figure 8 shows the simulated sensitivity values near the vessels wall for case[1] using electrode pairs 1 and 4. The metallic rod was rotated through 32 points at the edge of the vessel ($r\approx$vessel radius) and the values of δV calculated as the difference between two voltage measurements, with and without the rod in the vessel. This data has been superimposed on the graph which shows an approximate correlation between the simulated function and the measured values. Due to the finite area of the rod, and its large conductivity change, and also because of 3-dimensional effects, the practical measurements averaged out most of the sensitivity peaks.

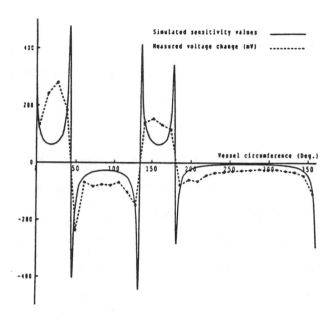

Figure 8; Simulated and measured sensitivity data

5   Conclusion

The results from this study clearly show that by taking account of the stirrers presence it
will not deteriorate the image quality. By taking advantage of its presence with additional
electrodes the image quality can be significantly enhanced.

6   Practical Comment

In practice it would be difficult to obtain accurate measurements from electrodes attached
to a rotating stirrer. A direct wire link would not be possible so information may have to
be accessed via radio telemetry or some other non-physical link. Electrodes could however
be more easily attached to a non-rotating sleeve surrounding the impellers drive shaft,
thus enabling a physical link to the electrodes. The effect on the flow regime within the
vessel will depend on the process being monitored. but will be very slight for low viscosity
newtonian mixing (e.g. water based) were the frictional forces on the vessel surfaces are
low.

The contents of the mixing vessel will give rise to a non-homogeneous field problem during
mixing, thus leading to field distortions within the vessel, an effect known as soft field.
It will be important to determine the susceptibility of the centrally mounted electrodes
to such effects in view of their close spacing. However such distortional phenomena also

affect the surrounding electrodes from which good images of mixing have been obtained, thereby introducing centrally mounted electrodes will still improve the quality of the images obtained.

Acknowledgement

This work was supported by a SERC Total Technology award in collaboration with ICI Chemicals and Polymers.

References

[1] Barber D C and Brown B H. 1984 *J.Phys E:Sci.Instrum,* **17** 723-33

[2] Brekon W R and Pidcock M K. 1987 *Clin.Phys.Physiol.Meas.,* **8** Suppl.A 77-84

[3] Dickin et al. 1992 *IEE proceedings-G,* **139** No.1 72-82

[4] Jossinet J and Kardous G. 1987 *Clin.Phys.Physiol.Meas.,* **8** Suppl.A.33-37

[5] Kotre C J. 1989 *Clin.Phys.Physiol.Meas.,* **10** No.3 275-281

[6] Seagar A D, Barber D C and Brown B H. 1987 *Clin.Phys.Physiol.Meas.,* **8** Suppl.A 13-31

[7] Vector fields Limited 1991 *PE2D Reference Manual-Version 8.3,* Vector fields limited, 24 Bankside, Kidlington, Oxford OX5 1JE

Recommendations for evaluation of performance criteria of electrical impedance data acquisition system for use in process tomography

X. J. Zhao. K. B. Tang, F. J. Dickin, R. C. Waterfall and M. S. Beck

Process Tomography Group. Department of Electrical Engineering and Electronics. UMIST, P.O. Box, 88. Manchester M60 1QD (U.K.)

Abstract

Criteria to evaluate the performance of an electrical impedance tomography (EIT) data collection system are presented. The main requirements of this system are: good measurement accuracy; high temperature stability; fast aperture time, high common-mode rejection ratio (CMRR); good signal to common-mode interference ratio (SCIR). The motivation for this paper is the need to make accurate and quantitative comparisons of different data collection systems. An evaluation of a system developed by the authors will be described.

1. Introduction

In recent years. development of electrical impedance tomography (EIT) has been carried out in many countries. EIT techniques promise an alternative technique with which to accommodate a variety of difficult measurement problems which cannot easily be solved by conventional methods. As the performance of both linear integrated circuits and microprocessors improves, the development of high speed, reliable, robust and cheap EIT systems for process industry become practicable.

An EIT system consists mainly of two parts: a hardware-based data acquisition system (DAS); and a software-based reconstruction algorithm. The overall performance of an EIT system is entirely dependent on a combination of the two parts. Both require separate criteria to evaluate their respective performance. Due to the increasing interest in EIT it is felt that an international criteria should be created to enable different EIT data acquisition system to be compared on a common basis. According to experimental results obtained during the development of the author's EIT system. a criteria covering the data acquisition has emerged.

2. Accuracy

Several papers have mentioned that the DAS may need an absolute accuracy of 0.1% for the measurement of peripheral voltage profiles (B. H. Brown and A. D. Seager 1987. D. Murphy and P. Rolfe 1988). However. no definition of the accuracy (A) for a DAS was presented. Estimates of the accuracy of some DAS's by referring to its signal-to-noise ratio (SNR) (A. M. Sinton et al 1991) is often ambiguous. As a measurement instrument, using accuracy to describe its performance is better than using its SNR. Signal-to-noise ratios are often quoted for amplifiers, such as those in audio and video equipment. The output signal to noise ratio (SNR_o) of a electronic system is comprised of the system noise coefficient F and the input signal's signal to noise ratio SNR_{in}, namely:

$$SNR_o = SNR_{in} + F$$

$$= SNR_{in} + F_1 + \frac{F_2}{A_1} + \frac{F_3}{(A_1 \cdot A_2)} + ... + \frac{F_i}{(A_1 \cdot ... \cdot A_i)} + ... \tag{1}$$

where F_i and A_i ($i = 1, 2,....$) are the noise coefficient and gain of the ith stage amplifier respectively. Input noise is mainly due to environmental noise such as electromagnetic radiation from radio transmitters, industrial equipment and electromagnetic coupling from the mains power supply. The noise coefficient F is caused by the DAS's internal components like: resistors (thermal noise); operational amplifiers (shot noise and finegrain noise). According to probability theory (S. M. Ross 1989), a reasonable assumption of the random noise is similar to Gaussian white noise. Thus the probability density function $p(x)$ of the total output noise of a DAS for ith independent measurement V_i would be

$$p(V_i) = \frac{1}{2\pi\sigma} e^{-\frac{(V_i - a_i)^2}{2\sigma^2}} \tag{2a}$$

$$a_i = \int_{-\infty}^{\infty} V_i \cdot p(V_i) dV_i \tag{2b}$$

$$\sigma = \sqrt{\int_{-\infty}^{\infty} (V_i - a_i)^2 p(V_i) dV_i} \tag{2c}$$

a_i is the mean value of the ith voltage measurement data of an DAS system and σ is the mean-square deviation. Thus, the probability of ± 3 mean-square deviation is given by:

$$P\{(a_i - 3\sigma) \le V_i \le (a_i + 3\sigma)\} \cong 0.995 \tag{3}$$

So, the signal to noise ratio for ith independent measurement (SNR_i) which is caused by random noise with credibility 99.5 percent would be

$$SNR_i = -20 \log(3\sigma / V_i) \text{ dB} \tag{4}$$

However, this specification only determines the random noise. Often, because of the gain error of the programmable gain amplifier (PGA) and common-mode voltage interference, the mean of the measurement may depart from the expected value. Fig.1 shows a diagram of a four electrode measurement protocol which employs the adjacent method (B. H. Brown and A. D. Seager 1987). The total number of electrodes is sixteen.

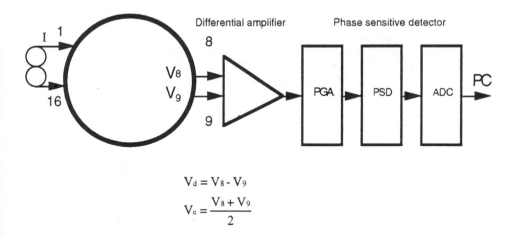

$$V_d = V_8 - V_9$$

$$V_c = \frac{V_8 + V_9}{2}$$

Fig.1 four electrode data collection method.

When a constant current I is injected at electrode pair 1, the differential voltage is measured at the pair 9, that is, between the electrode 8 and 9. Supposed the accurate value of the differential voltage should be 5mVpp, but the system always indicated it would be 6mVpp. It means that the system has a gain error, even if no random noise and common-mode interference is presented. This error would strongly affect images reconstructed using quantitative algorithms. The signal to noise ratio does not include the system gain error. During the development of the first UMIST EIT system, it was felt that to use the conception of accuracy rather than SNR would be more clear and precise, which would include the random noise, common-mode interference and gain error. One suggestion is defined as follows.

Accuracy: A

$$A_i = \frac{V_i - U_i}{U_i} \cdot 100\%$$

$$A = \max(A_1, A_2, ..., A_i, ..., A_m) \qquad \left[m = n(n-3)/2 \right]$$

(5)

Average accuracy: A_a

$$A_a = \sqrt{\frac{1}{n(n-3)/2} \sum_{i=1}^{n(n-3)/2} \left[\frac{V_i - U_i}{U_i} \right]^2} \cdot 100\%$$

here V_i is the voltage measured from the ith independent measurement, U_i is the expected value. n is the number of system electrodes.

3. Common-mode rejection ratio (CMRR) and signal to common-mode interference ratio (SCIR)

In a typical DAS, the differential voltage V_d as shown in fig.1 is quite small, common-mode voltage V_c is higher than the V_d. Most DAS's use a common-mode rejection ratio to measure the ability of system amplifier against the interference of the common-mode voltage. The CMRR is defined as follows:

$$CMRR = 20 \log \frac{K_{Vd}}{K_{Vc}} \text{ dB} \qquad (7)$$

here K_{Vd} and K_{Vc} are the gain of a DAS for differential and common-mode voltages respectively. The CMRR is mainly determined by the first stage in a DAS and is fixed. Often, the differential voltage to be measured exhibits a dynamic range of over 30dB, however, the common-mode voltages are almost at the same level. Thus, the same CMRR can produce different effects on the system accuracy to different measurements. So, it is more obvious to define a differential signal to common-mode interference ratio (SCIR) instead of using the CMRR to measure the immunity of a DAS to common-mode interference. The SCIR is defined as follows:.

$$SCIR = 20 \log \frac{V_d}{V_{ce}} \text{ dB} \qquad (8)$$

V_d is the differential signal, V_{ce} is the equivalent error which is caused by the common-mode voltage. Since the SCIR is proportional to differential signal V_d, using the smallest signal of V_d will be suitable to represent a DAS's ability against common-mode interference.

4. Stability

Stability is also a important criteria of a DAS especially when the EIT system is used in an industrial environment. The accuracy of a good DAS should not drift despite ambient temperature change and component ageing. It is recommended that the temperature coefficient (TC), short-term stability (S_{st}) and middle-term stability (S_{mt}) are used to determine the stability of a DAS, which is defined below:

Temperature coefficient:
$$TC_i = \frac{V_{i,T_1} - V_{i,T_2}}{T_1 - T_2} \bullet 100\%$$
$$TC = \max(TC_1, TC_2,....TC_i,....TC_m) \qquad [m = n(n-3)/2] \qquad (9)$$

Similarly, $V_{i,T1}$ is the voltage of the ith independent measurement when the ambient temperature is T_1. The V_{i,T_2} is the one when the temperature changes to T_2.

Short-Term stability:

$$S_{st,i} = \frac{V_{0.25,i} - V_{12,i}}{V_{0.25,i}} \, 100\%$$

$$S_{st} = \max(S_{st,1}, S_{st,2},...,S_{st,i},...,S_{st,m}) \quad [m = n(n-3)/2]$$

(10)

Again, the $V_{0.25,i}$ is the ith unique measuring voltage after an DAS has been operating in constant ambient condition for 15 minutes. $V_{12,i}$ is the measurement after a period of 12 hours. The definition of a middle-term stability (S_{mt}) is similar to the short-term one except the time interval is 100 hours. That is,

Middle-Term stability:

$$S_{mt,i} = \frac{V_{0.25,i} - V_{100,i}}{V_{0.25,i}} \cdot 100\%$$

$$S_{mt} = \max(S_{mt,1}, S_{mt,2},...,S_{mt,i},...S_{mt,m}) \quad [m = n(n-3)/2]$$

(11)

According to feedback theory (B. K. Jones 1986) in the electronics, when a DAS is in a maximum gain and measuring the smallest signal, its stability is in most adverse condition, which is caused by ambient temperature drift and component ageing. So, using the smallest independent measurement to assess the stability of a DAS is a reasonable simplification.

Aperture time Ta is the time taken by the DAS to capture a complete 'frame' of measurements. Other specifications such as isolation, leakage current, insulation strength of DAS between electrodes and mains power, work temperature, mean time between failure (MTBF) etc. are similar to conventional electronic instruments which can be referred to international standards.

5. Practical performance assessment of a DAS

A standard phantom is required for assessing a DAS. Giffiths (1988) constructed a resistor phantom with $\pm 1\%$ tolerance and ± 50ppm/°C temperature coefficient. Since the phantom element have $\pm 1\%$ tolerance, it only can assess a DAS the accuracy of which is below $\pm 1\%$. During the developing of UMIST EIT Mk.1a system, a phantom was built with a precision resistor network ($\pm 0.1\%$, 15ppm/°C). The resistor phantom can provide a differential signal with high common-mode voltage and an equivalent output-input impedance which are similar to that produced by a homogeneous medium in a vessel. Because the resistor values of the network are known, the differential signals between every two electrodes (terminal) and common-mode voltages can be obtained by using circuit theory or by experiment (employing DC which can be measured very accurately). Because the topographies of every terminal are the same, the ratios between the differential voltage which have the same electrode interval are fixed and equal. The resistor phantom was connected to the UMIST EIT Mk.1a system. The measurement protocol was the adjacent method. The differential signals were measured at three frequencies (12.5kHz, 25kHz, 50kHz) with two exciting currents (2.5mApp, 5mApp). To estimate the stability, the second set of data was measured after about 12 hours. During both of experiments, the ambient temperature changed by about 6°C . From the experimental results and according to the definition given in the previous section, the average accuracy (A_a) of the system is 0.5%. The short-term stability is about 0.2%. The temperature coefficient TC is ±0.2%/20°C . To measure the CMRR, two electrodes were connected together to render the differential signal zero, but the common-mode voltage was almost the same. The outputs of the DAS were read and the equivalent differential voltage Vce was calculated. The CMRR is 126dB. The signal to common-mode interference ratio (SCIR) is 70dB.

6. Conclusion

Some recommendations for the performance criteria to evaluate a DAS are presented here. Apparently, to appreciate the full property of an EIT system is very complicated because of the varying of number of electrodes and different measurement protocols. For example, in a DAS, 0.1 % accuracy can be relatively easily achieved by the opposite measurement method but not the adjacent one. The specification should give in a clear definition and define the measurement method, frequency, injection current and conductivity of the object to be measured.

7. References

A.M. Sinton, et al (1991): "Noise and spatial resolution of a real-time electrical impedance tomograph". CAIT conference, York.

B. H. Brown and A. D. Seager (1987): "The Sheffield Data Collection System". Clin. Phys. Physiol. Meas., Vol. 8 a, 91--97.

B. K. Jones (1986): "Electronics for Experimentation and Research". Prentice-Hall International, Englewood Cliffs.

D. Murphy and P. Rolfe (1988): "Aspects of Instrumentation Design for . Impedance Imaging". Clin. Physiol. Meas., Vol. 9 A, 514.

H. Griffiths (1988): "A Phantom for Electrical Impedance Tomography''. Clin. Phys. Physiol. Meas. 9 Suppl A, 1520.

J. G. Webser (1990): "Electrical Impedance Tomography" Adam Hilger, Bristol and New York.

S. M. Ross (1989): "Introduction to Probability Models". Academic Press, Inc. Boston.

Chapter 2

Data Processing, Mathematical Techniques and Simulation

Implementation of Iterative Algorithms for Image Reconstruction on Parallel Architectures

António Adrego da Rocha - António Jorge Pinto - António Rui Borges

Departamento de Electrónica e Telecomunicações
Universidade de Aveiro
3800 Aveiro, Portugal.

ABSTRACT: This paper makes an assessment of the performance of ART algorithms for X-ray transmission tomography and single photon emission tomography. Results related to their rate of convergence and quality of the reconstructed images are presented. It is also shown how one may explore the intrinsic parallelism they have in order to get efficient computer implementations on parallel architectures.

1. INTRODUCTION

Generally speaking, tomographic reconstruction consists in finding the spatial distribution (2 or 3D) of an object's internal physical property from a finite set of measurements taken outside at well-defined positions. It is a typical example of what is usually called an inverse problem, where one tries to determine the value of a function from a given set of functionals which in some way or another are related to it.

In practice, solving the problem always means representing the spatial distribution of the object's physical property as an image in some display system.

Two main strategies may be used to accomplish this.

In the first, the transform methods' strategy, a closed formula for the analytical solution of the problem is known. Reconstruction algorithms are then produced by discretizing this formula for computer implementation.

In the second, the series expansion methods' strategy, the problem is treated as a discrete one from the very beginning. The function is replaced by a discretized version on an appropriate rectangular grid and the integral equations that model the measurement process are converted to summation equations. As a result, we get to solve a system of simultaneous equations where the unknowns are the different function elements.

Although transform methods are usually more computationally efficient than series expansion methods, they are also a lot more restrictive. Most of their attractive characteristics are lost when the scanning geometry is not simple and regular or the physical model of data collection deviates rather strongly from the evaluation of line integrals along straight lines.

Series expansion methods, on the other hand, enabling an easy incorporation into the coefficients of the different equations of the details concerning the scanning geometry and the physics of data collection, are quite flexible. Moreover, since most of the time the system of equations is inconsistent due to measurement errors and imperfections in the adopted model of data collection, it is possible to impose an optimization criterion that makes the solution converge to a class with desirable features.

In this paper, we make an evaluation of some ART algorithms for X-ray transmission tomography and single photon emission tomography, presenting results about their rate of convergence and quality of the reconstructed images.

Finally, we will show how their intrinsic parallelism may be explored in order to get efficient computer implementations on parallel architectures.

2. DISCRETIZATION MODEL

Let $f(x,y)$ represent the object's physical property we want to determine and display as an image. To achieve this, one has to replace it by a discretized version which can be obtained using the following procedure.

Assume a rectangular grid of N square picture elements, pixels, covering the whole object's region of interest and also that each pixel value, f_j, is constant and equal to the function's average value inside it, figure 1.

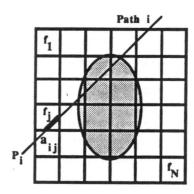

Figure 1 - Discretization model

Let $\{b_j(x,y): j = 1, ... , N\}$ be the set of basis functions where each element $b_j(x,y)$ is equal to 1 if the point (x,y) belongs to the pixel j and 0 otherwise.

Any well-behaved function $f(x,y)$ which we may wish to consider, can then be approximated by the picture function $\underline{f}(x,y)$ that is defined by the linear combination of basis functions presented below:

$$f(x,y) \approx \tilde{f}(x,y) = \sum_{j=1}^{N} f_j \cdot b_j(x,y) \ . \tag{1}$$

On the other hand, let $\{T_i: i = 1, \dots, P\}$ be the set of linear and continuous functionals which model the measurement process that was carried out. Their application to function $f(x,y)$ can now be approximated by (Herman 1980, Viergever 1988)

$$R_i f(x,y) \approx R_i \tilde{f}(x,y) = \sum_{j=1}^{N} R_i b_j(x,y) \cdot f_j \approx \sum_{j=1}^{N} a_{ij} \cdot f_j \approx p_i \ , \text{(with } i = 1, \dots, P), \tag{2}$$

where a_{ij} and p_i represent, respectively, the approximation to $R_i b_j(x,y)$ used in numerical implementations and the measured estimate of $R_i f(x,y)$.

In matrix form, the algebraic system of equations described in (2) can be written as

$$p \approx A \cdot f \tag{3}$$

where $p = (p_i) \in R^P$ is the measurement vector, $f = (f_j) \in R^N$ is the image vector and $A = (a_{ij}) \in (R^P \times R^N)$ is the projection matrix, embodying in each specific case the physical model of data collection.

In a more accurate formulation, one may introduce on the right-hand side of last equation a new term, $e = (e_i) \in R^P$, usually called the error vector, to take into account the differences between both sides due to measurement errors, image discretization and approximations to the adopted model of data collection and to $R_i b_j(x,y)$

$$p = A \cdot f + e \ . \tag{4}$$

Thus, the reconstruction problem may be stated in the following way: given A and p, estimate f, minimizing e.

In X-ray transmission tomography, $f(x,y)$ represents the linear attenuation coefficient of the object at a given energy and $R_i f(x,y)$ describes its line integral along the path i: $\int_{L_i} f(x,y)dL$. Therefore, $R_i b_j(x,y)$ corresponds here to the intersection length of the integration path i with pixel j and (3) is converted into a system of linear equations.

In single photon emission tomography, $f(x,y)$ represents the concentration of a radioisotope inside the object and $R_i f(x,y)$ describes its weighted line integral along the path i: $\int_{L_i} f(x,y)e^{-\int_{D_i(x,y)} \mu dD} dL$, where μ is the linear attenuation coefficient of the object at the energy of the emitted photons and the exponencial weighting factor is the attenuation suffered by photons from their emission point to the object boundary along the propagation path.

Under this formulation, the inversion problem is strongly ill-posed but some simplifications can be made to make it more amenable to computation. In many cases, one may assume the object to be homogeneous, having an effective linear attenuation coefficient μ close to its average real value. In this way, $R_i b_j(x,y)$ will correspond to the intersection length of the integration path i with pixel j multiplied by the factor $e^{+\mu d_{ij}}$, where d_{ij} is the distance from the pixel j center to the object boundary, and (3) is now converted into a system of nonlinear equations.

In order to compute coefficients a_{ij}, one has to know the values of the different d_{ij}'s beforehand. This, however, can be achieved since the object shape may be inferred from measured data through the use of a large spectrum window at the detector side collecting events from Compton scattering inside the object.

3. ITERATIVE ALGORITHMS

According to the notation previously used, solving a system of equations in an iterative way means devising a method to produce a sequence of vectors $f^{(k)}$ which we expect will converge to f. A good review of this class of algorithms can be found in (Censor 1983).

ART (the Algebraic Reconstruction Technique) is a special example of this class. It was introduced to image reconstruction by Gordon et al (1970) and was later shown to be a generalization of the Kaczmarz projection method for solving systems of equations.

It starts with an initial guess $f^{(0)}$ for the image vector (usually the zero vector). Then, at each iteration step, the current vector $f^{(k)}$ is updated to a new vector $f^{(k+1)}$ by taking into account a single equation, say the ith, and changing the components of the image vector connected with pixels intersected by the integration path. In each case, the amount of change is proportional to the difference between measured data p_i and the computed projection $\sum_{j=1}^{N} a_{ij} f_j^{(k)}$. In algebraic notation, we have

Initialization $f^{(0)}$ is arbitrary

Iteration step $f^{(k+1)} = f^{(k)} + \lambda \cdot \left(\dfrac{p_i - \langle a_i, f^{(k)} \rangle}{\langle a_i, a_i \rangle} \right) \cdot a_i$, (with $i = k \bmod P + 1$) (5)

where $<,>$ stands for the dot product of two vectors.

Actually, this is already a modified version of the algorithm because the so-called relaxation factor, parameter λ, was introduced to speed up the convergence rate. If the system of equations is consistent, vector $e = (0)$ in equation (4), it can be proved that the iterative process will converge to the solution, for $0 < \lambda < 2$ (Tanabe 1971, Herman et al 1978).

A very clear and simple presentation of this method can be found in (Kak and Slaney 1988). The basic idea is to look upon the image vector as a point in an N-dimensional space and to every equation as an hyperplane in this space. Then, the solution of a consistent system of equations represents the intersection point of all the hyperplanes and each iteration step turns out to be no more than the orthogonal projection of the previous image vector estimate upon a specific hyperplane, figure 2.

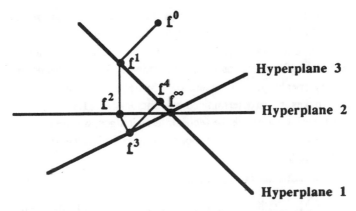

Figure 2 - Geometric illustration of convergence towards the solution in ART
without relaxation (λ equal to 1)

A whole family of ART-like algorithms can be developed if image vector updating is performed after processing groups of equations instead of only one (Herman et al 1988). In the limit situation, where all the equations are processed first, we get the well-known SIRT algorithm. As another example, we can consider the case where all equations related to the same principal direction of integration (what is usually called a projection) are processed as a group. This leads to an algorithm with a global organization very similar to the one described in (Kak and Slaney 1988) and named SART.

In the general case, we have

Initialization $f^{(0)}$ is arbitrary

Iteration step $\displaystyle f_j^{(k+1)} = f_j^{(k)} + \frac{\sum_{r=1}^{L}\left[\lambda \cdot a_{ij} \cdot \dfrac{\left(p_i - \langle a_i , f^{(k)} \rangle\right)}{\langle a_i , a_i \rangle}\right]}{\sum_{r=1}^{L} a_{ij}}$,   (6)

(with $i = L .(k \bmod (P/L)) + r$ and $j = 1, \dots , N$) .

According to Herman and Levkowitz (1988), for choices of L corresponding to groups made up of several projections, algorithms with better performances than those obtained with ART are to be expected. However, due to the extra memory required for the processing of each group, they tend to be less efficient in SIMD implementations.

4. PERFORMANCE ASSESSMENT

The standard image used in our simulations, known as Herman head phantom, is due to Herman (1980). The image was discretized on a 255 x 255 pixels grid. The results presented were obtained using a simulation package we developed, which is described elsewhere (Rocha et al 1990), and run on a Digital DECstation 3100.

All values refer to a X-ray transmission tomography case, using a parallel scanning geometry, where 320/640 projections were collected with 361 samples per projection. This gives rise, roughly speaking, to a system of $2.3 \times 10^5 / 1.2 \times 10^5$ equations with 6.5×10^4 unknowns which makes it overdeterminated by a factor of $3.6/1.8$.

As figures of merit to compare the reconstructed images, we use the norms defined by Herman (1980): namely, the normalized root mean square distance (d) and the normalized mean absolute distance (r)

$$d = \sqrt{\frac{\sum\limits_{u=1}^{L} \sum\limits_{v=1}^{L} \left(f_{u,v} - h_{u,v}\right)^2}{\sum\limits_{u=1}^{L} \sum\limits_{v=1}^{L} \left(f_{u,v} - \underline{h}\right)^2}} \qquad\qquad r = \frac{\sum\limits_{u=1}^{L} \sum\limits_{v=1}^{L} \left|f_{u,v} - h_{u,v}\right|}{\sum\limits_{u=1}^{L} \sum\limits_{v=1}^{L} \left|f_{u,v}\right|} \qquad (7)$$

where $\underline{h}$ is the average value of Herman head phantom and L is equal to $\sqrt{N}$.

Unless otherwise stated, the presented values are associated with images which are visually very close to the original Herman head phantom.

The first fact to bear in mind about the rate of convergence of iterative algorithms is that they are extremely dependent upon the value used for the relaxation factor and upon the ordering of the equations treated in succession.

The reason why this latter aspect is so important becomes apparent after considering again figure 2. The more orthogonal the hyperplanes associated with successive equations are, the faster the computed estimates will reach the region where the solution is. Hence, since two hyperplanes are orthogonal if and only if the associated equations describe integration paths which do not cross the same pixels, it is easy to devise an ordering that keeps orthogonality while processing the equations related to the samples of each projection.

When considering next successive projections, this rule can be almost fulfilled by selecting projections whose principal directions of integration are about $\pi/2$ apart. Ordering 1 in figure 4 has such a feature and produces in just one macro iteration (one cycle of processing all the equations) an image with very good quality. However, provided the rule is kept for the first half of the computations, it is not necessary to keep it as strongly for the rest, as ordering 2 described in figure 3 illustrates. The image obtained after one macro iteration has about the same quality as the one produced in ordering 1.

Orderings 3 and 4, also described in figure 3, take advantage of symmetric properties the measurement process presents to reduce the computational complexity. For each a_{ij} that is evaluated, three others are deduced; which means that four equations belonging to four different projections are processed simultaneously. Still, there is a price to be paid: four macro iterations in the former case, and three in the latter are required to obtain an image with similar quality to the ones mentioned before.

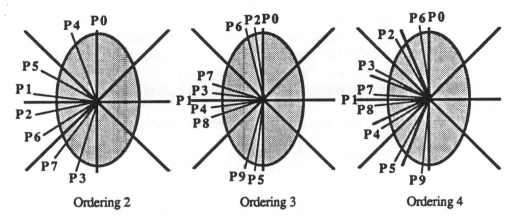

Figure 3 - Different ways of ordering the projections during the processing
sequence for fast rate of convergence

On the other hand, we found that the optimum value for the relaxation factor is very
much dependent upon the scanning geometry and the rate of convergence. So the best way
to determine it is to proceed by trial and error, using standard data to obtain reconstructed
images for different values and then choosing the one that seems to be the best.

Figure 5 presents an example where two parallel geometries are studied: the number of
samples per projection is the same, but the number of projections is 320 in one case and
640 in the other. Reconstructions were made for values of λ between 0.1 and 1. As can be
seen the optimum value belongs in each case to a different range of λ.

The influence of the rate of convergence, on the other hand, can be appreciated from
the fact that the best values of λ for the orderings presented in figure 4 are 0.3, 0.3, 0.075,
0.1, respectively, for orderings 1, 2, 3 and 4. Which means that the faster the algorithm
converges, the higher the relaxation factor should be.

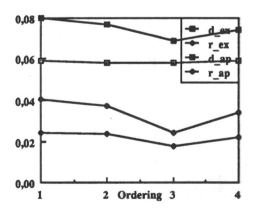 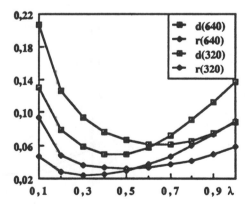

Figure 4 - Dependency of the rate of
convergence on the ordering
of equations

Figure 5 - Scanning geometry influence
on the optimum value for λ

When the system of equations is huge as in the present case, the elements a_{ij} of the projection matrix cannot be stored and have to be evaluated on line. This represents the major computational task of ART execution. The usual way of dealing with this problem is replacing their exact computation by a simplified one based on a binary decision: a one is assigned if the integration path crosses the pixel central part, otherwise a zero will be assigned.

In effect, the iteration step (5) is substituted by the following one

$$\text{Iterative step} \quad f^{(k+1)} = f^{(k)} + \lambda \cdot \left(\frac{p_i}{L_i} - \frac{Q_i}{N_i} \right), \quad \text{(with } i = k \bmod P + 1) \tag{8}$$

where N_i is the number of pixels whose a_{ij} were changed to one, Q_i is the sum of the pixel values where this change took place and L_i is the total integration path length. Note that the ratio p_i/L_i can be calculated beforehand and so is not generally accounted for during the actual algorithm execution.

Obviously, this simplification will introduce further noise in the reconstructed image but the resulting degradation is not too significant. This fact is illustrated in figure 4 where for each ordering of equations referred above, two reconstruction images were produced: one using the exact coefficients, its figures of merit have the suffix ex, and another implementing the equation (8), its figures of merit have the suffix ap.

Up to now, all presented results assumed the system of equations to be consistent. In order to examine the performance of the algorithm in the presence of noise, a noise vector with zero mean and variance modelled according to the X-ray transmission case was added up to the simulated measurement data.

Figure 6 presents the results both for the exact and the simplified algorithm using ordering 2. A typical real situation corresponds to N_i equal to 10^6 (number of photons emitted by the X-ray source during each measurement) and for it they both perform rather well. Even for N_i equal to 10^5, the basic image features can still be recognized.

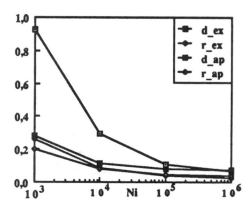

Figure 6 - ART behaviour under the presence of noise, modelling
an X-ray transmission tomography situation

5. IMPLEMENTATION EXAMPLE ON A PARALLEL ARCHITECTURE

It is not easy to devise efficient parallel algorithms to run ART in computer systems of the MIMD-type. The reason for this comes from the fact that each iteration step requires the updating of the image vector after processing every single equation. In this sense, the most one may hope for is ordering the equations in such a way that some of them are processed simultaneously because their correspondent integration paths do not share common pixels.

In fact, this kind of architecture only becomes really attractive when ART-like algorithms of the type described by the iteration step (6) are considered.

Here, we are going to describe an implementation on a computer system of the SIMD-type where the above mentioned restrictions do not affect the algorithm performance.

The GLiTCH (Storer et al 1988) is a parallel associative processor array currently being developed at Bristol University. It has 64 processor elements per chip (PEs), each one with 64 bits of Content Addressable Memory (CAM), 4 subset bits (that can be used as an extra matching condition) and a 1-bit arithmetic and logic unit (ALU).

An instruction broadcast to the array is followed by a description of the pattern which signals the intended processors to execute it. The PE's which are to perform the operation are identified by matching all or part of their contents to the given pattern. All other processors remain inactive during that operation.

Figure 7 presents a block diagram of its architecture. It also shows how a typical computer system based on those chips would look like.

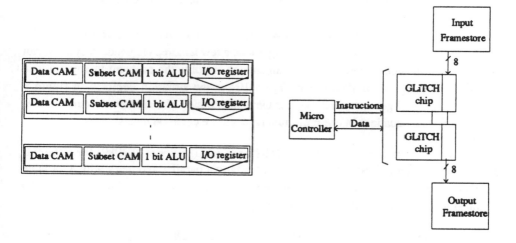

Figure 7 - The GLiTCH chip architecture and a linear chain of GLiTCH chips.

GLiTCH chips can be cascaded together to form a linear chain. An 8 bit wide shift register capable of transferring data in and out of the framestores (memories where data is stored) runs the entire length of the chain, moving data along it simultaneously with the processing of internal data carried out by the different processor elements.

In general, two main approaches can be followed to conceive an image reconstruction algorithm in parallel. Either the image vector is permanently stored in an accessible way to the different processors of the system and the measurement data is kept coming in when required - the pixel driven approach; or, on the contrary, it is each measurement vector that is kept accessible as long as required and image data is moving in and out - the projection driven approach, figure 8.

Obviously, the reasons detailed in the beginning of the section for explaining why ART could not be efficiently implemented in MIMD machines makes one reject the pixel-driven approach. Even if those reasons did not apply, this approach would always be totally unfeasible because any reasonable-sized image would require a system with an enormous number of chips.

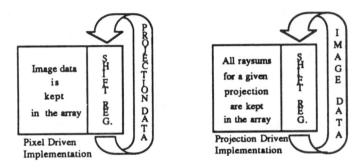

Figure 8 - Main approaches for ART implementation in the GLiTCH

The projection-driven approach, however, turns out to be rather promising since the size of the measurement vector is never larger than a few hundred elements. A system with just a few chips would then be more than enough to solve the problem in any realistic situation. The algorithm sketched in figure 10 for the situation depicted in figure 9 considers a parallel geometry and requires the preprocessing of measurement data in order to ensure that all equations in one projection do not share common pixels.

This algorithm was run on the GLiTCH simulator (Duller et al 1989) for different-sized image vectors (8 bits of resolution), assuming a parallel geometry with a variable number of projections and samples per projection (16 bits of resolution). The results obtained per macro iteration were the following:

Image size	64x64	128x128	256x256
N. of projections	128	256	512
N. of samples / projection	64	128	256
N. of required GLiTCH chips	1	2	4
Total Execution time (ms)	118	532	3,620
• Data Shifting time (ms)	54	426	3,375
• Computation time (ms)	116	494	2,208

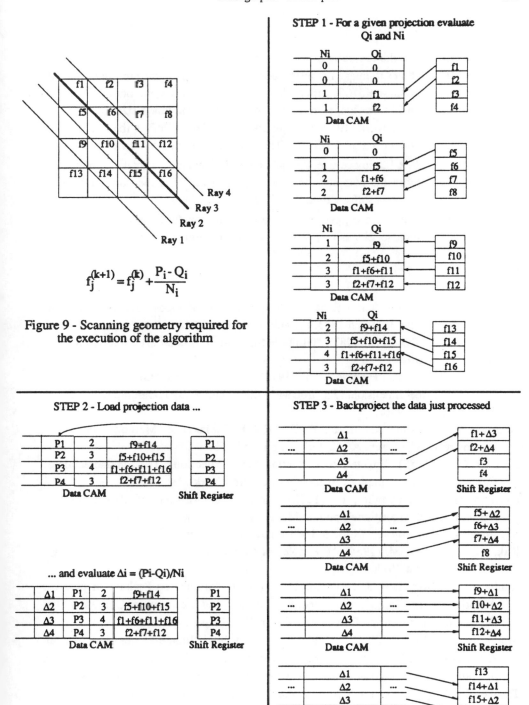

STEP 1 - For a given projection evaluate Qi and Ni

Ni	Qi
0	0
0	0
1	f1
1	f2

Data CAM

f1
f2
f3
f4

Ni	Qi
0	0
1	f5
2	f1+f6
2	f2+f7

Data CAM

f5
f6
f7
f8

Ni	Qi
1	f9
2	f5+f10
3	f1+f6+f11
3	f2+f7+f12

Data CAM

f9
f10
f11
f12

Ni	Qi
2	f9+f14
3	f5+f10+f15
4	f1+f6+f11+f16
3	f2+f7+f12

Data CAM

f13
f14
f15
f16

$$f_j^{(k+1)} = f_j^{(k)} + \frac{P_i - Q_i}{N_i}$$

Figure 9 - Scanning geometry required for the execution of the algorithm

STEP 2 - Load projection data ...

P1	2	f9+f14
P2	3	f5+f10+f15
P3	4	f1+f6+f11+f16
P4	3	f2+f7+f12

Data CAM

P1
P2
P3
P4

Shift Register

... and evaluate Δi = (Pi-Qi)/Ni

Δ1	P1	2	f9+f14
Δ2	P2	3	f5+f10+f15
Δ3	P3	4	f1+f6+f11+f16
Δ4	P4	3	f2+f7+f12

Data CAM

P1
P2
P3
P4

Shift Register

STEP 3 - Backproject the data just processed

Δ1	
Δ2	...
Δ3	
Δ4	

Data CAM

f1+Δ3
f2+Δ4
f3
f4

Shift Register

Δ1	
Δ2	...
Δ3	
Δ4	

Data CAM

f5+Δ2
f6+Δ3
f7+Δ4
f8

Shift Register

Δ1	
Δ2	...
Δ3	
Δ4	

Data CAM

f9+Δ1
f10+Δ2
f11+Δ3
f12+Δ4

Shift Register

Δ1	
Δ2	...
Δ3	
Δ4	

Data CAM

f13
f14+Δ1
f15+Δ2
f16+Δ3

Shift Register

Figure 10 - General overview of ART implementation in the GLiTCH

6. CONCLUSION

The achieved results are quite promising and seem to validate the use of general-purpose SIMD machines to image reconstruction. An optimized algorithm run on a RISC serial machine, DECstation 3100, with a clock rate similar to the one on the GLiTCH, takes between 40 and 50 times longer to execute for the 256 x 256 image size situation.

However, a lot of work still has to be done in order to define the architecture requirements for a wider class of algorithms. This is apparent in two different ways:

- above the 128 x 128 image size, the main factor influencing the total execution time is not any more the computation time ($O(N)$, where N is the number of pixel values), but the data shifting time ($O(N^{3/2})$);
- for divergent geometries, part of the regulality on transfering pixel values to and from each processor element CAM is lost and the execution becomes less efficient.

REFERENCES

Censor, Y. (1983). "Finite Series-Expansion Reconstruction Methods", Proceedings of the IEEE, Vol. 71, Nº 3, March 1983, pp. 409-419.

Duller, A. W. G. , Storer, R. (1989). "GLiTCH Simulation Version 2.1", Internal Report, University of Bristol.

Gordon, R. , Bender, R. , Herman, G. T. (1970). "Algebraic Reconstruction Techniques (ART) for Three-dimensional Electron Microscopy and X-ray Photography", J. Theor. Biol. 29, pp. 471-482.

Herman, G. T., Lent, A. , Lutz, P. H. (1978). "Relaxation Methods for Image Reconstruction", Comm. ACM, Vol. 21, pp. 152-158.

Herman, G. T. (1980). "Image Reconstruction from Projections. The Fundamentals of Computerized Tomography", Academic Press, New York.

Herman, G. T., Levkowitz, H. (1988). "Initial Performance of Block-iterative Reconstruction Algorithms", pub. in Mathematics and Computer Science in Medical Imaging, Ed. Viergever, M. A. & Todd-Pokropek, A. Springer Verlag, Berlin.

Kak, A. C. , Slaney, M. (1988). "Principles of Computerized Tomographic Imaging", IEEE Press, New York.

Rocha, A. A. , Borges, A. R. , Almeida, A. F. (1990). "Simulation Package of Iterative Algorithms for Tomographic Reconstruction", 2nd Portuguese Conference of Biomedical Engineering - Bioeng´ 90, Aveiro 1990 (in portuguese).

Storer, R. , Duller, A. W. G. , Dagless, E. L. (1988). "Image Generation with an Associative Processor Array", Proc. of CG International 88, published as New Trends in Computer Graphics, Ed. Magnenat-Thalmann N. & Thalmann D, Springer-Verlag.

Tanabe, K. (1971). "Projection Method for Solving a Singular System of Linear Equations and its Applications", Numer. Math., Vol. 17, pp. 203-214.

Viergever, M. A. ,(1988). "Introduction to Discrete Reconstruction Methods in Medical Imaging", pub. in Mathematics and Computer Science in Medical Imaging, Ed. Viergever, M. A. & Todd-Pokropek, A. Springer Verlag, Berlin.

Reconstruction from Limited Data with A-priori Knowledge

A Wernsdörfer

Institut für Meß- und Regelungstechnik, Universität (TH) Karlsruhe, Germany

ABSTRACT: An iterative reconstruction/restoration method for reconstructing a velocity vector field of a fluid from limited data is described. This procedure makes it possible to incorporate the conservation laws of fluidmechanics as a-priori knowledge, so that the quality of the reconstruction is improved.

1. INTRODUCTION

In many practical applications of computerized tomography, due to technical restrictions, it is not possible to sample an object with a sufficient number of views. But also reasons of cost saving and a slightly instationary behaviour of the object lead to a reduction of the measured projection data. The resulting limited set of data causes a deterioration of the quality of the reconstruction. Thus, it is necessary to improve the quality by additional knowledge about the object, the so-called a-priori knowledge. This a-priori knowledge can originate from different sources. For the reconstruction of a two-dimensional velocity field of a fluid by vector tomography the equations of mass, momentum and energy conservation of fluidmechanics offer such further informations. In the following it is described how these physical laws can be incorporated. The process of reconstruction is divided into two steps. The first step consists of the well-known reconstruction by ART (algebraic reconstruction technique), disregarding the physical laws. The imperfect result of the first step is then restored, utilizing the above mentioned laws, by operators of the projections onto convex sets (POCS). Thus an iterative procedure is proposed which converges to a solution, complying with both the measured projection data and the constraints, given by the laws of fluidmechanics.

2. RECONSTRUCTION METHOD

The reconstruction algorithm used is the vectorized algebraic reconstruction technique (VART) (Hauck, 1990) which is an extension of the scalar ART (Herman, 1980). In the following only the principles of this method are briefly explained. For VART the vector field is assumed to be of discrete nature. So, the object is presented by a n x n rectangular grid of so-called pixels. The value of any pixel is constant and equal to the value of the object at the center of the pixel.

Essential to vector tomography is a directed interaction between the vector field and the rays used. There is a distinction between the transversal interaction (orthogonal to the direction of propagation of the ray) and the longitudinal (tangential to that direction). For the longitudinal interaction the projection of the vector field $\underline{V}$ can be written as:

$$p(\theta, \ell) = \int_a^b \underline{V}(x,y)\,\underline{t}\;ds = \int_a^b (V_x(x,y)\,(-\sin\theta) + V_y(x,y)\,(\cos\theta))\,ds. \qquad (1)$$

Fig. 1 explains the expressions of (1).

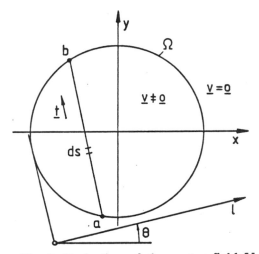

Fig. 1: Projection of the vector field $\underline{V}$.

Here it is assumed that the vector field $\underline{V}$ vanishes outside the circular space Ω. For VART the integral (1) turns into a sum

$$p(\theta, \ell_j) = \sum_i^{n^2} (V_{xi}\,(-\sin\theta) + V_{yi}\,(\cos\theta))\,a_{ij}. \qquad (2)$$

In this formulation both vector components V_x and V_y are written in a $(n^2 \times 1)$ dimensional vector in lexicographical order, respectively. a_{ij} is an weighting factor which describes the contribution of the i-th pixel to the j-th raysum. If $M = P \cdot N$ projections are measured (P $\triangleq$ number of views, N $\triangleq$ number of rays per view), the result will be a system of M linear equations with $2 \cdot n^2$ unknowns. This underdetermined system has no unique solution but by the iterative calculus proposed by Hauck (1990) one obtains the minimum least square solution as follows:

$$V_{xi}^{k+1} = V_{xi}^{k} + \lambda\,\frac{p(\theta, \ell_j) - \hat{p}(\theta, \ell_j)}{\underline{a}_j\,\underline{a}_j}\;a_{ij}\,(-\sin\theta) \qquad (3)$$

$$V_{yi}^{k+1} = V_{yi}^{k} + \lambda\,\frac{p(\theta, \ell_j) - \hat{p}(\theta, \ell_j)}{\underline{a}_j\,\underline{a}_j}\;a_{ij}\,(\cos\theta)$$

with

k $\triangleq$ number of iteration

$$\hat{p}(\theta, \ell_j) = \sum_i^{n^2} (V_{xi}^{k}\,(-\sin\theta) + V_{yi}^{k}\,(\cos\theta))\,a_{ij} \qquad (4)$$

λ ≙ the relaxation parameter to influence the convergence rate of the algorithm.

It is obvious that after each step of VART an image v_x^k, v_y^k is available to correction in the sense of the a-priori knowledge. Only after the restoration the image serves as the basis of the next step.

3. RESTORATION METHOD

The proposed restoration method ranks among the projections onto convex sets (POCS). The theory of POCS is described in the work of Youla et al. (1982). In this section only the principles are reviewed. Considering all functions $f(x,y)$ of a Hilbert space H square-integrable in the space Ω, with an adequate definition of the inner product and norm, all elements of this Hilbert space H complying with a particular property form a subset C_i. An element fulfilling m such properties is an element of the intersection C_o of the m subsets C_i:

$$f \in C_0 = \overset{m}{\underset{i}{\cap}} C_i . \tag{5}$$

The problem of image restoration consists in finding an element of the set C_o starting with an arbitrary element f^o. To reach this aim, first of all an operator P_i is applied to the image f so that the result g complies with the desired property of the subset C_i:

$$g = P_i f \rightarrow g \in C_i . \tag{6}$$

To obtain at least one image complying with all m properties the different operators P_i are successively applied to the new image, respectively. This results in the sequence:

$$f^{k+1} = (P_m \ P_{m-1} \ ... \ P_2 \ P_1)_\ell \ f^k \tag{7}$$

$$\ell \quad = 1+k \bmod m.$$

This sequence will converge to an element of C_o if two conditions are fulfilled:

1. The subsets C_i are convex.
2. The operators P_i present orthogonal projections.

In this case orthogonal projection means that any element of the subset C_i has a smaller distance to the previous image f than that one obtained by the operator P_i. This must not be mixed up with the projection of the vector field (1) which represents the measured data.

Mathematically this condition is expressed by:

$$g = P_i f \quad \underline{and} \quad ||g-f|| = \text{Min} \left\{ ||g_j-f||, \ \forall \ g_j \in C_i \right\}. \tag{8}$$

The distance $||\cdot||$ is defined by the norm of the Hilbert space H, here the euclidian norm is chosen. Fig. 2 shows this relation graphically for m = 3.

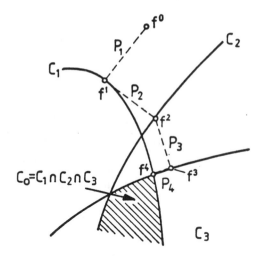

Fig. 2: Convergence to an element of the intersection C_0.

The convergence rate of the procedure can be influenced by introducing a relaxation parameter λ_i for each operator P_i. If the property of the elements of C_i can be expressed as

$$C_i(f) = 0 \qquad\qquad\qquad (9)$$

there will be a possibility of obtaining the operator P_i by solving the following optimization problem:

$$||g-f|| + w(C_i(g)) \rightarrow Min \qquad\qquad\qquad (10)$$

with w a Lagrange multiplier.

The calculation of the operator strongly depends on the constraint C(f). Thus, it is not possible to find a closed solution for any constraint. However, POCS has a remarkable quality in connection with VART because it can be shown that the reconstruction algorithm VART presents a POCS operator by itself. Therefore, the sequence

$$f^{k+1} = (P_m P_{m-1} \cdots P_2 P_1 P_{VART})_\ell f^k \qquad\qquad\qquad (11)$$

$$\ell = 1 + k \bmod m$$

certainly converges to an element which complies with the measured data $p(\theta, \ell)$ and the desired properties C_i, $i = 1, \ldots m$. The entire procedure is shown in the diagram of Fig. 4:

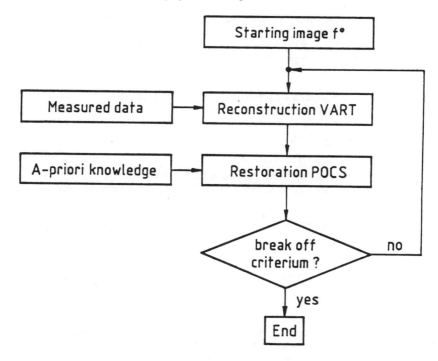

Fig. 4: Iterative reconstruction/restoration by VART and POCS.

4. LAWS OF CONSERVATION OF FLUIDMECHANICS

In this section an application of the proposed method is presented. The problem consists in reconstructing the two-dimensional velocity field of a fluid by vector tomography.

In this case the differences $\Delta T = T_{a\vec{b}} - T_{b\vec{a}}$ in the time of flight of ultrasonic impulses are measured between two US-transducers each alternatively acting as receiver and transmitter. The difference ΔT results from the acceleration of the ultrasonic beam by components of the velocity field in direction of sound propagation and from the retardation in the counter-direction (Hauck, 1990). This measured ΔT is the basis of the reconstruction. Of course, the considered velocity field is subject to the conservation laws of fluidmechanics. In the following it is shown how the different laws can be formulated as operators of POCS. First, it is necessary to make some assumptions in order to simplify the problem.

4.1 CONSERVATION OF MASS

The general formulation of the law of mass conservation is

$$\frac{\partial \rho}{\partial t} + \mathrm{div}\, \rho \,\underline{V} = 0. \qquad\qquad \rho \triangleq \text{ density of the medium} \qquad (12)$$
$$t \triangleq \text{ time.}$$

Assuming only stationary flows and an incompressible medium it follows

$$\text{div } \underline{V} = \frac{\partial V_x}{\partial x} + \frac{\partial V_y}{\partial y} = 0. \tag{13}$$

Consequently, the constraint (9) can be written as

$$C_D(\underline{V}) = \text{div } \underline{V} = 0. \tag{14}$$

The reconstructed flow field has to comply with this condition at each pixel of the discrete grid. In the following the discrete gradients are defined by

$$\frac{\partial V_x}{\partial x} = \tfrac{1}{2} \cdot (V_x(2,2) - V_x(1,2) + V_x(2,1) - V_x(1,1)) \tag{15}$$

$$\frac{\partial V_y}{\partial y} = \tfrac{1}{2} \cdot (V_y(2,2) - V_y(2,1) + V_y(1,2) - V_y(1,1)) \, .$$

1,2	2,2
1,1	2,1

It is of no use trying to vary simultaneously all $2n^2$ elements of the vector field so that the condition is fulfilled at each point. In order to avoid the large number of variables only the eight elements of a 2x2 mask are varied at first. This is the smallest mask which is necessary to calculate the condition (13). Then this mask is moved over the entire image as long as the condition is fulfilled at each point.

Simard et al. (1988) derived the operator P_D for such a mask solving the optimization problem (10) with the constraint (14)

$$\sum_{i}^{5} \left[\left(V_{xi}^{k+1} - V_{xi}^{k} \right)^2 + \left(V_{yi}^{k+1} - V_{yi}^{k} \right)^2 \right] + w \cdot \text{div } \underline{V}^{k+1} \to \text{Min} \, . \tag{16}$$

4.2 CONSERVATION OF MOMENTUM

For an incompressible medium the conservation of momentum is expressed by the Navier-Stokes differential equations

$$\frac{d\underline{V}}{dt} = -\frac{1}{\rho} \nabla p + \underline{g} + \eta \Delta \underline{V} \tag{17}$$

$p \triangleq$ pressure
$\underline{g} \triangleq$ volumetric forces
$\eta \triangleq$ dynamic viscosity
$\Delta \triangleq$ Laplace-Operator
$\nabla \triangleq$ Nabla-Operator

After a short straight-forward calculation and the substitution

$$\underline{\omega} = \text{rot } \underline{V} = \left(\frac{\partial V_z}{\partial y} - \frac{\partial V_y}{\partial x}, \ \frac{\partial V_x}{\partial z} - \frac{\partial V_z}{\partial x}, \ \frac{\partial V_y}{\partial x} - \frac{\partial V_x}{\partial y} \right) \tag{18}$$

one can combine the three differential equations to

$$\frac{\partial \omega}{\partial t} + \underline{V} \text{ grad } \underline{\omega} = \underline{\omega} \text{ grad } \underline{V} + \eta \Delta \underline{\omega}. \tag{19}$$

Now we assume a stationary, frictionless plane flow field and hence (18) is reduced to

$$\underline{V} \text{ grad } \underline{\omega} = 0 \rightarrow \underline{V} \text{ grad rot } \underline{V} = 0. \tag{20}$$

So the constraint (9) reads

$$C_w(\underline{V}) = \underline{V} \text{ grad rot } \underline{V} = 0. \tag{21}$$

In order to evaluate this constraint, derivatives of second order are necessary, hence the smallest mask is a 3x3 mask, resulting in an optimization problem of 19 variables. This number can be reduced considering (13). It follows

$$\frac{\partial V_x}{\partial x} = -\frac{\partial V_y}{\partial y} \qquad \begin{aligned} \frac{\partial}{\partial y} \rightarrow \frac{\partial^2 V_x}{\partial x \, \partial y} &= -\frac{\partial^2 V_y}{\partial y^2} \\[2mm] \frac{\partial}{\partial x} \rightarrow \frac{\partial^2 V_x}{\partial x^2} &= -\frac{\partial^2 V_y}{\partial y \, \partial x} . \end{aligned} \tag{22}$$

If (22) is applied to (21) only ten variables remain in a mask consisting of five pixels. Finally (10) becomes

$$\sum_i^5 \left[\left[V_{xi}^{k+1} - V_{xi}^k \right]^2 + \left[V_{yi}^{k+1} - V_{yi}^k \right]^2 \right] + w \cdot \underline{V}^{k+1} \text{ grad rot } \underline{V}^{k+1} \rightarrow \text{Min} . \tag{23}$$

For this problem the operator P_w is evaluated analytically. This mask is moved over the entire image till all points of the grid comply with (21).

4.3 CONSERVATION OF ENERGY

A stationary flow field of an incompressible, frictionfree medium is fully determined by the conservation of mass and of momentum. Thus, the energy constraint can not supply further information to the problem. Nevertheless, the possibility of evaluating this constraint should be briefly discussed. With the previous simplifications, and assuming additionally an adiabatic isobaric flow, the conservation of energy is formulated as

$$\underline{V} \text{ grad } \frac{||\underline{V}||^2}{2} = 0. \tag{24}$$

The energy constraint is reduced to the conservation of the kinetic energy and presents a kinematic relation. The problem is highly nonlinear and a simplification similar to the momentum conservation is not possible. Attempts of leading the elements of the smallest 3x3 mask to the minimum of (10) by a numerical optimization method succeeded but proved to be very time consuming. The image quality of the other operators could not be achieved. Thus, in the following presentation of simulation results only the first two operators P_D and P_W are taken into consideration.

5. SIMULATIONS

In this section the performance of the proposed method is demonstrated by a simple flow field. As a test-function the velocity field of the centric Oseen vortex is chosen which represents an exact solution of the Navier-Stokes differential equations

$$\underline{V}(r,\varphi) = \begin{bmatrix} V_x(r,\varphi) \\ V_y(r,\varphi) \end{bmatrix} = \frac{\Gamma_\infty}{2\pi r} \left[1 - \exp\left[-\left(\frac{r}{C}\right)^2 \right] \right] \begin{bmatrix} \sin\varphi \\ -\cos\varphi \end{bmatrix} \tag{25}$$

$\Gamma_\infty \triangleq$ total circulation

$C \triangleq$ parameter of the distribution of the circulation.

To simulate the condition of adhesion at the wall of pipe $(\underline{V}(R,\varphi)=0)$, a second velocity field is superposed, which is restricted to a thin layer close to the wall. The resulting flow field is presented in Fig. 5. Here and in all following figures the magnitude of the plotted vectors are normalized. The image is discretized on a 36x36 grid. The field is numerically projected with $P=3$ views ($\theta_1 = 0°$, $\theta_2 = 60°$, $\theta_3 = 120°$) and $N=36$ rays per view. Such a small number of views means a severe limitation of data.

The results of the following simulations will be discussed:

S1 : $\underline{V}^{k+1} = P_{VART} \underline{V}^k$, $\lambda_{VART} = 1.0$

S2 : $\underline{V}^{k+1} = P_D P_{VART} \underline{V}^k$, $\lambda_{VART} = 1.0, \lambda_D = 1.5$

S3 : $\underline{V}^{k+1} = P_W P_{VART} \underline{V}^k$, $\lambda_{VART} = 1.0, \lambda_W = 1.0$

S4 : $\underline{V}^{k+1} = P_W P_D P_{VART} \underline{V}^k$, $\lambda_{VART} = 1.0, \lambda_D = 1.5, \lambda_W = 1.0$

For the entire iterative procedure $I = 20$ iterations are chosen, except for S4, here the number of iterations is $I = 40$. For the movement of the masks of the operators P_D and P_W $I = 30$ iterations are chosen, respectively. The simulation S3 of the operator P_W is individually given, although it was derived in connection with condition (13) in order to demonstrate the performance of the operator, even condition (13) is not exactly fulfilled.

The error criterium is defined as

$$E = \frac{||\underline{V}_{true} - \underline{V}_{Rec}||}{||\underline{V}_{true}||} \cdot 100 \ \% \ . \tag{26}$$

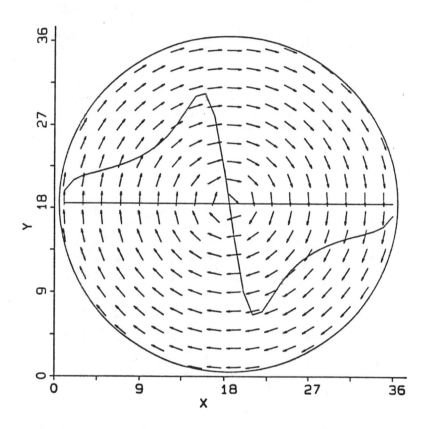

Fig. 5: True velocity field $\underline{V}$.

In Tab. 1 the error E is evaluated for the different simulations:

	S1	S2	S3	S4
E	42,1 %	35,2 %	37,8 %	4,1 %

Tab. 1: Error criterium of S1 → S4.

Considering the error without any restoration (S1) a comparison of the errors shows that by the operators P_D (S2) and P_w (S3) an improvement is already achieved. But the connection of these two operators (S4) leads to a dramatic improvement. This becomes obvious comparing Fig. 6 and Fig. 7. Fig. 6 points out the velocity field of S2 and Fig. 7 the result of S4. In Fig. 6 the vector field is disturbed by strong artefacts of the magnitude and orientation. These artefacts almost completely vanished by the restoration (Fig. 7). Fig. 8 compares a slice through the 15th row of the magnitude $||\underline{V}||$ of the true flow field with S1 and S4, respectively.

No numerical instabilities could be observed in any simulation. This is due to the fact that POCS is ideally complementing VART, as stated above. The very good performance of the combination of P_D and P_W can be explained by the fact that the flow field considered here is fully determined by the mass and conservation laws. The measured data serve as a kind of boundary values. Therefore, this method will yield similar results even for more complicated flow fields.

Although the programs used were not optimized, the calculations were made within a reasonable computation time because very small masks were used. Since the problem lends itself to be vectorized the computation time can be limited even for much finer discretizations.

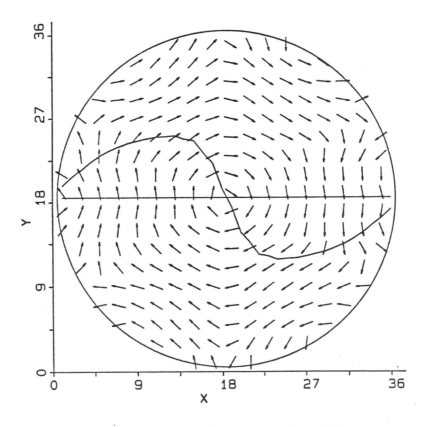

Fig. 6: Velocity field without restoration (S1).

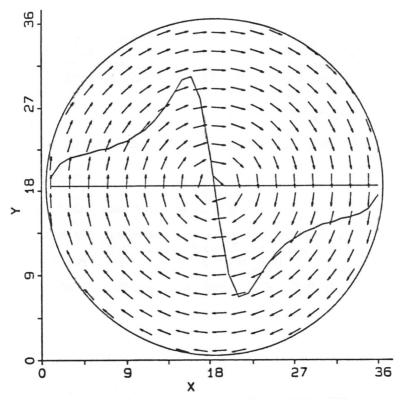

Fig. 7: Velocity field restored by P_D and P_W (S4).

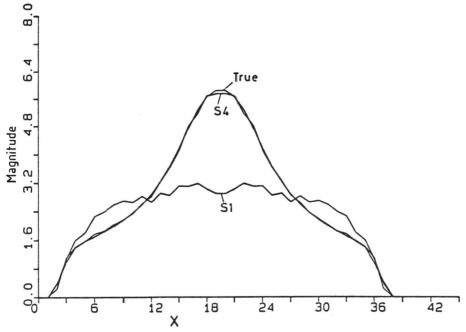

Fig. 8: Slice through the magnitude $||\underline{V}||$.

6. CONCLUSIONS

In this paper a very efficient method of reconstruction of a two-dimensional velocity field is proposed which incorporates the laws of mass and momentum conservation of fluidmechanics as a-priori knowledge by an iterative reconstruction/ restoration procedure. This yields very good results even if the available data are limited.

ACKNOWLEDGEMENT

This work is financially supported by the Deutsche Forschungsgemeinschaft (DFG), Bonn.

REFERENCES

Hauck A 1990, *Tomographie von Vektorfeldern*, VDI-Forschrittsberichte, Reihe 8, No. 220 (Düsseldorf: VDI)
Herman G T 1980, *Image Reconstruction from projections - the Fundamentals of Computerized Tomography* (New York: Academic Press)
Simard P Y, Mailoux G E 1988, *IEEE Trans. on Pattern Analysis and Machine Intelligence*, 10, No. 2, pp. 248
Youla D C, Webb H 1982, *IEEE Trans. on Medical Imaging*, MI-1, No. 2, pp. 81

Quantitative algorithm and computer architecture for real-time image reconstruction in process tomography

M. Zaid Abdullah, Stuart V. Quick, and Fraser J. Dickin

Process Tomography Unit, UMIST,
Department of Electrical Engineering & Electronics,
P.O. Box 88, Manchester. M60 1QD.

Abstract

A finite element based quantitative image reconstruction algorithm, employing a modified Newton-Raphson (MNR) technique to rapidly iterate to a final acceptable solution, is described. The algorithm was fed data from a flexible data collection system when connected to: a) a saline-filled laboratory phantom containing objects of known size, conductivity and location; and b) a simulated cyclonic separator instrumented with sixteen non-invasive electrodes conveying saline. Reconstructed images from both experiments produced by the algorithm will be discussed. Consideration is also given to the most computationally intensive aspects of the MNR algorithm, namely the inversion of large matrices. A parallel multi-processor computer architecture, dedicated to the task of optimising such operations, will be outlined.

1. Introduction

There is a strategic requirement to procure quantitative information from electrical impedance tomography (EIT) image reconstruction algorithms in order to update existing details used, for example, by computational fluid dynamics models. One approach to this requirement has been to use an iterative image reconstruction algorithm based on the modified Newton-Raphson (MNR) or Gauss-Newton matrix minimisation technique to solve the inverse problem (i.e. determining internal conductivity distributions from boundary voltage measurements). The electrode voltages induced by the application of electric currents are a highly non-linear function of the conductivity distribution. Consequently, due to the ill-posedness of the inverse problem, errors in the measured voltages on the boundary electrodes are translated into large errors in the calculated conductivity distribution. Also, errors in the predicted electrode voltages from the forward finite element-based model are converted into erroneous conductivity distribution updates which corrupt the reconstructed images. It is therefore imperative that measurements made by the data acquisition system (DAS) via electrodes attached to the vessel are accurate. Details of the DAS are given elsewhere (Wang *et al* 1992). Section 2 will address the mathematical aspects associated with the reconstruction algorithm and will describe the approaches taken to alleviate some of its shortcomings when applied to EIT problems. Results from the MNR algorithm for two case studies are given in Section 3.

The complexity of the MNR algorithm is manifest in the time taken to reconstruct an image. For a finite element mesh composed of 104 triangular elements, (see Figure 1) where each element represents one of the independent measurements from a vessel fitted with 16 electrodes utilising the 4-electrode measurement method, 7.1 million floating point operations are necessary in order to perform a single iteration of the algorithm. On average, a minimum of four iterations are required to reduce an error constraint below a predefined value. A single iteration consumes almost one hour of CPU time on a 16 MHz i386sx-based PC precluding its use for on-line real-time visualisation. The authors have implemented their MNR algorithm, written in the 'C' language, on a vector co-processor board based on an Intel i860 RISC processor with a clock speed of 25 MHz and have been able to attain one iteration approximately every four seconds. However, biomedical researchers, who have implemented a mesh with over 400 elements modelling a 32-electrode system, have indicated that the reconstruction time is exponentially proportional to the number of elements. The RPI group reported their 496-element iterative algorithm as consuming 6 minutes of IBM3090 CPU time and over 30 seconds of Cray X/MP 4 CPU time (Goble & Gallagher 1988). With the envisaged future demand for higher spatial resolutions, requiring more electrodes and consequently bigger finite element meshes, there is a need for a computer architecture optimised to perform the time consuming parts of the reconstruction algorithm. Section 4 assesses the structure of the MNR algorithm by profiling the whole program to determine the amount of CPU time spent in each subroutine. A list of requirements to enable real-time, i.e. a minimum of 10 frames per second, image reconstruction is given and subsequently, one parallel computer architecture which is most suited to this task is described.

The mathematical notation adopted in the following analysis employs a bold lower case letter to represent a vector and an uppercase bold letter for a matrix. The symbol ^{T} is used to denote mátrix transposition and $^{-1}$ to denote matrix inversion.

2. Qualitative image reconstruction algorithm

The image reconstruction algorithm can be separated into two distinct stages. Firstly, for a given distribution of element conductivities and injected boundary currents, the *forward* problem is solved using the finite element method (FEM) to yield a set of boundary voltages. The second stage is the solution of the *inverse* problem using the MNR algorithm, whereby the distribution of unknown element conductivities is determined from a measured set of boundary voltages and known injected currents. The following subsections describe both stages.

2.1 The forward problem

The model of a source free conducting inhomogeneous body Γ, with conductivity distribution σ, into which steady-state current is injected and the corresponding voltage V is measured, is governed by the following generalised Maxwell equation (Weber 1950):

$$\nabla \cdot \{\sigma \, \nabla V(x,y)\} = 0 \qquad \text{in } \Gamma \qquad (1)$$

Equation (1) is a second order partial differential in V which, for inhomogeneous current distributions, can only be solved numerically. For a unique solution to exist, sufficient boundary conditions must be specified. These conditions can be in the form of boundary potentials - Dirichlet conditions, or current densities crossing the boundary - Neumann conditions, or a mixture of both. Also, for a unique solution to exist, at least one potential must be specified in the model as a reference (eqn. (2)). For laboratory studies on Perspex vessels no current crosses the boundary between the electrodes (eqn (3)). The term I in equation (3) describes the applied current over the electrodes surface and n denotes the outward unit normal to vessel.

$$V = 0 \quad \text{at reference point} \qquad (2)$$

$$\int \sigma \frac{\delta V}{\delta n} = +I \quad \text{on source (input) electrode} \qquad (3a)$$

$$\int \sigma \frac{\delta V}{\delta n} = -I \quad \text{on sink (output) electrode} \qquad (3b)$$

By employing the FEM, for which many libraries of software subroutines exist, equation (1) is reduced to a set of simultaneous equations describing the behaviour of each of the 104 elements in Figure 1. The number of equations is proportional to the number of nodes in the mesh. In Figure 1 there are 69 nodes and these are assembled to form a stiffness matrix Y which has 69 x 69 entries. The 69 unknown nodal potentials form a vector v and the Neumann boundary (current) conditions are also formed into a vector c. Thus, the forward problem is to determine the components of v given those of c and Y as described by equation (4), whereas the inverse problem is to find σ given c and a limited v.

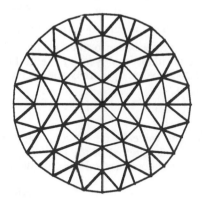

Figure 1 Layout of the 104-element, 69-node mesh used to reconstruct quantitative images using the adjacent electrode pairs data collection method

Forward problem $\qquad\qquad v = Y^{-1} c \qquad\qquad\qquad\qquad$ (4)

The positive definiteness of Y is guaranteed by the conservation of energy theorem. Matrix Y is also sparse, symmetrical and doubled centred, characteristics which enable its inversion to be computed using a Cholesky decomposition algorithm. Hence, the inverse of Y can be represented by the following relation:

$$Y^{-1} = (L^{-1})^T (L^{-1})\qquad\qquad (5)$$

where L represents the real-valued lower triangular matrix of Y.

Once the system of equations describing the mesh elements is factorised in the form of equation (5), they can be solved using the forward and back-substitution methods. Using equation (5), Y^{-1} need only be formed once and then repeatedly multiplied by c for every permutation of current injection known as a *projection* (p) to yield different v's. For a 16-electrode EIT system, utilising the simplest data collection which measures voltage between adjacent electrodes having injected current at two different adjacent electrodes in a 4-electrode configuration, 14 projections are performed. Hence, 14 sets of v are determined and these can be rearranged into a 14 x 69-long vector v' given by:

$$v' = (v_1^T, v_2^T, v_2^T, ..., v_{14}^T)^T\qquad\qquad (6)$$

Equation (6) yields the nodal potential for each of the 69 nodes with respect to the reference node (at the centre of the mesh). However, for the inverse problem, only the voltages at the nodes corresponding to boundary electrodes can be utilised. Thus, a transformation matrix T, the columns of which contain only two non-zero entries (± 1) corresponding to the nodes of interest, is used to extract the 104 independent voltages (stored in a column vector f) from v':

$$f = T v'\qquad\qquad (7)$$

2.2 The inverse problem

As mentioned at the start of this section, the inverse problem attempts to determine the conductivity (or resistivity (ρ), which is simply its inverse) distribution from a finite number of boundary voltage measurements and current boundary conditions. Yorkey (1987) first described the use of a modified form of the well known Newton-Raphson mathematical technique for reconstructing EIT images. In essence, the modified Newton-Raphson algorithm iterates to a final solution by updating an initial (guessed) resistivity distribution in response to an error (φ), formed by comparing the results from the forward problem to the measured values. If φ, defined as half the sum squared difference between the calculated and measured voltages, is less than a prescribed error limit (ε) the resultant resistivity distribution is deemed acceptable. The algorithm employed by the authors to update the resistivity distribution is identical to the one devised by Yorkey and is given by :

$$\Delta \rho_i = - \left\{ [\, f\,'(\rho)^T \, f\,'(\rho)\,]^{-1} \, [\, f\,'(\rho)\,]^T \, [\, f(\rho) - v_m\,] \right\} \qquad (8)$$

where $\Delta \rho_i$ is the resistivity update value for the ith iteration, $f\,'(\rho)$, referred to as a Jacobian matrix, represents the sensitivity directional of the forward solution for a given resistivity distribution, and v_m is the measured boundary voltages for all projections.

The derivative of the forward function f to form $f\,'$ was performed and assembled using a standard differentiation technique (Yorkey 1987). The product of the transposed Jacobian by itself, the first expression on the right hand side of equation (8), forms a Hessian matrix, which exhibits an ill-conditioned characteristic making its inverse both difficult to calculate and sensitive to measurement errors. Ill-conditioning arises from the non-linear behaviour of the resistivity distribution with respect to the measured boundary voltages, since resistivity changes in elements situated at the centre of the model produce an almost insignificant change in boundary voltage. Furthermore, the positive definiteness of the Hessian matrix suffers due to numerical rounding errors and also if the initial 'guess' of ρ is too far from the actual distribution. In such instances, the algorithm will begin to diverge and results in negative values of resistivity. One approach to improve the Hessian conditioning is to employ the Marquardt method (Marquardt 1963), in which a normalised Hessian matrix (denoted by *) is treated with a smoothing operation to guarantee its positive definiteness and therefore the existence of its inverse. The normalisation procedure is performed by multiplying all of the Hessian's row elements and then all of its column elements by $1/\sqrt{h_{ii}}$ which leaves all of the diagonal elements equal to 1. The smoothing operation performed on the normalised matrix by adding all of the diagonal elements (h_{ii}) to a smoothing factor λ_i. Thus $\Delta \rho_i$ in equation (8) now becomes,

$$\Delta \rho_i = - \left\{ [\, (\, f\,'(\rho)^T \, f\,'(\rho)\,)^* + \lambda_i I\,]^{-1} \, ([\, f\,'(\rho)\,]^T \, [\, f(\rho) - v_m\,])^* \right\} \qquad (9)$$

where I is the identity matrix.

For noise-free simulation studies, normalisation improves the accuracy of the reconstructed resistivity distribution. However, data acquired from the DAS includes noise which further introduces errors into the reconstruction to an extent where ρ cannot be faithfully reconstructed (Abdullah 1992a).

Values of λ_i, exhibiting rapid convergence properties of the algorithm, were obtained empirically, its value being decreased by a single order of magnitude per iteration once the algorithm begins to converge. This order of magnitude decrease is necessary since the quadratic convergence property of the MNR becomes more pronounced as the distance between the estimated and actual resistivity distribution decreases. For the reconstructed images from the MNR algorithm shown in Section 3, the initial value of λ_i is normally 0.1. The overall strategy encompassed by the quantitative MNR reconstruction algorithm is summarised in the following flow-chart shown in Figure 2 below:

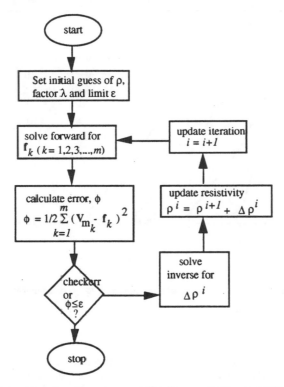

Figure 2 Flow-chart describing the modified Newton-Raphson (MNR) quantitative reconstruction algorithm employed for EIT image reconstruction.

3. Case study results

The MNR algorithm, as mentioned in Section 1, is coded in 'C' and run on an i860-based co-processor board with 8 Mbytes of linearly addressable RAM. The board, available commercially, was supplied with a Greenhills C compiler which operates in a Unix-like environment. The 25 MHz i860 has a theoretical peak performance of 25 million floating-point operations per second (MFLOPS) on double precision arithmetic. Unfortunately, due to the poor design of the board and its associated software development environment, (for example, the assembler cannot assemble the full i860 instruction set) a sustainable performance of just over 4 MFLOPS was achieved. This performance equates to one iteration taking 3.86 seconds on the i860 compared to over 52 minutes on a 'standard' 16 MHz i386sx-based PC. From data acquired using the UMIST Mk.1b DAS, 4 to 5 iterations are normally required to produce a final image. The initial value of resistivity fed into the MNR algorithm is that of the bulk resistivity (ρ_b) of the inhomogeneous material inside the vessel which, in almost all cases, is within ±40% of the final solution imperative for convergence. Hence, the convergence of the solution is governed only by the choice of λ_i. The relationship between the normalised reconstruction error, (φ^*), and the number of iterations taken for different values of λ_i, is given in Figure 3. For decreasing values of λ_i Figure 3 indicates that the descent towards the actual resistivity distribution ρ_a requires fewer iterations. However, if λ_i is decreased beyond a threshold limit (i.e. $\lambda_i \leq 10^{-6}$ in this situation), the algorithm fails to converge to ρ_a.

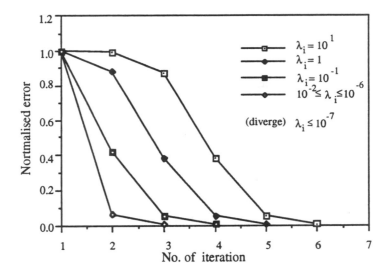

Figure 3 Variation in the normalised reconstruction error ϕ^* versus number of iterations for different values of λ_1.

3.1 Reconstruction accuracy study

To assess the accuracy of the reconstructed image a simulation study was performed using the FEM to model an object with a known resistivity. The model, shown in Figure 4a, depicts a circular object of 4.5 cm diameter and 400 Ω cm resistivity placed at the centre of a 9 cm diameter phantom. Objects placed at this location are known to be less easily detectable for the adjacent electrode pairs data collection method since any variation of resistivity in this region produces a minimal change in the measured potential difference on the periphery (Patel 1990). Figure 4b shows the reconstructed image with an initial guessed resistivity of 200 Ω cm corresponding to the background resistivity.

To enable quantitative characterisation of the reconstructed image, the average and maximum percentage error was calculated using mathematical formulae similar to the ones proposed by Dines and Lytle (1981). For the reconstructed image shown in Figure 4b, the average percentage error between the reconstructed and actual resistivity of the object is less than 1% as expected and the maximum error is around 5%. Also, it is apparent that, due to numerical computation errors, the resistivity of some pixels is caused to 'oscillate'. The oscillation error varies from 2 to 6% for the object while, for pixels not associated with the object, the error is less than 1%.

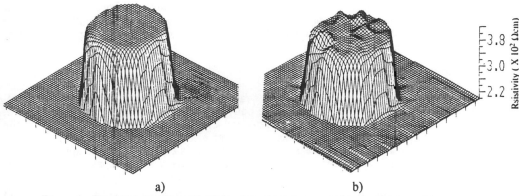

Figure 4   Simulated object from the finite element mesh representing the phantom a) true
image and, b) reconstructed image.

In order to validate these results experimentally, a 4.8 cm diameter object was made from
solidified non-nutrient agar and saline to a resistivity of 200 Ω cm and placed into the 9 cm
phantom. The phantom was fitted with 16 equi-spaced point-sized silver palladium electrodes
filled with saline of 400 Ω cm resistivity.

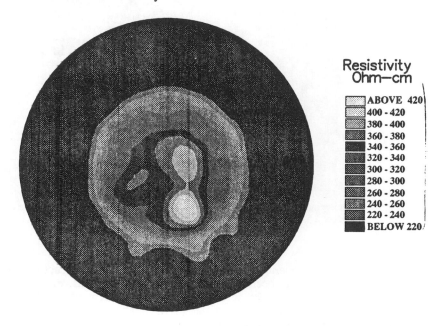

Figure 5   Two dimensional reconstruction from the MNR algorithm for a 4.8 cm diameter
200 Ω cm agar disc placed at the centre of a 9 cm diameter 400 Ω cm saline-
filled phantom

From Figure 5 it can be seen that, if the contrast between the object resistivity and the
background resistivity is maintained at a ratio of 2:1 or lower, the object's resistivity can be
determined. However, for larger contrast ratios such as 100:1, the instabilities caused by the
propagation of numerical errors throughout the iterative procedure will saturate into the
pixels representing the object and affect their resistivity. For very large contrast ratios,
produced when both highly conducting (e.g. aluminium) and highly insulating (e.g. Perspex)

materials are inserted into the vessel, the iterative reconstruction algorithm is terminated after 4 to 5 iterations in order to avoid over-contaminating the image pixels with cumulative numerical artefacts. A practical example of an extreme contrast ratio occurring in the process industry is described in the following subsection.

3.2 Cyclonic separator study

A 4.4 cm diameter Mozeley hydrocyclone was instrumented with 16 rectangular nickel-plated brass electrodes in the top-half of the body, as shown in the photograph in Figure 6. The motivation for using relatively large-sized electrodes covering over 90% of the circumference of the cross-section of interest is given elsewhere (Abdullah 1992b). It is suffice to say that the sensitivity of the measurement electrodes is enhanced by this approach for a small diameter vessel. An extreme range of practical resistivities encompassing both the air core and a conducting slurry was simulated by placing an insulating Perspex rod and a conducting aluminium rod both of 6 mm diameter into the hydrocyclone filled with a 525 Ω cm resistivity saline solution. The reconstructed image shown in Figure 7 shows the location of both rods near the periphery of the hydrocyclone. The authors hope to be able to acquire future images from the same separator when inserted into a test rig and fed with a controllable experimental slurry.

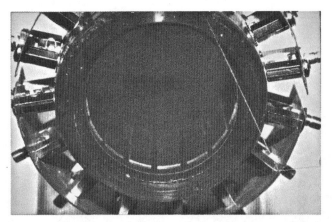

Figure 6   Photograph showing the location of 16 plate electrodes fabricated into the top-part of a 5 cm diameter Mozeley hydrocyclone separator.

3.3 Summary

The MNR algorithm has been successfully implemented to reconstruct two-dimensional quantitative resistivity profiles occurring inside experimental process vessels. The resolution of the images are relatively low due to the small number of elements used to discretise the vessel. The number of elements is proportional to the number of independent measurements M acquired from the n electrodes governed by the following equation:

$$M = \frac{n(n-3)}{2} \tag{10}$$

Therefore, to improve spatial resolution of the image, it is necessary to increase the number of electrodes. However, increasing the number of electrodes not only extends the time taken to acquire the data but also deleteriously affects the image reconstruction time as highlighted in Section 1. The authors' feel that a relatively low-cost dedicated parallel array processor could be employed to perform the most time consuming parts of the reconstruction algorithm thus obviating the need for a trade-off between the image reconstruction time and number of electrodes. This proposal is examined in the following section.

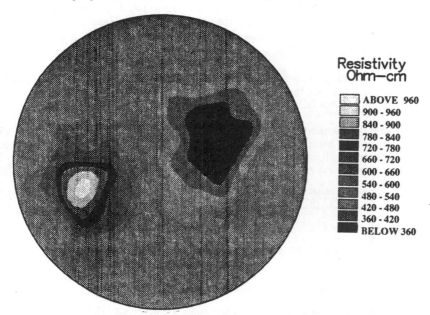

Figure 7 Two dimensional reconstruction from hydrocyclone shown in Figure 6 with both a Perspex rod and an aluminium rod of 6 mm diameter used to simulate an extreme range of practical resistivities.

4. The need for a dedicated image reconstruction computer architecture

As stated in Section 3 above, the quantitative image reconstruction algorithm is computationally demanding. The computational burden on the processor is expected to increase almost exponentially as the number of electrodes and hence the number of mesh elements increases due to the need for higher spatial resolution. The main factors affecting the performance of the present optimised MNR algorithm, which utilises sparse matrix techniques, have been examined by the authors who feel that a dedicated parallel architecture can be harnessed to perform the large matrix operations in real-time. The remainder of this section describes the structure of the time consuming subroutines within the MNR algorithm and outlines one possible approach for performing these routines on a dedicated parallel computer architecture.

4.1 Profile of the MNR algorithm

Using standard software profiling tools to examine the amount of CPU time spent performing each function within the MNR program the following simplified table (Table 1) was compiled:

Time (%)	No. of calls	Function
43.6	8	Y_inverse
27.0	4	Hessian
19.6	4	Jacobian
7.0	8	Cholesky
2.8	-	Other functions

Table 1 Profile of percentage CPU time consumed by functions within MNR algorithm for a complete image reconstruction taking 4 iterations.

Each of the functions correspond to:

Y_inverse : LU decomposition of **Y** matrix to form its inverse for the forward problem (eqn. (5)) *and* the inverse of the **Y** matrix for the inverse problem (eqn. (9)).

Hessian   : the transpose of the Jacobian and the calculation of the Hessian (eqn. (9)).

Jacobian   : the calculation of the derivative $f'(\rho)$.

Cholesky : the Cholesky decomposition of the **Y** matrix.

The majority of the 'other' functions incorporate sparse matrix techniques which, in comparison to the previous four functions, have a minor cumulative effect on the algorithm's performance and thus will not be considered further.

In order to highlight the number of matrix multiplication operations performed by the CPU a further function called 'Matrix_Multiply' was included by incorporating the matrix multiplication routines performed in both the 'Y_inverse' and 'Hessian' functions. The results from performing a new profile on the same data are shown in Table 2 below:

Time (%)	No. of calls	Function
54.6	12	Matrix_Multiply
19.6	4	Jacobian
8.8	4	Hessian
7.2	8	Y_inverse
7.0	8	Cholesky
2.8	-	Other functions

Table 2   New profile of percentage CPU time consumed by functions - highlighting the amount of time spent performing matrix multiplication's.

Since the matrix multiplication function is a superset of all floating-point calculations within the MNR algorithm, any improvement made to this routine will result in an improved performance in all other dependent functions.

The number of floating-point arithmetic operations F for a single matrix multiplication of order N is given by:

$$F = [N + (N-1)]*N^2 \qquad (11)$$

For N = 104, $F \approx 2.24 \times 10^6$ floating-point operations. This value is reduced in practice by employing sparse matrix procedures to avoid performing multiplications on matrix elements containing zeros. If the number of electrodes is doubled from 16 to 32 the corresponding value of N is more than quadrupled to 464. For N = 464, $F \approx 200 \times 10^6$ which , even allowing for sparse matrix techniques, would require several tens of minutes of CPU time on the present i860 system.

Another important factor affecting the performance of the reconstruction algorithm is the amount of information, i.e. data, passed between the floating-point memory and the processing unit. A large volume of 'traffic' data necessitates a wide memory bandwidth into and out of the floating-point memory. As a 'worst case' example, consider the following calculations to determine the memory bandwidth; assuming that 32-bit single precision floating-point numbers are utilised, the loading and storage requirements for each of the multiply and addition variables is 3 words (12 bytes) and N = 104. The total amount of data transferred during a single matrix multiplication is;

$$[3N + 3(N-1)]*N^2 = [312 + 309] \times 104^2 = 6,716,736 \text{ words} = 26.87 \text{ Mbytes}$$

Thus, if the algorithm is to be performed in real-time, say at a minimum of 10 images per second, the required CPU performance and the input/output (I/O) transfer rate can be extrapolated from the details above:

Required CPU performance = $10 \times 12 \times 2.24 \times 10^6$ = 268.8 MFLOPS

Required floating-point memory bandwidth = $10 \times 12 \times 17.9$ Mbytes = 2150 Mbytes per second.

The above calculations are somewhat simplified since they do not include statistics for the core instructions needed to implement the entire functions. It should also be noted that this figure can be reduced by utilising a large register set within the processor. However, as a first estimate based solely on floating-point performance figures, they yield a good indication of the required CPU performance and associated bus bandwidth to facilitate real-time image reconstruction.

4.2 Determination of parallel processor architecture

In order to ensure that the MNR algorithm can be performed by a computer architecture in real-time a number of key issues must be satisfied which include the following:

a) The aggregate floating-point performance must match or better the theoretical floating-point throughput. For a given matrix manipulation routine, vector processors will be necessary which are optimised to performing sum-of-products operations by employing cascaded floating-point and addition units.

b) The I/O memory bandwidth must match or better the theoretical memory bandwidth. This requirement encompasses both floating-point and instruction traffic. Floating-point numbers must be loaded into the processor quickly since, in the case of high level language arrays, memory index calculations can be time consuming.

c) Matrix calculations in the MNR algorithm are usually performed on globally accessible data since all previously calculated information must be available in order to proceed with the next stage of processing.

The above issues severely constrain the number of computer architectures that can be used to achieve the required image reconstruction rate. In particular, to attain the above level of floating-point performance, i.e. more than 268 MFLOPS, it is necessary to utilise multiple vector processors. One such suitable architecture is the wavefront array processor which is described briefly in the next subsection.

4.3 Wavefront array processors - structure and projected performance

Wavefront array processors represent an optimal solution for performing matrix calculations quickly due mainly to their use of multiple processing elements (PEs) each capable of fast floating-point operations. For such applications, the architecture of a wavefront processor (see Figure 8) is that of a square array of PEs. Each PE typically consists of the following: memory - usually a small amount (a few kbytes) of fast-access (ns) RAM; a control unit; and a fast floating-point arithmetic logic unit. A full description of the function of this architecture is beyond the intended scope of the paper. The interested reader is referred to Hwang (1985).

For a simple N^{th} order matrix multiplication, the minimum number of clock cycles necessary to perform a complete matrix calculation is $2N - 1$. Once the calculation is completed, a further N clock cycles are required to remove all the data from the array. Thus, the minimum total time T for a full solution to be made available from the array is given by,

$$T = T_t N + (C_t + T_t)(2N - 1) \tag{12}$$

where: T_t is the time taken to transport an operand from a PE to its nearest neighbour PE via a link; C_t is the vector calculation time within each node i.e. the time taken by the PE to perform a single sum-product operation.

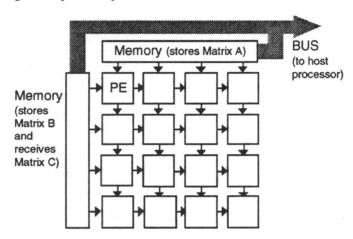

Figure 8 Generalised diagram of a wavefront array computer architecture for 16 processing elements (PEs).

Equation (12) assumes that one PE is assigned to every element in the matrix. For the types of matrix described in Section 2.2 above, relatively large numbers of PEs would be required. For example, for a 104 x 104 array, exactly 10,816 PEs would be needed, which, solely from a financial standpoint, is unacceptable. To overcome this problem, a matrix partitioning technique is employed whereby every PE is responsible for several matrix entries which are in-turn a square subset of the full matrix. In implementing this modification, the PE must pass a group of values, as opposed previously to a single value, to its neighbour. Equation (12) must be modified to reflect the additional data transfers:

$$T = \left[\frac{N}{n}\right] T_t N + \left(\left[\frac{N}{n}\right]^2 C_t + \left[\frac{N}{n}\right] T_t\right)(2N - 1) \tag{13}$$

where: n is the number of processing elements.

A simple simulation was performed, using data taken from manufacturers data sheets, on two popular microprocessors in order to determine the what effect increasing the number of PEs has on the overall performance. The microprocessors chosen were: a) a 25 MHz Intel i860XR costing £178 and; b) a 25 MHz INMOS T805 transputer costing £236. The times in ns for the variables T_t and C_t were extrapolated from manufacturers data: for the i860 $T_t = 300$ and $C_t = 300$; for the T805 $T_t = 4000$ and $C_t = 3000$. The main difference between the microprocessors in the simulation was that the i860 has 32-bit parallel links whereas the T805 has 10 Mbit/s serial links. Table 3 below shows the results for 16 and 64 PEs, *i.e.* n = 4 and 8 for both microprocessors from a simulation for N = 104.

Microprocessor	n^2	T (ms)
i860	16	1.5
	64	0.8
T805	16	15
	64	8.8

Table 3 Results from simulated wavefront array processor for N = 104 on two popular microprocessors using manufacturers data.

It can be seen from Table 3 that, despite a four-fold increase in the number of PEs, there is no corresponding decrease in T. In the case of the i860 there is a 55% improvement whilst for the T805 an approximately 59% improvement. Also, it can be seen that the T805 array is approximately ten times slower than the i860. It is apparent that a 'trade-off' between I/O bandwidth, physical size and cost constraints must be achieved before implementing a wavefront array processor architecture. The following guidelines must therefore be adhered to:

a) The array must be kept physically small for several reasons which include: cooling, power requirements, portability, fault-finding, and manufacturing cost.

b) The PEs must be fast, especially in small, i.e. $n^2 = 16$, arrays, since they are required to perform correspondingly more operations due to the partitioning ratio N/n.

c) Transfer of operands must be performed quickly between PEs. This becomes an important consideration for smaller arrays whose links are more heavily loaded.

d) Certain parts of the algorithm such as the assembly of the master matrix cannot be performed efficiently on a wavefront array architecture and therefore have to be performed on a connected host processor. In order to achieve optimum data transfer between the host processor and the wavefront array, the array should be viewed as a set of content-addressable processors by the host.

4.4 Recommendations and future investigations

In order to avoid the protracted and expensive development costs outlined in Section 4.3 by designing and building 'suitable' wavefront array processors, the authors believe that a comprehensive generic parallel architecture simulator can be employed to eliminate inefficient designs. Existing commercial simulators do not, however, appear to enable parallel computer architecture designers to incorporate important processor-orientated criteria such as: instruction pipelines; memory traffic and bandwidth performance; and also cache coherency and cache hit rates. The results from the simulator, after testing a number of interesting configurations, will yield the most promising architecture meeting all of the requirements listed above as well as any financial and component availability restrictions.

5. Conclusion

A quantitative iterative image reconstruction algorithm based on a modified Newton-Raphson technique capable of producing complete images at a rate of one every 24 seconds, for a vessel fitted with 16-electrodes, has been described. The algorithm is susceptible to errors in the voltages measured on the periphery of the process vessel and is therefore dependent on being fed signals with optimal signal-to-noise ratios from the associated data acquisition system. The algorithm is CPU intensive and spends over 50% of its time performing matrix multiplication functions. A parallel computer architecture based on a wavefront array was analysed and found to be a good vehicle for improving the performance of the algorithm. The wavefront array processor is suited to high volumes of information transfer which the MNR algorithm was categorised as and not, as was commonly thought, solely a matter of processing information rapidly.

6. Acknowledgements

The work described in Sections 2 and 3 is supported by the European Coal and Steel Community and UMIST under agreement number 7220/EA/829. The authors also gratefully acknowledge the help of Mr. W.F. Conway in designing and constructing the EIT phantoms.

7. References

Abdullah, M.Z., Dickin, F.J., Zhao, X.J. and Waterfall, R.C., (1992a), "Use of the modified Newton-Raphson algorithm for quantification in electrical impedance tomography", Malaysian Journal of Physical Science, (in press).

Abdullah, M.Z., Conway, W.F., Dyakowski, T., and Waterfall, R.C., (1992b), "Investigation of electrode geometries for use in cyclonic separators", (in this volume).

Dines, K.A., and Lytle, R.J., (1981), "Analysis of electrical conductivity imaging", Geophysics, **46**, 7, pp. 1025-1036.

Goble, J.C., and Gallagher, T.D., (1988), "A distributed architecture for medical instrumentation: an electric current computed tomograph", Proc. Annu. Int. Conf. IEEE Engineering in Medicine and Biology Society, **10**, pp. 285-6.

Hwang, K., and Briggs, F.A., (1985), "Computer architecture and parallel processing", Chapter 10, McGraw-Hill, New York.

Marquardt, D.W., (1963), "An algorithm for least-sqaures estimation of non-linear parameters", SIAM J. Appl. Math., **11**, pp. 431-441.

Patel, A., (1990), "Data collection methods", Chapter 4, in "Electrical Impedance Tomography", ed. Webster, J.G., Adam-Hilger, Bristol.

Wang, M., Dickin, F.J., and Beck, M.S., "Improved electrical impedance tomography data collection system and measurement protocols", (in this volume).

Weber, E., (1950), "Electromagnetic fields - Theory and applications Volume 1: Mapping of fields", John Wiley & Sons, New York.

Yorkey, T.J., Webster, J.G., Tompkins, W.J., (1987), "Comparing reconstruction methods for electrical impedance tomography", IEEE Trans. Biomed. Eng., **BME-34**, pp. 843-852.

Algorithm for Tomography with Incomplete Data on Binary Objects

J. Landauro, P. Dugdale, *R.G. Green, A.J. Hartley and R.G. Jackson

School of Engineering, Bolton Institute of Higher Education, Bolton BL3 5AB, U.K.
*Department of Engineering I T, Sheffield City Polytechnic, Sheffield S1 1WB, U.K.

ABSTRACT: This paper discusses the development of reconstruction software written in Occam 2 for execution in a transputer system. The Bolton optical process tomography system imposes physical and cost constraints on the information available. To cope with this, a novel iterative algorithm has been developed that is capable of processing four projections and reconstructing a two phase flow image with approximately 80-90 per cent accuracy in less than two seconds. The algorithm processes only two values (0 and 1). A 16x16 grid image is used and it is assumed that the parallel beams cut the centre of each pixel in the image.

1. INTRODUCTION

The classic 2D reconstruction problem is essentially to reconstruct a cross section (ie $f(x,y)$) of a 3D object (ie $F(x,y,z)$) from its 1D projections (ie $g(s,\theta)$) or views. In order to obtain the views the object is acted upon by various probes, including x-rays, gamma rays, visible light, microwaves, electrons, protons, neutrons, heavy ions, sound waves, and by nuclear magnetic resonance (Herman [1980], Deans[1983]).

The reconstruction methods presently used are very well established in the scientific and industrial community (medical scanning and pattern and image reconstruction) and they may be classified in four categories: (1) Convolution back-projections, (2) Filtered back-projections, (3) Direct Fourier transform, and (4) Algebraic Reconstruction Techniques (ART). The advantages and disadvantages of the above methods can be found in detail elsewhere(Bates, Garden, and Peters [1983]). The mathematical foundation of Computerized Tomography is discussed by Natterer [1986].

Unfortunately, the above methods require that the number of projections be equal or greater than the numbers of pixels resulting from the discreteness of the image. For applications in two-phase fluid flow the opposite seems to be the norm. There are signal and mathematical constraints (Natterer [1986]) that strongly determine the quality of the image (ie resolution). Crewe and Crewe[1984] have shown that a very good approximation may be obtained for binary or Boolean objects using a stochastic reconstruction technique which utilizes a limited number of projections. According to this paper, the method takes a considerable amount of computing time by way of repeatedly calculating probability matrices to converge to an approximate image. Their method is fully based in a form of attenuation law (or mass balance).

Applications of Computerized Tomography for fluid flow pattern recognition including ultrasound and electrical impedance have been published. Electrical impedance tomography for two phase flow has been investigated by Huang, Plaskowski, Xie and Beck [1989] by using a capacitance sensor system assembled in situ. The apparatus was tested using static physical models to simulate the flow of a two-phase system. The results showed a limited resolution of the discrete constituent phases, because of a reduced number of capacitance electrodes and a simplified reconstruction algorithm. Capacitance imaging has also been studied by Halow, Fasching and Nicoletti [1990] for high speed non-intrusive maps of void fraction distribution within fluidized bed reactors. Furthermore, Weigand and Hoyle [1989] simulated a two-phase flow and by using ultrasound tomography determined a 2D image of the flow which forms the basis for the deduction of the void fraction.

In the present paper we will modify the ART method in such a way that it will process only binary variables (ie 1 and 0). The algorithm is still in essence Kaczmarz's method for solving iteratively a linear system of equations (Gordon [1974]). However, the set of resulting linear equations are constrained by some physical law that describes the absorption or attenuation of the incident beams when passing through the object. Furthermore, It is assumed that the beams cut the centre of each pixel. Crewe and Crewe [1984] have demonstrated by extensive computing tests that it is possible to approximate an image by using not less than four projections (ie 0°, 90°, 45°, and 135°) when the parallel beams cut the centre of each pixel in the image.

The novelty of this paper is the introduction of Kaczmarz's method to converge to the image instead of the cumbersome approach of Crewe and Crewe[1984].

2. FUNDAMENTALS

Kaczmarz's method is a variant of the SOR (Succesive Over-Relaxation) method of numerical analysis. The reconstruction problem is formulated as a general image restoration problem and is solved as a set of simultaneous linear equations [Gordon [1974]). By ART we mean the application of Kaczmarz's method to Radon's integral equation. Depending on how the discretization is carried out we come to different versions of ART.

Given a set of known projections for an image, Kaczmarz's method for image reconstruction may be stated as follows:

[1]   Start with an arbitrary initial image,
[2]   For the current θ, take the projection of the image and subtract it from the known projection to obtain an array of correction values,
[3]   Backtrace the correction values over the image, and
[4]   Increment θ, and go to step[2].

In this manner, one iterates around the image until convergence to the solution is reached.

Numerous papers on ART and its variants have been published since 1970. A development for the computing implementation of ART can be found in Kak[1984].

2.1   **The reconstruction problem as a set of linear equations.** Suppose f(x,y) is approximated by a finite series,

$$f(x,y) \approx \hat{f}(x,y) = \sum_{i=1}^{I} \sum_{j=1}^{J} a_{ij} \, \phi_{ij} \, (x,y) \tag{1}$$

where $\{\phi_{ij} \, (x,y)\}$ is a set of base functions. Then

$$g(s,\theta) \approx \Re \hat{f}(x,y) = \sum_{i=1}^{I} \sum_{j=1}^{J} a_{ij} \, [\Re \phi_{ij}] = \sum_{i=1}^{I} \sum_{j=1}^{J} a_{ij} \, h_{ij} \, [s,\theta] \tag{2}$$

Here, $h_{ij}(s,\theta)$ is the Radon transform of the ϕ_{ij} which can be computed in advance.

When the observations are available on a discrete grid (s_m, θ_n), we can write

$$g(s_m,\theta_n) \approx \sum_{i=1}^{I} \sum_{j=1}^{J} a_{ij} \, h_{ij} \, (s_m,\theta_n), \quad 0 \le m \le M-1, \; 0 \le n \le N_\theta -1 \tag{3}$$

which can be solved for a_{ij} as a set of linear simultaneous equations via least squares, generalized inverse, or other methods directly from Eq(1).

A particular case arises when f(x,y) is digitised, for example, an I x J grid and if f(x,y) is assumed to be constant in each pixel region, then $a_{ij} = f_{ij}$; where f_{ij} is a sample value of f(x,y) in the (i,j)th pixel, and

$$\phi_{ij}(x,y) = \begin{cases} 1 \text{ inside the } (i,j)\text{th pixel region} \\ \\ 0 \text{ otherwise} \end{cases}$$

Furthermore Eq (3) becomes

$$g(s_m, \theta_n) \approx \sum_{i=1}^{I} \sum_{j=1}^{J} f_{ij} h_{ij}(s_m, \theta_n), \quad 0 \le m \le M-1, \quad 0 \le n \le N_\theta - 1 \tag{4}$$

mapping f_{ij} into a $Q = (I \times J)$ vector f by row (or column) ordering, one gets

$$g = H f$$

where g is a $P = (M \times N_\theta)$ vector, and H is a $(P \times Q) = (M \times N_\theta) \times (I \times J)$ arrays (matrix) respectively. A more realistic observation equation is of the form

$$g = H f + \eta$$

where η represents noise. The reconstruction problem now is to estimate f from g.

The above approach has the advantage of being independent of the scanning modality (eg parallel beam versus fan beam). Also, the observation mode can easily incorporate a more realistic projection gathering model, which may not approximate well the Radon transform.

2.2   **Algebraic Reconstruction Technique (ART).**   A subset of iterative reconstruction algorithms have been historically called ART. These algorithms iteratively solve a set of P equations. Let's define

$$<h_p, f> = h_p^T f = g_p \qquad p = 0, 1, \dots, P-1$$

where h_p is the pth row of H (^{T} means transpose) and g_p is the corresponding element of g. The algorithm, originally due to Kaczmarz, has an iteration that progresses cyclically as

$$\bar{f}^{(k+1)} = f^{(k)} + \frac{g_{k+1} - <h_{k+1}, f^{(k)}>}{|h_{k+1}|^2} h_{k+1}, \quad k=0,1,\dots,$$

$$\tag{5}$$

where $\tilde{f}^{(k+1)}$ determine $f^{(k+1)}$, depending on the constraints imposed on f.

A numerical illustration of iterative reconstruction (ART) follows. We use a simple 2x2 grid of values and the associated measured projections (see Fig F1):

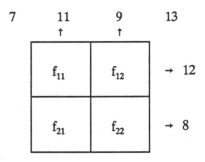

Fig. F1 Original object and six ray-sum

All six projection measurements, including the two verticals, two horizontal, and two diagonal, have been made. We assume these projection measurements are all that is available and, from these the matrix of elements shown must be reconstructed. We begin the process arbitrarily by setting all values to zero, calculating the resulting projections, and comparing them to the measured projections. The process is usually halted when the difference between the measured and calculated projections is acceptably small. Thus

$$H = \begin{bmatrix} 1 & 0 & 1 & 0 \\ 0 & 1 & 0 & 1 \\ 1 & 1 & 0 & 0 \\ 0 & 0 & 1 & 1 \\ 0 & 1 & 1 & 0 \\ 1 & 0 & 0 & 1 \end{bmatrix}$$

where

$f^T = [f_{11}, f_{12}, f_{21}, f_{22}], \; g^T = [11, 9, 12, 8, 13, 7]$
$P = 2x2 + 2x1 = 6$ (i.e. $M \times N_\theta$), $Q = 2x2 = 4$ (i.e. $I=2 \; J=2$)
$P \times Q = 6 \times 4$
$h_1 = [1010], h_2 = [0101]$ and so on,
$\|h_{k+1}\|^2 = 2$ for any k
$< h_{0+1}, f^{(0)} > = h_1^T . f^{(0)} = 0$ for $k = 0$, and $f^{(0)} = 0$.

The calculations following the following steps

$$\bar{f}^{(1)} = \begin{bmatrix} 0 \\ 0 \\ 0 \\ 0 \end{bmatrix} + \frac{11-0}{2} \begin{bmatrix} 1 \\ 0 \\ 1 \\ 0 \end{bmatrix} = \begin{bmatrix} 0 \\ 0 \\ 0 \\ 0 \end{bmatrix} + \begin{bmatrix} 5.5 \\ 0 \\ 5.5 \\ 0 \end{bmatrix} = \begin{bmatrix} 5.5 \\ 0 \\ 5.5 \\ 0 \end{bmatrix}$$

$$\bar{f}^{(2)} = \begin{bmatrix} 5.5 \\ 0 \\ 5.5 \\ 0 \end{bmatrix} + \frac{9-0}{2} \begin{bmatrix} 0 \\ 1 \\ 0 \\ 1 \end{bmatrix} = \begin{bmatrix} 5.5 \\ 0 \\ 5.5 \\ 0 \end{bmatrix} + \begin{bmatrix} 0 \\ 4.5 \\ 0 \\ 4.5 \end{bmatrix} = \begin{bmatrix} 5.5 \\ 4.5 \\ 5.5 \\ 4.5 \end{bmatrix}$$

$$\bar{f}^{(3)} = \begin{bmatrix} 5.5 \\ 4.5 \\ 5.5 \\ 4.5 \end{bmatrix} + \frac{12-10}{2} \begin{bmatrix} 1 \\ 1 \\ 0 \\ 0 \end{bmatrix} = \begin{bmatrix} 5.5 \\ 4.5 \\ 5.5 \\ 4.5 \end{bmatrix} + \begin{bmatrix} 1 \\ 1 \\ 0 \\ 0 \end{bmatrix} = \begin{bmatrix} 6.5 \\ 5.5 \\ 5.5 \\ 4.5 \end{bmatrix}$$

$$\bar{f}^{(4)} = \begin{bmatrix} 6.5 \\ 5.5 \\ 5.5 \\ 4.5 \end{bmatrix} + \frac{8-10}{2} \begin{bmatrix} 0 \\ 0 \\ 1 \\ 1 \end{bmatrix} = \begin{bmatrix} 6.5 \\ 5.5 \\ 5.5 \\ 3.5 \end{bmatrix} + \begin{bmatrix} 0 \\ 0 \\ -1 \\ -1 \end{bmatrix} = \begin{bmatrix} 6.5 \\ 5.5 \\ 4.5 \\ 3.5 \end{bmatrix}$$

$$\bar{f}^{(5)} = \begin{bmatrix} 6.5 \\ 5.5 \\ 4.5 \\ 3.5 \end{bmatrix} + \frac{13-10}{2} \begin{bmatrix} 0 \\ 1 \\ 1 \\ 0 \end{bmatrix} = \begin{bmatrix} 6.5 \\ 5.5 \\ 4.5 \\ 3.5 \end{bmatrix} + \begin{bmatrix} 0 \\ 1.5 \\ 1.5 \\ 0 \end{bmatrix} = \begin{bmatrix} 6.5 \\ 7.0 \\ 6.0 \\ 3.5 \end{bmatrix}$$

$$\bar{f}^{(6)} = \begin{bmatrix} 6.5 \\ 7.0 \\ 6.0 \\ 3.5 \end{bmatrix} + \frac{7-10}{2} \begin{bmatrix} 1 \\ 0 \\ 0 \\ 1 \end{bmatrix} = \begin{bmatrix} 6.5 \\ 7.0 \\ 6.0 \\ 3.5 \end{bmatrix} + \begin{bmatrix} -1.5 \\ 0 \\ 0 \\ -1.5 \end{bmatrix} = \begin{bmatrix} 5 \\ 7 \\ 6 \\ 2 \end{bmatrix}$$

and the answer is shown in Fig. F2

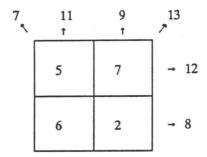

Fig. F2 Original object with pixel values

In this example, the reconstruction after one iteration is perfect.

3. ART FOR BINARY GREY LEVEL OBJECTS

The optical tomography approach -as a means to describe two-phase fluid flow in a pipe- is faced with some special problems. For example, reconstruction using x-ray tomography depends upon obtaining a large number of projections at precisely known angular intervals. Because of physical constraints in the experimental probe (which should be the case for any real-time industrial application) it is not possible to comply with the requirement of a large number of projections. Therefore, in this paper we are not concerned with finding a precise mathematical, solution, but instead we are looking for an approximate answer which will contain the principal features of a more exact solution.

In general, if we have a grid I^2 and if we use the method in this paper we require $(6I-2)$ projections points or equations. For example, for a grid $16\times16=256$ pixels (or variables) it is possible to obtain with four views 94 points values (or equations). According to the relation, $I^2-(6I-2)\leq0$, it is only possible to have an un-ambiguous solution if $I\leq5$. For values of $I>5$ the solution is ambiguous.

Because we are experimenting with water-air mixtures, we are not so much interested in variations or average of some physical parameters (eg density) as the presence or absence of water in the pipe. The fluid flow can be adequately described using binary coding, a one (1) indicating water and zero (0) indicating air. Therefore, our version of the reconstruction problem simplifies to that of recovering a Boolean image from its projections.

The basic step in the process is to consider a rectangular array of lattice points which have either a 1 or 0 at each location. Four projections are made, in orthogonal pairs at 45°. Using only the data in these four projections we then attempt to reconstruct a cross section of the water-air mixture. In a grid of 16 x 16 and having each beam passing through the pixel's centre we may have two extreme situations. Each pixel of the array could be 1 if the pipe is full of water (ie 256 1's), and each pixel of the array could be 0 if the pipe is full of air. For water-air mixtures the array will have a number of 1's and a number of 0's.

Another step is the mapping of the output digital byte of the intensity beams (ie 0-255) onto values with range 0-16, and simultaneously obey some implicit law (eg attenuation law). We have developed a look-up table that performs this mapping, and it was based on the assumption that the incident beams (eg IR) obeys approximately the attenuation model of x-ray. Thus,

$$I = I_0 \exp\left[-\int_L f(x,y)\, du\right] \tag{6}$$

where I_0 is the initial intensity of the incident beam, L is the path of the ray and u is the distance along L (see Fig. F3).

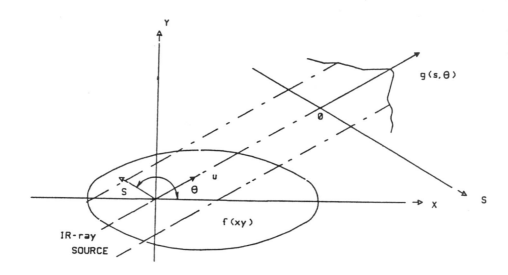

Fig. F3. Projection imaging geometry in CT scanning

By definition,

$$g = \ln\left(\frac{I_0}{I}\right) \tag{7}$$

and a linear transformation is obtained as

$$g = g(s,\theta) = \Re\; f(x,y) \equiv \int_L f(x,y)\; du \quad -\infty < s < \infty,\; 0 \le \theta \le \pi \tag{8}$$

where $g(s,\theta)$ represent the coordinates of the beam (ie IR) relative to the object, and $\Re$ is the Radon transform.

4. COMPUTATIONAL TRIALS FOR TEST MODEL

In order to test this approach, we choose to work with an array of zeros and ones that resembles a human face (see Fig F4). Arrays of various sizes that represent letters from the alphabet have been tried and the reconstruction has been very good indeed. This computing experiment merely serves to indicate that the program is producing reasonable results using four projection sums. The computer output of the human face in Fig F4 is shown in Fig F5.

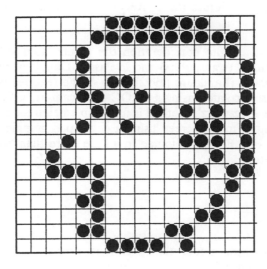

Fig F4. Human face for computational test

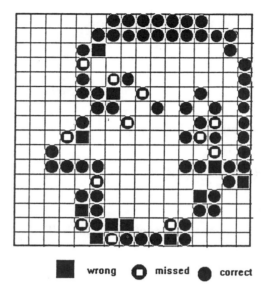

■ wrong   **◯** missed   **●** correct

Fig F5. Computer output of human face

The original pattern in Fig F4 is made of 74 points. The computer output shown in Fig F5 has 73 points, with 11 points wrongly located. For this example, the accuracy of the prediction is greater than 80 per cent. The error seems to depend upon the complexity of the pattern. For example letters from the alphabet can be reconstructed with one hundred per cent accuracy.

Furthermore, tests using different modes of projections have shown that some projection orderings accelerate the convergence of the image by using a smaller number of iterations.

An algorithm that takes into consideration the points discussed above has been developed in Occam 2 (transputers) and in Pascal. Datails of the algorithm itself can be found elsewhere (Landauro [1992]) One of the features of the algorithm is that the matrix H is calculated using a PROC in Occam or a Procedure in Pascal and it is called once. Kaczmarz's method is fully implemeted for image convergence. Final values are output to the screen using a developed graphic Occam program. The human face in Fig F5 was obtained in a little more than two seconds using a single T800 transputer.

5. DISCUSSION

There seems to be little doubt that this reconstruction method can produce reasonable results when using four projections or more. The algorithm is flexible enough to allow the use of realistic pixel values from experimental observation. The mapping look-up table can be adjusted to comply with experimental results.

Furthermore, the algorithm was tested using data from a file, but this is not a restriction for capturing information directly from the probe. Because the experimental probe has not been fully completed the algorithm has not been tested in real-time yet. However, preliminary tests have been done by using a simplified algorithm and two projections and the results are encouraging.

Nomenclature

f	image function (2D)
F	body function (3D)
g	Radon transform ($\Re$) of function f
N_θ	number of projections
M	number of samples in each projection
x	variable on the x-axis
y	variable on the y-axis
s	orthogonal distance from the x-y axis origin to beam
I	intensity of beam
θ	angle between y-axis and beam
u	distance along a beam
η	noise
< , >	dot product
$\| \ \|^2$	Euclidean length
H	matrix (ART)
h	row vector of H

Superscript

~	approximate
^	analytical function
T	transpose

Subscript

θ	angular displacement
p	row

6. REFERENCES

Bates R H T, K L Garden and T M Peters [1983]. *Overview of computerized tomography with emphasis on future developments*. Procc IEEE, 71(3):356-372.

Crewe A V, D A Crewe [1984]. *Inexact reconstruction from projections*. Ultramicroscopy, 12:293-298.

Dean S R [1983]. *The Radon Transform and some of its Applications*, Wiley, New York.

Gordon R [1974]. *A tutorial on ART*. IEEE Trans Nucl Sci, NS-21:78-93.

Halow J S, G E Fasching and Nicoletti [1990]. *Preliminary capacitance imaging experiments of a fluidized bed. Advances in Fluidization Engineering*. AIChE Symposium Series, 86(276): 41-50.

Herman G T [1980]. *Image Reconstruction from Projections*, Academic Press, New York.

Huang S M, A Plaskowski, C G Xie, M S Beck [1989]. *Tomographic imaging of two-component flow using capacitance sensors*. J Phys E:Sci Instrum. 22:173-177.

Landauro J [1992]. *Optical tomography for two-phase fluid flow*. MPh, School of Engineering, BIHE, UK.

Natterer, F [1986]. *The mathematics of computerized tomography*, Wiley, New York,

Weigand F and Hoyle B S [1989]. *Real-time parallel processing in industrial flow measurement using transputer arrays*. IEEE. Trans on Ultrasonics, Ferroelectrics, and Frequency Control, 36(6):652-660.

Electric Field Interaction and an Enhanced Reconstruction Algorithm In Capacitance Process Tomography

Q Chen, B S Hoyle, and H J Strangeways

Department of Electronic and Electrical Eng, University of Leeds, Leeds, LS2 9JT, UK.

ABSTRACT: This paper presents an enhanced reconstruction technique for capacitance-sensed process tomography based upon the linear backprojection algorithm. The aim is to overcome limitations inherent in linear backprojection when significant field interaction between the sensing electrodes and the process material occurs. The general problem of this field interaction is examined followed by a description of the new reconstruction method.

1. INTRODUCTION

Capacitance tomography involves taking a set of capacitance measurements from electrodes situated around the circumference of an imaging plane, and using the measurements to generate an image of the material lying within the imaged area. The process of generating an image from a measurement set is called image reconstruction, and is a solution of the *inverse problem*; where the *forward problem* would involve a computation of the set of capacitance values from a known material distribution. In this case the resulting image is of the permittivity distribution of a cross-section, and from this the material profile can be deduced. However, if the permittivity distribution is not uniform, the electric field distribution is distorted from that arising from the uniform permittivity case. If this distortion effect is not considered an error is produced in the reconstructed image called the *soft-field* error.

The main emphasis of this research is to investigate image reconstruction in terms of the static electric fields existing within the image plane. The relationship between the permittivity distribution, the electric field distribution and the flow regime is studied, as well as the effect of the soft-field error on image reconstruction. When solving the inverse problem it is necessary to consider that the electric field distribution depends upon the permittivity distribution.

It is intended to use an iterative reconstruction algorithm that is able to compensate to some extent for the soft-field effect. Part of this reconstruction algorithm involves simulating the capacitance measurement process using a numerical model. This requires a solution of the forward problem that involves generating a set of capacitance values from a material distribution.

2. ELECTRIC FIELD INTERACTION IN CAPACITANCE PROCESS TOMOGRA-PHY

The measurement data produced by a capacitance tomography system consists of a set of inter-electrode capacitance values C_{ij} that are related to the electric field $\vec{E}(x,y)$ and to the permittivity distribution $\varepsilon(x,y)$ by the electric energy function:

$$W_e = \frac{1}{2} C_{ij} V_0^2 = \frac{1}{2} \int_{s(x,y)} \varepsilon(x,y) \, |\vec{E}(x,y)|^2 \, dx \, dy \qquad (1.1)$$

such that:

$$C_{ij} = \frac{1}{V_0^2} \int_{s(x,y)} \varepsilon(x,y) \, |\vec{E}(x,y)|^2 \, dx \, dy \qquad (1.2)$$

where $s(x,y)$ is the sensing area between the electrodes i and j.

In equation (1.2) the inter-electrode capacitance value is related to the permittivity and electric field distributions. In practice the electric field distribution $\vec{E}(x,y)$ is not a linear function of the permittivity distribution, and the theoretical expression relating the two may be obtained through Laplace's equation. It is of interest to investigate what happens to the electric field in two-phase flows, because the permittivity distribution affects the electric field distribution, and therefore the image reconstruction must account for this. A thorough study of this field interaction is therefore important in generating a workable solution to the inverse problem.

Figure 1 below shows the electric field intensity and equipotential lines between electrodes to which a potential difference has been applied, for air/oil and air/water permittivity distributions respectively.

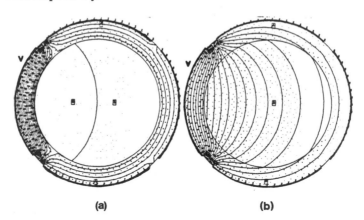

(a)   (b)

Fig.1. Electric field intensity and equi-potential
line for core flow of: (a) air(A)/water(B), and (b) air(A)/oil(B).

Figure 1b is the air/oil case where the electric field lines and equi-potentials are not significantly distorted with respect to the case of a single homogenous medium. Figure 1a shows the fields when water is present. Water has a much higher relative permittivity than either air or oil, and the electric field intensity within water is thus much lower than in oil or air. The equipotential lines are spaced further apart in water relative to their spacing in oil or air.

This work has concentrated upon two-phase flows such as air/water and oil/water. The problem that arises in these cases is demonstrated in figure 1 where a uniform electric field is distorted when a non-homogeneous dielectric distribution is introduced. In simple terms for a dual permittivity system, if one of the permittivity values is much larger than the other, there will be significant distortion of the electric field distribution. In a high permittivity area the equi-potentials will be spaced further apart and the electric intensity distribution has lower relative values. This property will be used later in an image reconstruction algorithm for display of the permittivity distribution of two-phase flows.

3. IMAGE RECONSTRUCTION

There are various approaches to the problem of image reconstruction ranging from simple techniques to sophisticated ones. Usually the simple techniques produce low quality image reconstructions in a short time, with more complicated algorithms producing acceptable quality images but at the expense of processing time. A commonly used algorithm for image reconstruction is *backprojection*, where a spatially varying function, whose shape depends on the source of a measurement, and whose amplitude depends on the measurement value, is projected over an image for each of the measurements in the set. The resulting image is the sum of the backprojected functions from all the measurements.

A system is presented which extends the simple backprojection method into an iterative technique that attempts to compensate for the distorting effects arising from high permittivity values in the permittivity distribution.

3.1. Reconstruction using a Sensitivity Distribution

The linear backprojection algorithm has been used as a solution for the inverse problem of capacitance tomography [Huang *et al* 1989]. Each capacitance measurement between an electrode pair is backprojected through a *sensitivity distribution*, which represents where each capacitance measurement is sensitive to changes in permittivity distribution. The image area is divided into a mesh of elements, and the sensitivity of each sensing electrode, for each backprojection, is then calculated by perturbing or changing the permittivity of one mesh element at a time in an otherwise homogenous medium. The sensitivity distribution is a relationship between the electric field distribution and the surrounding electrode capacitance measurement distribution. Previous research [Xie *et al* 1992] assumes a uniform permittivity throughout the imaged area in order to calculate the sensitivity distribution. However, if the effect of the non-uniformity of permittivity distribution in flow regimes is not taken into account in the calculation of the sensitivity distribution, any field distortions in high permittivity areas may be expected to lead to soft-field errors in the reconstructed image. A non-uniform sensitivity distribution will usually be closer to the ideal than that for a uniform distribution. A calculation of the sensitivity distribution that takes into account the permittivity distribution is investigated below.

The non-uniform sensitivity distribution is found from:

$$\text{if } \varepsilon(x,y) = \varepsilon_1 : \quad S_{ij}(x,y) = \frac{C_{ij}(\varepsilon(x,y) \leftarrow \varepsilon_2) - C_{ij}}{C_{ij\,\varepsilon_2} - C_{ij\,\varepsilon_1}} \qquad (2.1)$$

$$\text{if } \varepsilon(x,y) = \varepsilon_2 : \quad S_{ij}(x,y) = \frac{C_{ij}(\varepsilon(x,y) \leftarrow \varepsilon_1) - C_{ij}}{C_{ij\,\varepsilon_2} - C_{ij\,\varepsilon_1}}$$

where $C_{ij}(\varepsilon(x,y) \leftarrow \varepsilon_x)$ is the total system capacitance when the permittivity of the element at (x,y) is set to ε_x (which is ε_1 when the actual permittivity at the element is ε_2 and *vice versa*).

However this method of calculation of the non-uniform sensitivity distribution is long and complicated and must be repeated for each flow-regime encountered. In a practical system the computation time required for re-calculation of the sensitivity distribution for each intermediate ε distribution is likely to be impractical.

Calculation of a non-uniform sensitivity distribution is not therefore useful for a practical system, although it is valuable for an analysis of the soft field effect in image reconstruction algorithms. A useful approach can be taken by using the ideas discussed in section 2, which describes how the permittivity distribution is related to the electric intensity and capacitance distributions. For two phase flows, where the two permittivity values are significantly different, the electric intensity distribution is closely related to the permittivity distribution, and the boundaries between permittivity areas may reasonably be assumed to be distinct. Furthermore for two phase flows, where there is a large difference in permittivity between the two materials, it is possible to replace the sensitivity distribution by the electric intensity distribution and use this as an alternative for backprojection, as described below.

Consider figure 2a which shows a uniform sensitivity distribution between adjacent electrodes, and figure 2b which shows the electric intensity sensitivity distributions resulting from bubble flow consisting of oil and water which have permitivity values of 3.0 and 80.0 respectively.

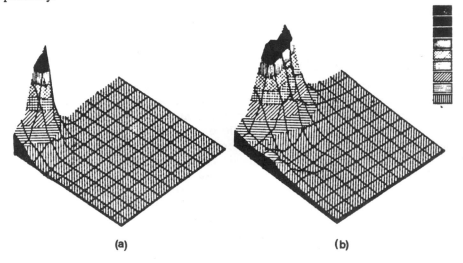

(a)   (b)

Fig.2. Sensitivity distribution (for adjacent electrodes)
corresponding to bubble flow of oil/water media is
(a) in uniform and (b) non-uniform permittivity distributions

It can be seen from these figures that the sensitivity distribution can in fact be non-uniform and is related to the flow regime since it is a function of the permittivity distribution.

3.2. Iterative Reconstruction Algorithm

An iterative method is proposed for reconstructing images which attempts to compensate for non-linearity in the sensitivity distribution. The iteration aims to correct the permittivity distribution at each iteration in order to give a better approximation to the non-linear solution. The algorithm for the iterative reconstruction method is shown in flowchart form in Figure 3.

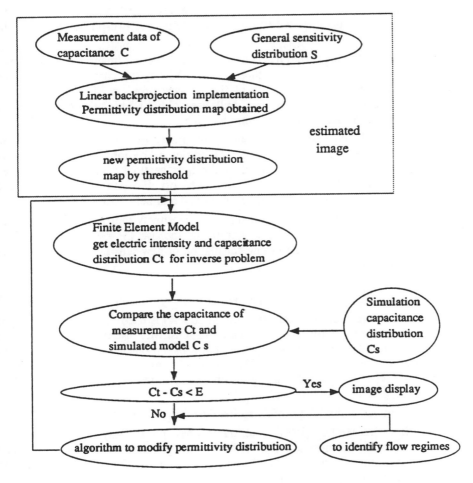

E -- accepted the small values

Fig.3. Flowchart of algorithm for the iterative backprojection method

To test the algorithm a set of simulated capacitance measurements are generated from a numerical model for a chosen permittivity distribution (flow regime). This is used in place of actual measurement data obtained from a physical system, although for the sake of clarity these will be referred to as the measured capacitance values.

The basic method is:

1) An initial approximate permittivity distribution is calculated. This may be done using a uniform sensitivity distribution in a backprojected algorithm. The general uniform sensitivity distribution is calculated using a finite-element model, such as the method described by Xie et al [1992]. This sensitivity distribution only needs to be calculated

once for a particular electrode configuration and making the assumption, for this calculation only, of a homogeneous dielectric. The permittivity distribution is then
reconstructed from the capacitance measurements, by linear backprojection of the
uniform sensitivity distributions, to obtain an initial estimated image. A permittivity
thresholding step is also included to take into account the two-phase nature of the
flow-regime.

2) To check whether the algorithm has converged to the correct image, the capacitance
measurements are compared with those obtained from the current reconstructed
permittivity distribution by a solution of the forward problem. If the discrepancy
between measured capacitance values and those obtained by solving the forward
problem is acceptably small, the algorithm terminates.

3) Depending upon the capacitance distribution, sensitivity area, and the current reconstructed permittivity image, the algorithm modifies and improves the permittivity
distribution using techniques described in the next sections. The algorithm then
repeats the second and third stages in an iterative loop. If no stable solution is found
then the algorithm must be terminated after a fixed number of attempts.

The method as described only needs to calculate the sensitivity matrix once for the uniform permittivity case, but is then able to iteratively improve the reconstructed result.
This has the advantage that time-consuming calculation of new sensitivity distributions at
each iteration step can be avoided.

3.3. Electric Intensity Method for Modifying the Permittivity Distribution

In this study an Iterative Electric Intensity Method (IEIM) is used to reconstruct images
which attempt to compensate for any non-linearity of sensitivity distribution. The electric
intensity distribution is now used as the function that is backprojected (instead of the sensitivity distribution) within the iteration. The estimated permittivity distribution is then
obtained from the result of backprojecting intensity distributions.

3.4. Boundary Iterative Method for Modifying the Permittivity Distribution

The Boundary Iterative Method (BIM) determines a new permittivity distribution which
is then used to generate the next solution to the forward problem. The aim is to reduce
the discrepancy between reconstructed and measured (by simulation) capacitance values
to an acceptably small level. This is done by using three items of information:

1) In two phase flows, the permittivity can take one of two values for the two materials.
The boundary between the two permittivity distribution can be obtained mathematically because at the boundary $\nabla \varepsilon$ (the gradient of the permittivity distribution) is at a
local maximum or minimum.

2) By analysing the capacitance distribution, the flow regime can also be identified
approximately.

3) Comparing the capacitance distribution of measurements C_{ij} and simulated values
C_{ij}^o, the maximum relative error of capacitance values indicates that the effect of the
field between the two electrodes i, j is at its highest, leading to the largest error. It is
therefore appropriate to change the permittivity distribution map in this field area in
which the maximum relative error of capacitance distribution occurs. This change is
implemented by using the information available concerning the phase boundaries
and the flow regime.

3.5. Choice of Permittivity Modification Method

Each iteration of the reconstruction uses one of the methods described in order to reduce the error between the capacitance measurements and the corresponding values calculated by the forward problem solution. Therefore, the image of the permittivity distribution is improved and becomes closer to the actual distribution.

It is possible to mix the methods used to modify the permittivity distribution within the iterative algorithm. Tests have been carried out using the IEIM for the second permittivity calculation, followed by BIM for subsequent iterations.

3.6. Simulations

Figure 4 shows results of simulations for two-phase oil/water stratified flow.

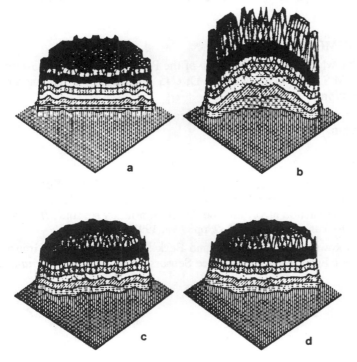

Fig.4. Image reconstruction of a stratified flow of oil/water media.

This system would normally be expected to yield a high soft field error if a backprojection reconstruction is employed which relies upon a sensitivity distribution computed assuming a homogenous permittivity distribution. Figure 4a shows the image corresponding to the reference model, obtained from the forward problem solution.

Figure 4b shows the result obtained when a simple linear backprojection is used for reconstruction; the large errors are clearly visible in this image.

The result of a second iteration of the new IEIM algorithm using electric field distributions is shown in Figure 4c. Comparing these results and the reference model shows that the result of the second iteration is markedly closer to the actual distribution. Figure 4d shows the result following the application of a second iteration using the new BIM algorithm, as mentioned above.

Clearly each iteration of the solution needs additional computation time; the results for this flow regime indicate that two interations would probably be adequate for current process tomography requirements.

4. CONCLUSIONS

A new process tomography image reconstruction technique has been developed which combines the backprojection algorithm with aspects of the electric field behaviour and derived knowlege of the flow regime. It is shown that, for certain types of flow regime, it is important to consider the effects of electric field distortion and to account for this in the reconstruction. Tests indicate that the algorithms would considerably enhance results in situations where large permittivity differences exist in flow regimes, such as mixtures of oil/gas and water.

ACKNOWLEDGMENTS

The authors acknowledge the collaboration of the Process Tomography Group at UMIST led by Professor M S Beck, in particular to Dr C G Xie and Dr S M Huang for discussions and useful suggestions.

This work is supported through a UK Overseas Research Scholarship and a Tetley and Lupton Scholarship.

REFERENCES

Xie C G, Huang S M, Hoyle B S, Thorn R, Lenn C, Snowden D and Beck M S, "Electrical Capacitance Tomography for flow imaging : system model for development of image reconstruction algorithm and design of primary sensors", *IEE Proceedings-G Circuits, Devices and Systems*, **139**, pp89-98, 1992.

Huang S M, Plaskowski A B, Xie C G, and Beck M S, "Tomographic Imaging of Two-Component Flow using Capacitance Sensors", *J.Phys. E: Sci. Instrum.*, **22**, pp173-177, 1989.

Capacitance Tomography: Reconstruction Based on Optimization Theory

Ø Isaksen and J E Nordtvedt[1]

Engineering Centre, Department of Physics, University of Bergen, Allégt. 55, N-5007 Bergen, Norway

ABSTRACT: In this paper, a new reconstruction principle for interpreting process tomography data is suggested. The proposed algorithm is evaluated using simulated data from a capacitance tomography system. The algorithm uses a numerical finite element solution of a mathematical model of a capacitance tomography system, capable of calculating the capacitances for different sensor configurations and flow regimes. The dielectric distribution is parameterized using, in these tests, only a few parameters, and an optimization algorithm is used to modify the parameters in order to obtain a dielectric distribution which gives the minimum discrepancy between estimated and measured capacitances. The method proves to be very promising, and a step towards quantitative capacitance tomography.

1   Introduction

Tomography is an international large and fast moving research field, still mainly due to the usefulness of the technique within medical diagnostics. However, since the first medical X-ray scanner was introduced in the early seventies (Hounsfield 1973), a lot of other interesting techniques as well as applications have emerged. For example, X-ray tomograhy has been used for Non-Destructive Testing purposes (*e.g.*, Persson and Östman, 1986a and 1986b), high energy X-ray tomography for steel NDT (Miyoshi *et al.* 1987), Nuclear Magnetic Resonance Imaging (*e.g.*, Rothwell 1985) and X-ray computerized tomography for petrophysical studies of reservoir rock and visualization of the flow process in the porous material (Rothwell and Vinegar 1985, Cromwell *et al.* 1984, Hove *et al.* 1987, Hunt *et al.* 1988). Further, electrical impedance tomography, γ-tomography and capacitance tomography have been used for industrial process monitoring and control (*e.g.*, Dickin *et al.* 1991, Hellesø 1989, Huang *et al.* 1989, Isaksen 1989, Xie *et al.* 1991).

In industrial process applications, such as studies of flow of oil/gas/water mixtures in pipes, the traditional CT equipment is not applicable, due to the high cost and the need for high data acquisition rate and portability. Hence, easy configurable sensor systems, such as an electrical impedance or a capacitance system, may be preferred. In this paper, we will be concerned with capacitance tomography, although the proposed method of reconstruction apply equally well for other sensor systems. In capacitance tomography, a number of electrodes are mounted circumferentially around the object of interest; in our particular application a flow pipe; see Fig.1. The capacitances between all combinations of electrode pairs are measured, and the dielectric distribution within the pipe is usually reconstructed using the Linear Back Projection (LBP) method (Xie *et al.* 1991). This system has proven to be a useful and efficient way of obtaining qualitative flow pattern information.

However, accurate quantitative information from such a system is quite hard to obtain, due to

---

1. Corresponding author

the following five problems associated with the capacitance technique:

1) In X-ray tomography, an simple expression exists relating the measured quantity (the intensity of the transmitted photons) and the parameter whose distribution is sought. In capacitance tomography, however, there is no simple relation expressing the dielectric distribution as a function of the measured capacitances.

2) In CT, the use of a narrow, collimated X-ray beam ensure that the region of sensitivity for a given measurement is well defined; in a capacitance system, the electric field between the source and detector electrodes determine the sensitivity region, which does not posses a sharp boundary.

3) For capacitance tomography, unlike the CT, the sensitivity for the measured parameters is not constant within the region of interest.

4) In X-ray CT, the measurements have negligible sensitivity for changes in the attenuation coefficient outside the region of measurement; in capacitance tomography, there may be regions of negative sensitivity, *i.e.*, if the dielectric constant is increased in the lower part of the pipe in Fig.1, there will be an increase in the capacitance between electrodes *1* and *2*.

5) The number of measurements is small in a capacitance system; this is because the electrode size cannot be decreased without limit, due to the finite resolution of the sensor electronics.

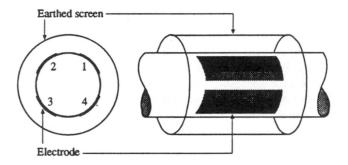

Fig.1.   Sketch of the sensor configuration for a four electrode capacitance tomography system.

Thus, the powerful reconstruction methods developed for X-ray tomography, cannot easily be adopted into a capacitance tomography system, and consequently, the LBP method has traditionally been used for solving the inverse problem. Although the problem of non uniform sensitivity may be accounted for by modifying the LBP algorithm, the method is in itself a "smoothing" algorithm and the number of measurements are very limited (*28* for an eight electrode system), hence smoothing of sharp transitions in the dielectric constant will always occur. Thus, the LBP method is not strictly suitable for obtaining quantitative results.

We have tried to overcome the above mentioned problems by applying optimization theory in developing a new reconstruction algorithm. In this method, a numerical simulator, capable of calculating the capacitances for a particular sensor configuration and flow regimes is used, together with a parameterization of the dielectric distribution and an optimization algorithm. The algorithm calculates the parameters in the representation, thus obtaining the dielectric distribution.

2   Theory

A sketch of the implicit estimation procedure is shown in Fig.2. The physical process is an eight electrode capacitance tomography system, in which the potential at the electrodes are altered in sequence in order to measure all the different capacitances possible (*e.g.*, Isaksen 1989). Thus, the experimental outputs are *28* capacitances. A mathematical simulator, capable of calculating the same capacitances for a given flow regime, defines the calculated outputs. The flow regime is defined by a set of parameters, and the parameters are modified in order to obtain least possible discrepancies between the measured and calculated capacitances.

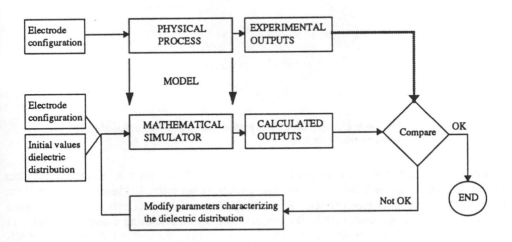

Fig.2.   The implicit estimation procedure.

Mathematical model

For a given dielectric distribution, electrode configuration, and boundary conditions, the potential inside the screen (see Fig.1) can be calculated by solving the Poisson's equation, given by:

$$\nabla \cdot (\varepsilon(\vec{x}) \nabla \Phi(\vec{x})) = -\rho(\vec{x}), \tag{1}$$

where $\varepsilon(\vec{x})$ is the dielectric constant, $\Phi(\vec{x})$ is the potential, and $\rho(\vec{x})$ is the charge distribution. The screen and all the electrodes except the source electrode are defined to be at zero voltage. Eq.1 has been solved numerical by the Finite Element Method, both in two (Isaksen 1989) and three (Tollefsen and Isaksen 1992) dimensions. The two dimensional mesh is shown in Fig.3. The electric field is found from

$$\vec{E} = -\nabla \Phi, \tag{2}$$

and hence the capacitance per unit length is then given by

$$C = \frac{1}{U} \oint_\Gamma \varepsilon_0 \varepsilon_r (\vec{E} \cdot \hat{n}) \, dl, \tag{3}$$

where $\varepsilon_0 = 8,8542 \cdot 10^{-12} F/m$, ε_r is the relative dielectric constant, Γ is a closed curve enclosing the detector electrode, U is the voltage between the source and the detector electrode, and $\hat{n}$ is the unit normal vector to Γ.

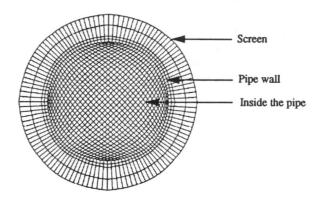

Screen

Pipe wall

Inside the pipe

Fig.3.   2D Finite Element Mesh. There are *900* elements inside the pipe and *1380* elements inside the screen.

The mathematical model has been verified using measured data for a four electrode system (see Fig.1), and with the following sensor construction parameters: *40°* between two adjacent electrodes, *41 mm* inner pipe diameter, *4 mm* thick pipe wall made of perspex, *60 mm* screen radius, and *250 mm* electrode length. The models have been tested using a number of different static flow regimes, *e.g.*, the pipe filled with oil ($\varepsilon_{oil} = 2.167$), the pipe filled with air, and different both stratified and annular flow regimes. All the measurements have been done by using a Hewlett Packard 4192A LF Impedance Analyzer. Fig.4 shows the errors of the calculated capacitances from the 2D and the 3D model in percent of the measured capacitances, for three different cases and *5* different flow regimes. The 3D model uses *1084* elements in *31* layers, *i.e.*, a total of *33604* elements. As can be seen from the figure, quite accurate results are obtained; the average error is approximately *2%*.

Parameterization

In order to be able to use an optimization procedure to calculate the dielectric distribution inside the pipe (*i.e.*, calculate the flow regime), the flow regime has to be represented by a set of parameters. A parameterization with only a small number of parameters, but of great flexibility to represent a number of different flow regimes, is wanted. Fig.5 show some possible flow regimes of two phase oil/gas flow in pipes. As can be seen from the figure, to represent all these flow regimes with only one single representation is indeed a difficult task. We have therefore, as a first approach, tested two different representations; one for idealized stratified flow and one for idealized annular flow; see Fig.6. For stratified flow, the vector for which we seek an estimate is given by $\vec{\beta}_1 = [\theta, d]^T$ (parameterization I), and for annular flow by $\vec{\beta}_2 = [x, y, r]^T$ (parameterization II). An algorithm capable of assigning correct dielectric constant to all the element in the mathematical model for a specified parameterization has been implemented.

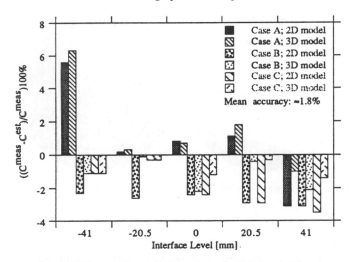

Fig.4. Calculated capacitances from the 2D and 3D mathematical model in percent of the measured capacitances using a HP Impedance Analyzer for static stratified flow regimes. Case A: The capacitance between electrode *1* and *2*; Case B: The capacitance between electrode *1* and *3*; Case C: The capacitance between electrode *1* and *4*. The horizontal axis shows the interface level in *mm* from the centre of the pipe, hence *-41* denotes only air in the pipe, *41* only oil in the pipe, and the three others represents levels with both oil and gas present.

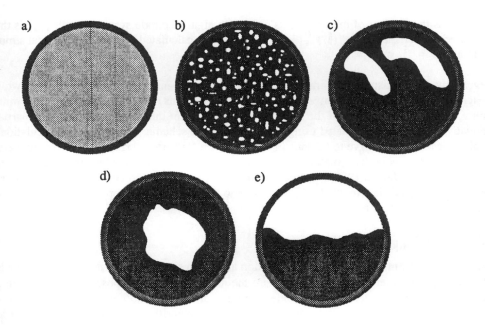

Fig.5. Five possible flow regimes of two phase flow in pipes; a) Homogeneous flow; b) Bubble flow; c) Slug flow; d) Annular flow; e) Stratified flow.

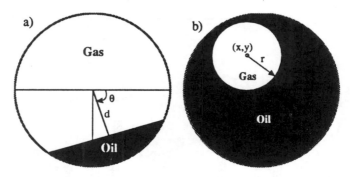

Fig.6.   Parameterization of the flow regimes. a) Stratified flow; b) Annular flow.

Optimization algorithm

An optimization procedure is, in principle, an algorithm capable of minimizing or maximizing a function defined by a set of independent variables, or parameters. Hence, in order to be able to use an optimization algorithm to solve the present problem, we have to define a function by the parameters in the representations given above and the measurements. Such a function, most commonly denoted as an object function, is in this work defined by the equation:

$$J(\vec{\beta}) = \frac{1}{M} \sum_{i=1}^{M} \left(\frac{F_i^{meas} - F_i^{est}(\vec{\beta})}{F_i^{meas}} \right)^2 \tag{4}$$

where M is the number of measurements (28 for an eight electrode system), $\{F^{meas}\}_{i=1}^{M}$ is the measured capacitances, $\{F^{est}(\vec{\beta})\}_{i=1}^{M}$ is the capacitances calculated by the mathematical simulator, and $\vec{\beta} = \vec{\beta}_1$ or $\vec{\beta} = \vec{\beta}_2$.

Several methods exists for minimizing Eq.4, and we have, initially, used the Gauss-Newton Levenberg-Marquardt algorithm (e.g., Gill et al. 1981). In this method the step towards a minimum for Eq.4 is a function of the first partial derivatives of the object functions. The partial derivatives of J is approximated using a finite difference scheme, hence, 3 and 4 calculations of all the capacitances have to be done in each iteration for parameterization I and parameterization II respectively. The method has been used with success in other application (e.g., Watson et al. 1987, Aga 1989, Nordtvedt et al. 1990), and proved to be a rather robust procedure. However, as a fast method is required due to the nature of this application, we are presently also testing other methods of optimization.

Linear Back Projection

We have implemented a Linear Back Projection algorithm similar to the one developed by Xie et al. (1992), in order to be able to compare the results from the proposed algorithm with a state-of-the-art procedure. The area inside the pipe is divided into 900 pixels; see Fig.3. Using 28 measurements (for an 8 electrode system) the LPB algorithm calculates the greylevel in each pixels. The greylevel for pixel k, $g(k)$, is given by

$$g(k) = \frac{\sum\limits_{i=1,7}\left[\sum\limits_{j=i+1,8}\left(\frac{C_{ij}^m - C_{ij}^{gas}}{C_{ij}^{oil} - C_{ij}^{gas}}\right)S_{ij}(k)\right]}{\sum\limits_{i=1,7}\left[\sum\limits_{j=i+1,8}S_{ij}(k)\right]} = \frac{\sum\limits_{i=1,7}\left[\sum\limits_{j=i+1,8}N_{ij}S_{ij}(k)\right]}{\sum\limits_{i=1,7}\left[\sum\limits_{j=i+1,8}S_{ij}(k)\right]}, \qquad (5)$$

where C_{ij}^m is the measured capacitance between electrode i and j, C_{ij}^{gas} is the measured capacitance between electrode i and j when there is only gas inside the pipe, k is the pixel index ($k=1,...,900$), C_{ij}^{oil} is the measured capacitance between the electrode i and j when there is only oil inside the pipe. $S_{ij}(k)$ indicates the sensitivity in C_{ij} due to a change in the dielectric constant in pixel k. $S_{ij}(k)$ is given by:

$$S_{ij}(k) = \left(\frac{C_{ij}^{(oil,k)} - C_{ij}^{gas}}{C_{ij}^{oil} - C_{ij}^{gas}}\right)\left[\frac{1}{\varepsilon_{oil} - \varepsilon_{gas}}\right]\frac{A_{max}}{A_k}, \qquad (6)$$

where $C_{ij}^{(oil,k)}$ is the capacitance when only pixel k is oil and the rest is gas, ε_{oil} and ε_{gas} is the dielectric constant for the oil and the gas, A_{max} is the area of the largest pixel, and A_k is the area of pixel k.

Due to the fact that the reconstruction is performed on a high resolution grid with few measurements, and due to the negative sensitivity areas, post processing on the grey levels has been proposed in order to improve the image (Xie *et al.* 1992). It has been suggested that N_{ij} should be truncated to unity whenever $N_{ij} > 1.0$ and else to perform the following threshold procedure:

$$g_{new}(k) = \left(\begin{array}{l} g(k) < \gamma \Rightarrow g_{new}(k) = 0 \\ otherwise \Rightarrow g_{new}(k) = g(k) \end{array}\right), \qquad (7)$$

where γ is given by $\gamma = (1-\alpha)\xi$, and where α and ξ is given by:

$$\alpha = \text{AVG}\left[|N_{ij}|; \{N_{ij} = 1 \text{ if } N_{ij} > 1\}\right]$$
$$\xi = \text{AVG}\left[g(k); \{\text{for } g(k) > 0\}\right].$$

AVG is the average operator. In this work, using an 8 electrode sensor system, the threshold procedure (Eq.7) was implemented. The truncation procedure only disturbed the image, and was therefore not used.

3   Results and Discussion

In principle, the errors made in the estimation of the flow regime may be divided into three categories (Kerig and Watson 1986): (1) modelling errors; (2) bias errors; and (3) variance errors. The modelling errors are due to inadequate mathematical description of the physical process, *e.g.*, a model with inaccurate location of electrodes or incorrect pipe wall thickness. Bias errors occur if the parameterization of the flow regime is not capable of representing the

"true" (although unknown) flow regime. Variance errors are due to the experimental uncertainties, and will always be present in the estimation. In estimating the flow regime, one would
like to minimize all these three types of errors, hence obtaining a best possible estimate. The
proposed algorithm has so far been tested using artificial data, i.e., data generated by a the
above described model using the parameterized flow regime. Thus, in the results shown in this
paper, a unique solution of the optimization problem exists, because neither modelling, bias,
nor variance errors are present in the problem. The reason for using this approach is that we
have addressed if the information content in the capacitance measurements, makes a unique
determination of the flow regime by optimization possible. For "true" flow regime calculated
by $\theta=90°$ and $d=10mm$, Fig.7 show the square root of the objective function (i.e., the Root
Mean Square value), as a function of both θ and d. As can be seen from the figure, a well
defined minimum exists for this surface at $\theta=90°$ and $d=10mm$, hence making a unique determination of the flow regime possible. To generate data we have used the 2D model of an 8
electrode system with sensor construction parameters as described for the 4 electrode system
above, except that number of electrodes is increased to eight, and that the angle between two
adjacent electrodes now is $10°$.

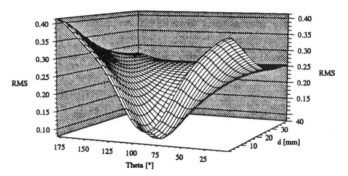

Fig.7.   The square root of the objective function (the RMS value) calculated
around a "true" solution given by $\theta=90°$ and $d=10mm$.

Figs.8a) and 9a) shows the "true" stratified and annular flow regimes respectively, for both
which we have calculated the 28 "measured" capacitances. We have used both the improved
Linear Back Projection and the optimization procedure to estimate the flow regimes. The
reconstruction using the LBP-algorithm (see Figs.8c) and 9c)) is clearly indicating both the
stratified as well as the annular flow regimes, but it is not easy to tell where the oil/gas-inter-
face is located. The reconstruction based on optimization is capable of finding the minimum of
J, hence good results are exhibited by Figs.8d) and 9d). Figs.8b) and 9b) shows how the
parameters (θ and d for the stratified case, and x, y, and r for the annular case) is converging
towards the solution, and Figs.8e) and 9e) show the number of simulation needed for convergence for a number of initial conditions.

The number of iterations used for convergence is approximately 7 for both cases, thus 21
respectively 28 simulations are needed for the stratified and the annular case. One single simulation, i.e., the calculation of 28 capacitances, used approximately 14 CPU-seconds on an
HP720 (a 17 MFLOPS RISC-based workstation). Hence, the time needed for the calculation
of the flow regime by the optimization algorithm is approximately 5 minutes, far too long for
all practical purposes. However, we do expect that combining the LBP method with the optimization algorithm, fast, as well as quantitatively good, estimates of the regimes may be
obtained.This can be done by selecting the correct parameterization and provide good initial

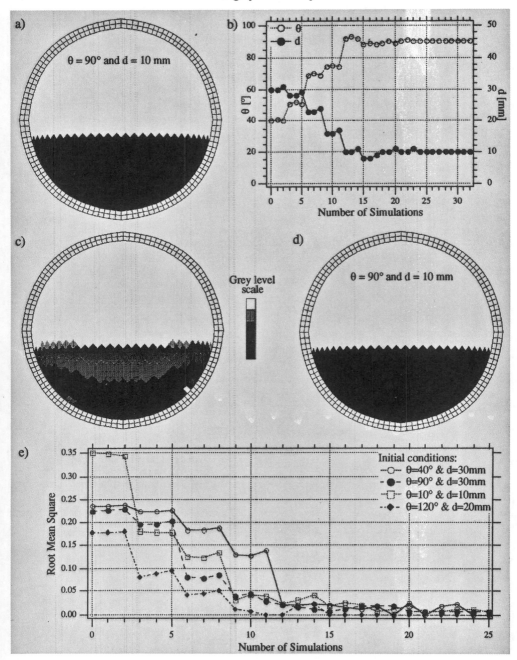

Fig.8. Estimation of stratified flow by the new algorithm and the LBP method. True flow regime is defined by $\theta=90°$ and $d=10mm$: a) The true oil/gas distribution; b) θ and d plotted as a function of number of simulations, initial values were $\theta=40°$ and $d=30mm$; c) Image reconstruction by using the improved LBP algorithm d) Image reconstructed by using the new algorithm, initial values were $\theta=40°$ and $d=30mm$; e) The RMS value of the estimate as a function of the number of simulations for different initial conditions.

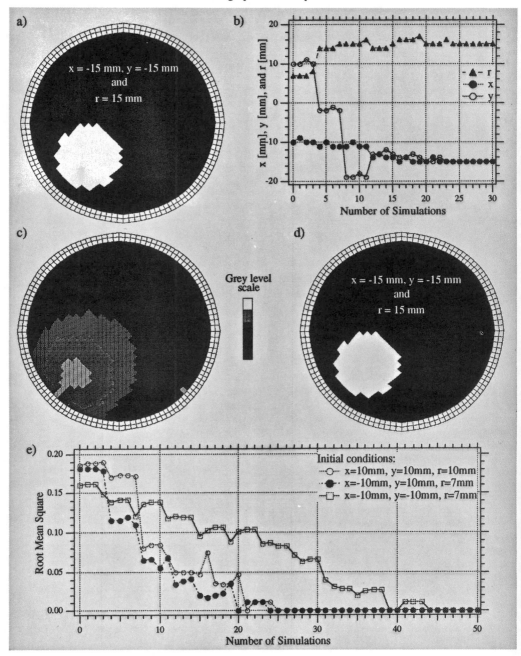

Fig.9. Estimation of annular flow by the new algorithm and the LBP method. True flow regime is defined by *x=-15mm*, *y=-15mm*, and *r=15mm*: a) The true oil/gas distribution; b) *x*, *y*, and *r* plotted as a function of number of simulations, initial values were *x=-10mm*, *y=10mm*, and *r=7mm*; c) Image reconstruction by using the improved LBP algorithm d) Image reconstructed by using the new algorithm, initial values were *x=-10mm*, *y=10mm*, and *r=7mm*; e) The RMS value of the estimate as a function of the number of simulations for different initial conditions.

values for the parameters by the LBP method, and use the optimization algorithm to improve the estimate of the flow regime.

In future studies, we will examine the influence of the bias errors on the estimate, *e.g.*, by calculating the "true" flow regime with a very fine mesh, and obtain estimates of the flow regime by the implicit procedure using a model with a coarser mesh. We are also working with new parameterization techniques, adding a higher flexibility into the estimation procedure, and last, but maybe the most important issue, we are presently comparing the LBP and the implicit algorithms using real experimental data.

4   Conclusions

In this paper, a new method for interpreting data from process tomography systems has been proposed. An algorithm has been developed capable of reconstructing the flow pattern in a pipe filled with oil and gas, using data from a capacitance tomography system. The method proves to be very promising, and a step towards quantitative capacitance tomography.

Acknowledgement

We are indebted to the Royal Norwegian Council for Scientific and Industrial Research for partially supporting this work. We would also like to thank Jarle Tollefsen, Dept. of Physics, University of Bergen, Norway, for providing 3D results which we could compare with our 2D capacitance model.

References

Aga M 1991 *Using the Levenberg-Marquardt Algorithm and the B-spline Representation to Determine the Characteristic Properties of the Porous Medium* MSc Thesis University of Bergen Norway.

Cromwell V, Kortum, D J, and Bradley, D J 1984 *The Use of Medical Computer Tomography (CT) System To Observe Multiphase Flow in Porous Media* Paper SPE 13098 presented at the 59th Annual Technical Conference and Exhibition Houston TX USA September 16-19

Dickin F J, Zhao X J, Abdullah M Z, and Waterfall R C 1991 *Tomographic imaging of industrial process equipment using electrical impedance sensors* Reviewed proceedings of the 5th Conference on Sensors and Their Applications (Bristol: Adam Hilgar) 215-220.

Gill P E, Murray W, and Wright M H 1981 *Practical Optimization* (London: Academic Press).

Hellesø O G 1989 *Two Phase Imaging og Pipe Flow Using γ-tomography* MSc Thesis University of Bergen Norway

Hounsfield G N 1973 *Brit. J. Radiol.* 46 1016-22.

Hove A, Ringen J K, and Read P A 1987 *Visualization of Laboratory Corefloods With the Aid of Computerized Tomography of X-rays* SPERE 2 No.2 148-154.

Huang S M, Xie C G, Thorn R, Snowden D, and Beck M S 1991 *Tomographic imaging of industrial equipment - design of capacitance sensing electronics for oil and gas based processes* Reviewed proceedings of the 5th Conference on Sensors and Their Applications (Bristol: Adam Hilgar) 197-202

Hunt P K, Engler P, and Bajsarowics C 1988 *Computed Tomography as a Core Analysis Tool: Applications, Instrument Evaluation, and Image Improvement Techniques*, Journ. of Petr. Techn. September 1988.

Isaksen Ø 1989 *Imaging Two-component Pipe Flow by Capacitance Sensors* MSc Thesis, University of Bergen, Norway

Kerig P D and Watson A T 1986 *Relative Permeability Estimation From Displacement Experiments: An Error Analysis* SPERE (March 1986) 175.

Khan S H and Abdullah F 1991 *Computer aided design of process tomography capacitance electrode system for flow imaging* Reviewed proceedings of the 5th Conference on Sensors and Their Applications (Bristol: Adam Hilgar) 209-215

Miyoshi S, Tanimoto Y, Uyama K, and Sano Y 1987 *The Evaluation of SCC Defects of Steel Pipe Using a High Energy X-ray CT Scanner*, Nuclear Engineering and Design **102** 275-287.

Nordtvedt J E, Mejia G, Yang P, and Watson A T 1991 *Estimation of Capillary Pressure and Relative Permeability Functions From Centrifuge Experiments* paper SPE 20805 accepted for publication in SPERE.

Persson S and Östman E 1986a *The Use of Computed Tomography in Non-destructive Testing of Polymeric Materials, Aluminium and Concrete: Part 1 - Basic Principles* Polymer Testing **6** 407-414.

Persson S and Östman E 1986b *The Use of Computed Tomography in Non-destructive Testing of Polymeric Materials, Aluminium and Concrete: Part 2 - Applications* Polymer Testing **6** 415-446.

Rothwell W P *Nuclear magnetic resonance imaging* Applied Optics **24** No.23 3958-3968.

Rothwell W P and Vinegar H J 1985 *Petrophysical applications of NMR imaging* Applied Optics **24** No.23 3969-3972.

Tollefsen J and Isaksen Ø 1992 *Two and Three Dimensional Modelling of Capacitance Sensors* to be published.

Watson A T, Kerig P D, Richmond P C, and Tao T M 1988 *A Regression-Based Method for Estimating Relative Permeabilities From Displacement Experiments* SPERE (March 1988) 3.

Xie C G, Huang S M, Hoyle B S, and Beck M S 1991 *Tomographic imaging of industrial equipment - development of system model and image reconstruction algorithm for capacitive tomography* Reviewed proceedings of the 5th Conference on Sensors and Their Applications (Bristol: Adam Hilgar) 203-208.

Xie C G, Huang S M, Hoyle B S, Thorn R, Lenn C, and Beck M S 1992 *Electrical Capacitance Tomography for Flow Imaging - System model for development of reconstruction algorithms and design of primary sensors* IEE Proceeding G **139** No.1 89-98.

Chapter 3

Equipment Design and Modelling

APPLICATION OF GAMMA-RAY TOMOGRAPHY TO GAS FLUIDISED AND SPOUTED BEDS

S J R Simons, J P K Seville, R Clift, W B Gilboy[+] and M E Hosseini-Ashrafi.

Department of Chemical and Process Engineering and [+]Department of Physics, University of Surrey, Guildford, Surrey, GU2 5XH.

ABSTRACT: Gamma-ray tomography has been used to obtain quantitative information on local time-averaged voidage distributions within fluidised beds, using conventional multi-orifice distributor plates, and with spouted beds (a variant of a fluidised bed in which most or all of the gas enters through a single orifice). Such information has not previously been determined with accuracy. The voidage profiles obtained by the gamma-ray technique clearly show the position and penetration of the gas jets, the presence of "dead" zones and the transition to the bubbling regime. The experiments carried out so far suggest that an instrument suitable for industrial sized applications and capable of producing high-speed images of complex flow systems could be developed.

1. INTRODUCTION

A fluidised bed consists of a mass of granular solids through which an upward fluid flow is passed at a superficial velocity (U) sufficient to support the weight of the bed. The velocity just necessary to do this is called the "minimum fluidisation velocity" (U_{mf}) and any further increase in the flow causes the bed to expand to accommodate the increase. In gas fluidised systems the increased gas flow passes through the bed in the form of bubbles, giving the bed the appearance of a boiling liquid (figure 1a). It is this bubbling action which causes the particles to mix continuously and hence promotes uniform bed temperatures and composition, although bubbling can also lead to excessive by-pass of unreacted fluidising gas; a compromise has often to be made between these conflicting features during system design.

Fluidised bed reactors are widely used in the process industries because of the good mixing and high rates of heat and mass transfer which can be obtained within them; notable applications are as combustors and gasifiers, catalytic reactors, agglomerators and driers. In such process operations it is conventional to support the bed on a plate or distributor containing a number of discrete orifices, nozzles or caps, so that the free area of the plate is relatively small (typically below 5 % of the total area of the plate). In these circumstances the bed is conveniently divided into two regions; the bubbling bed (as described above) and the "jet" region, immediately above the distributor, where the gas and particle velocities and the void fractions are much higher immediately above each orifice than in the regions between them or in the bubbling bed. In applications where no fluidising gas is introduced between these orifices, unfluidised "dead"

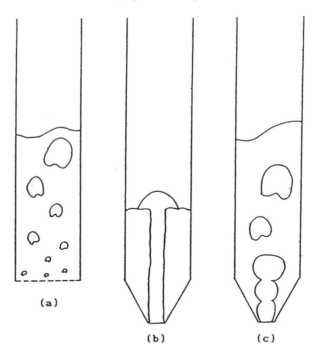

(a)

(b)   (c)

Figure 1. Variations of fluidised beds;
    a) fluidised bed with flate plate distributor
    b) spouted bed
    c) spout-fluidised bed.

zones may form. Hence, the extent and structure of the jet region, which is
determined by the distributor design, will have a marked effect on such
parameters as reactor performance (Grace and de Lasa, 1978) and particle
attrition (Seville et al., 1992a).

An alternative form of gas-solid contacting device, where the fluidising
gas is injected into the bed via a single orifice to form a high velocity
jet or "spout", can be used in applications where the constituent particles
are too coarse or non-uniform (in size, shape or density) for good
fluidisation or where particle agglomeration needs to be inhibited. In such
cases the bed is said to be "spouted" or, where there is sufficient bed
depth for bubbles to form and break away from the top of the jet,
spout-fluidised (figure 1, b and c). The presence of the high velocity jet
induces solids circulation by the entrainment of solids into the jet along
its length, whilst the motion of bubbles through the main part of the bed
induces solids mixing primarily by the solids-carrying capacity of the
bubble wake and by the displacement of surrounding solids. The behaviour of
the jet region is therefore far more critical to the resulting reactor
performance of such systems than to those of conventional fluidised beds.

A good knowledge of the hydrodynamics and structure of the jet and bubble
regions in fluidised and spouted beds is essential if adequate design
procedures and process models are to be developed. For instance, the
variety of qualitative descriptions of jetting behaviour and the influence
of particle size and density, gas velocity and density and orifice size
have led to numerous empirical correlations, which tend to be ambiguous as

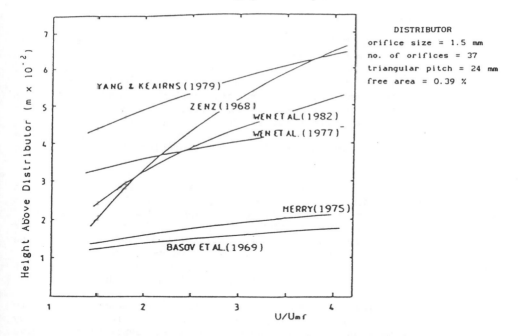

Figure 2. Comparison of predictions of jet penetration length in a bed
of quartz sand (300 - 355 μm), fluidised by atmospheric air,
from several correlations (for refs. see Seville et al., 1986).

far as the definition of jet penetration length is concerned. The matter is
complicated by the wide variety of gas and solid flow patterns in jets
which have been observed. A good review of jet behaviour is given by
Massimilla (1985), who also tabulated the most important correlations for
jet penetration length; figure 2 indicates the discrepancies which can
occur between these correlations.

Measurement of the height of the jet region and the transition to the
bubbling regime is not straight forward. The only techniques which have
achieved significant results are X-ray imaging (Rowe et al., 1979), direct
observation of "two dimensional" or semi-cylindrical beds (see, for
instance, Kececioglu et al., 1988) and an indirect method based on
evaluation of the solids velocity and collision frequency with an impact
probe (Donsi et al., 1980). X-ray imaging gives an instant-in-time snapshot
of jet behaviour but is expensive to use and the resulting images require
some skill in interpretation. The indirect method is complex and
necessarily invasive to the process, whilst the use of semi-cylindrical
beds has occasioned much debate (Rowe et al., 1979; Whiting and Geldart,
1980) as to whether the central dividing wall is responsible for
stabilising an otherwise unsteady jet. Recent work carried out in the
United States has used multi-electrode capacitance tomography for the
real-time imaging and measurement of the voidage distributions within
cold-models of fluidised coal beds (Halow and Fasching, 1990), but such
systems currently suffer from poor spatial resolution and require large
contrasts in the phase conductivities. In this paper a similar non-invasive
technique, that of gamma-ray tomographic imaging, is described in which
local time-averaged voidage distributions within fluidised and spouted beds
can be obtained in an accurate, readily interpretable manner.

2. EXPERIMENTAL TECHNIQUES

Radiation imaging using Computer-Aided Tomography (CAT) is probably best known for its role in medical diagnostics, although industrial applications are fast growing in importance. The technique involves the stepping of a collimated beam of radiation (X-rays in the medical application) across the object being scanned and measuring the attenuation of the beam at each position. The object or the source/detector assembly itself is then rotated through a predetermined angle about an axis perpendicular to the scanning plane and a further set of attenuation measurements is made. The sequence is repeated until the object or the source/detector axis has rotated through $180°$.

There are various techniques available (Brooks and Di Chiro, 1976) for the reconstruction of tomographic, cross-sectional images of scanned objects from sets of attenuation measurements. Conventionally the image consists of a square matrix of picture elements, or pixels, whose grey-level (or colour) varies according to the linear attenuation coefficient of the object at the corresponding point in the cross-section. The linear attenuation coefficient itself depends on the density and atomic number of the material and the energy of the incident radiation at each point.

Although the technique has considerable potential for measuring density profiles in multiphase flows, X-rays themselves are unsuitable for many non-medical applications since they have insufficient penetration to give adequate contrast with the high density, high atomic number materials commonly encountered and they are not mono-energetic. Tomographic systems using mono-energetic gamma radiation are therefore preferred for quantitative analysis of industrial applications.

2.1 TOMOGRAPHIC IMAGING OF FLUIDISED BEDS

The early work on the application of gamma-ray tomography to gas fluidised beds conducted at the University of Surrey utilised a scanning assembly developed by the Radiation Physics Group of the Department of Physics (Gilboy et al., 1982). The system is shown schematically in figure 3. A single collimated photon beam of 5 mm diameter from a 100 mCi Am source (prominent peak of 59.6 keV) and a single NaI detector were used to produce the tomographic images. The source and detector were aligned on an optical bench with the object to be scanned (a miniature fluidised bed) rotated and translated through the beam by a series of stepper motors. For these experiments 40 x 2 mm steps were taken at 30 x $6°$ intervals with 1000 photons/ray-sum collected at each position. This led to sample times of several seconds and total scan times of 6 to 7.5 hours. The resulting voidage distributions were therefore long time-averages of the gas/solid activity within the beds.

The complete apparatus was controlled by a microcomputer and the reconstructed images were made up of 5 mm square pixels. The reconstruction technique, termed "filtered back-projection", is described fully by Brooks and Di Chiro (1976). Calibration between attenuation and voidage was achieved by scanning a settled bed of material and obtaining a single attenuation coefficient, averaged over the whole cross-section. Without disturbing the bed, the interstitial voids were then slowly filled with water and a second average attenuation coefficient obtained. From the known attenuation coefficient of water, the voidage of the settled bed and hence the attenuation coefficient of the particles were obtained.

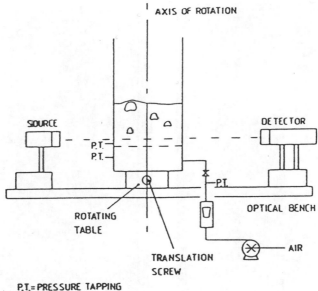

Figure 3. Early gamma-ray tomography experimental apparatus (after Seville et al., 1986).

Initial investigations were centred on a 51 mm diameter perspex fluidised bed, 200 mm in height (figure 4), which could be fitted with two interchangeable distributors; a solid brass plate containing a central 2 mm diameter tapered orifice and a porous sintered bronze plate with the same axial orifice but with a separate connection from the orifice for background gas flow through the plate. The bed was fluidised using compressed air with the flowrate controlled by rotameters. The static bed depth was 60 mm and the bed was scanned at heights 14 to 40 mm above the distributor. The principal objectives of the experiments were to examine the effects of both background fluidisation and particle shape on the axial and radial bed voidage profiles. Figure 4 (a) and (b) show the dramatic effect background fluidisation can have on bed behaviour. Typical tomograms and line scans obtained during the investigations (figure 5) clearly indicate that an increase in background fluidisation causes an increase in the radial extent of the high voidage (jet) region coupled with a decrease in the axial penetration of the jet. These observations are consistent with the conclusion that both background fluidisation and high particle sphericity enhance particle mobility and, hence, entrainment into the jet, thereby dissipating the jet momentum over a shorter distance (Kececioglu et al., 1988). Results of these investigations are discussed more fully by Seville et al., 1992b.

Separate experiments, using a larger, 146 mm diameter fluidised bed fitted with a multi-orifice distributor but the same tomographic scanning equipment, were carried out by Seville and co-workers (1986) to investigate the effect of increasing gas velocity on jetting and bubbling behaviour. The bed particles were quartz sand (300 - 355 μm, U_{mf} = 0.92 m/s) and the settled bed depth was 150 mm. The distributor was a flat plate with 37 discrete orifices of 1.5 mm diameter on a 24 mm triangular pitch, giving a free area of 0.39 %. Three different scanning heights were used (20, 30 and

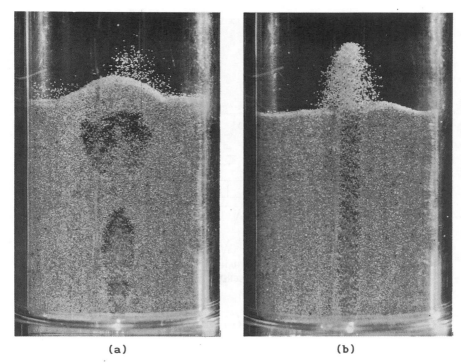

(a)   (b)

Figure 4. 51 mm diameter semi-cylindrical fluidised bed of quartz sand
(300 - 355 μm) with (a) and without (b) background fluidisation.

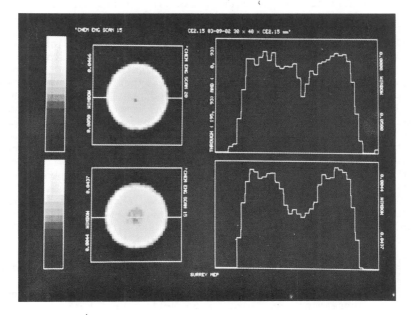

Figure 5. Typical tomograms with associated line scans of the bed shown in
fig. 4; with (bottom) and without (top) background fluidisation.

40 mm above the distributor) at three gas velocities (1.38, 2.30 and 3.22 m/s).

To facilitate comparison between the tomographic images, an attenuation threshold value was chosen (0.03 mm^{-1} corresponding to a voidage fraction of 0.525) below which all pixels were set to black, with the remainder to white. Figure 6 shows the resulting binary images for each of the nine combinations of experimental conditions. Regions of high average voidage are apparent at 20 and 30 mm above the distributor orifices with U/U_{mf} = 3.5 and are also discernible at 20 mm with U/U_{mf} = 2.5. Such images clearly show a decrease in order of the structure with increase in scan height above the distributor (i.e. as the jetting region degenerates into bubble flow) and an increase in structural detail at all heights as the velocity is increased (i.e. an increase in jet penetration length with increasing gas velocity). Indeed, the excellent resolution of the images allowed Seville et al. (1986) to compare the jet penetration lengths determined by the gamma-ray technique with those predicted using several well-known correlations.

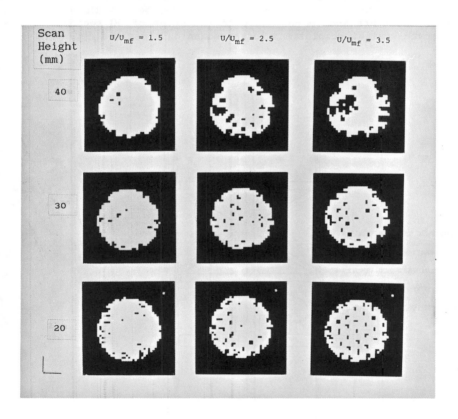

Figure 6. Reconstructed binary bed cross-sections, threshold value = 0.525 (after Seville et al., 1986).

2.2 TOMOGRAPHIC IMAGING OF SPOUT-FLUIDISED BEDS

The single source/detector scanning arrangement used in the earlier work cited above unfortunately led to long data acquisition times and was limited in application to small-scale objects. The tomographic scanner instrumentation has therefore been recently updated and refined in order to overcome these constraints.

The scanner now employs an array of six ^{153}Gd (Gadolinium) sources in conjunction with six collimated CsI scintillation detectors, all mounted on a fixed gantry with a circular opening through which a 100 mm (maximum) diameter cylindrical column can be lowered and raised (figure 7). Instead of rotating the object to be scanned through the beam, the scanner ring is moved laterally in steps of 1.0 mm each followed by a rotation of 1.5° around the object until a full 180° rotation is obtained (Hosseini-Ashrafi and Tüzün, 1992). This results in reconstructed images made up of a 155 mm square grid of 1.0 x 1.0 mm pixels. Because of the multiplication of sources and detectors, each scan can be performed in 1/6 th of the steps required for the single source/detector system described earlier. The shortest total scan time achieved so far has been with a 2 mm wide collimator aperture and is currently in the order of 90 seconds. However, for improved spatial resolutions longer scanning times are necessary.

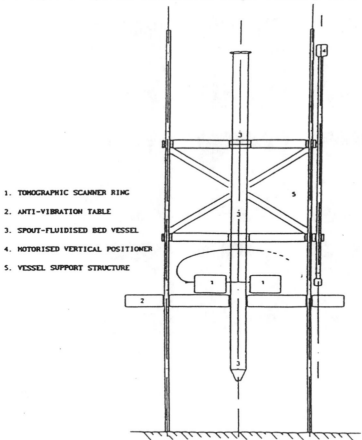

1. TOMOGRAPHIC SCANNER RING

2. ANTI-VIBRATION TABLE

3. SPOUT-FLUIDISED BED VESSEL

4. MOTORISED VERTICAL POSITIONER

5. VESSEL SUPPORT STRUCTURE

Figure 7. Up-dated gamma-ray tomography experimental apparatus (after Hosseini-Ashrafi and Tüzün, 1992).

The conical/cylindrical vessel used in these experiments consisted of a 100 mm diameter cylindrical section with a conical base having an inlet orifice of 22 mm diameter. The bed material was activated carbon (U_{mf} = 0.19 m/s, cumulative mean size 906 μm) and the bed depth was 550 mm. A superficial gas velocity of 0.37 m/s ensured that the bed operated in the slugging mode (i.e. with gas bubbles of a diameter comparable to that of the column) and scanning heights of 35, 70 and 200 mm above the orifice were selected to provide images of the cone/jet and bubbling/slugging regimes. The experimental objective was to obtain sufficient data on the bed hydrodynamic behaviour to assist in the development of modelling procedures. In order to study the effects of particle cohesion on bed structure (Seville, 1992), which can lead, for instance, to disastrous defluidisation in high-temperature coal gasifiers, a non-volatile viscous oil (200/50 cs) was added to the bed material in an amount equivalent to 13.6 % of the particle volume.

The total scan time at each height was approximately 4 hours (equivalent to a lateral scan time of 4 seconds/mm) to ensure high resolution image reconstruction. Figure 8 (a to d) shows examples of the tomographic images of the dry and cohesive beds taken at 35 and 70 mm above the orifice. Only limited information can be obtained by visual inspection of the tomograms, although the jet (depicted as a dark region in the centres of the figures)

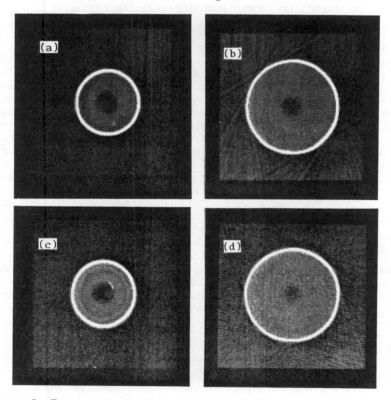

Figure 8. Tomograms of spout-fluidised bed
   a) at 35 mm and b) 70 mm from orifice, dry solids
   c) at 35 mm and d) 70 mm from orifice, cohesive solids.

is clearly discernable in both the dry and sticky cases and a ridge of high voidage (adjacent to the jet) to low voidage (towards the vessel wall) exists in the cone region of the cohesive bed. More quantitative analysis can be achieved using the calibrated line scans of each image. These are depicted as left to right diametric voidage profiles in figure 9 (a to d). The differences in the voidage profiles at each plane are now more clearly defined. The average annular voidage fraction of the static bed is higher with the cohesive material (figure 9, b and c) than for the dry case (figure 9, a and b), since the pendular liquid bridges of the former can support the component particles in a more open structure.

The presence in the cone of a ridge of denser material adjacent to that immediately surrounding the jet (corresponding to a "dead" zone) is more apparent in the cohesive bed than with the dry material. At 70 mm the annular region in the dry bed is slightly more expanded than at 35 mm and the jet width has decreased, indicating that the scan has taken place near the top of the jet. An increase in solids content in the core of the jet is also shown. A similar pattern occurs with the sticky material - no "dead" zone has been detected at 70 mm, indicating that the cone region is of prime importance in the defluidisation process (Kececioglu et al., 1984). Both scans at 200 mm (not shown here) indicate a more chaotic voidage distribution and a lowering in the average solids content, which is indicative of a transition to the bubbling/slugging regime.

3. CONCLUSIONS

The application of gamma-ray tomography to the study of the voidage distributions within fluidised and spout-fluidised beds has been demonstrated, the local time-averaged voidage profiles clearly showing the position and penetration of the gas jet, the presence of "dead" zones and the transition to the bubbling/slugging regime. While the time-averaged nature of the measurements means that rapid events such as bubble motions cannot be followed individually, the excellent accuracy and resolution of the technique enables new features of the bed to be observed. The experiments carried out so far in our laboratories suggest that gamma-ray tomography is suitable for process modelling studies and that further development of the instrumentation will enable imaging of industrial sized applications.

ACKNOWLEDGEMENT

The purchase of the tomography equipment described in Section 2.2 was made possible by a grant from the Science and Engineering Research Council Specially Promoted Programme in Particulate Technology. The work described was partially funded by the University of Surrey Research Committee and the British Coal Corporation.

REFERENCES

Brooks R A and Di Chiro G 1976 *Phys. Med. Biol.* 21 689
Donsi G Massimilla L and Colantuoni L 1980 "The dispersion of axi-symmetric gas jets in fluidized beds", in Fluidization eds J R Grace and J M Matsen (Plenum: New York)
Gilboy W B Foster J and Folkard M 1982 *Nucl. Inst. and Meth.* 193 209
Grace J R and deLasa H I 1978 *Am. Inst. Chem. Engr. J.* 24 364
Halow J S and Fasching G E 1990 *A.I.Ch.E. Symp. Series* 276, 86 '41-50
Hosseini-Ashrafi M E and Tüzün U 1992 *Chem. Eng. Sci.* in press

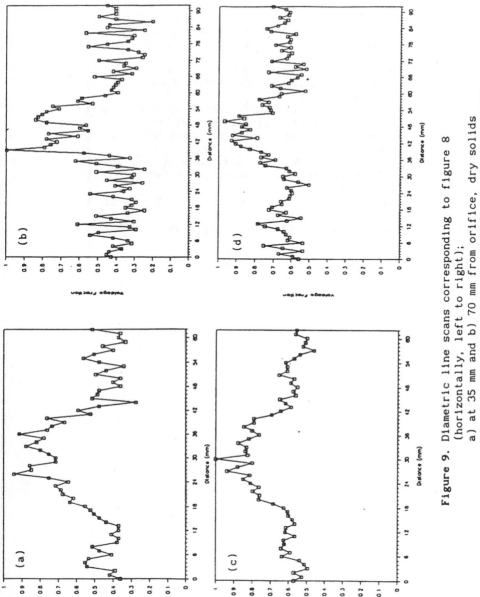

Figure 9. Diametric line scans corresponding to figure 8 (horizontally, left to right);
a) at 35 mm and b) 70 mm from orifice, dry solids
c) at 35 mm and d) 70 mm from orifice, cohesive solids.

Kececioglu I Yang Y-C and Keairns D L 1984 *A.I.Ch.E.J.* **30** (1) 99–110.

Massimilla L 1985 "Gas jets in fluidised beds", in Fluidization eds J F
    Davidson R clift and D Harrison (Academic Press 2nd ed: London) 133

Rowe P N MacGillivray H J and Cheesman D J 1979 *Trans. Inst. Chem. Eng.* **57**
    194

Seville J P K 1992 "Fluidisation of wet particles", in the Proceedings of
    the 5th European Symposium on Particle Characterization, PARTEC,
    Nüremberg, **2** 801–810

Seville J P K Morgan J E P and Clift R 1986 "Tomographic determination of
    the voidage structure of gas fluidised beds in the jet region", in
    Fluidization V eds k Østergaard and A Sørensen (Engineering Foundation:
    New York) 87–94

Seville J P K Mullier M A Hailu L and Adams M J 1992a "Attrition of
    agglomerates in fluidised beds", to be presented at FLUIDIZATION VII,
    Broadbeach, Australia.

Seville J P K Rojo V Wood M P MacCuaig N Clift R and Gilboy W B 1992b
    (submitted)

Whiting K J and Geldart D 1980 *Chem. Eng. Sci.,* **35** 1499–1501

Process Engineering Studies using Positron-based Imaging Techniques

D J Parker[*], M R Hawkesworth[*], T D Beynon[*] and J Bridgwater[+]

[*]School of Physics and Space Research,
[+]School of Chemical Engineering,
        The University of Birmingham, Birmingham B15 2TT

ABSTRACT: This paper is concerned with two closely related positron-based 3D imaging techniques now available for studying industrial processes - positron emission tomography (PET) and positron emission particle tracking. The availability of robust and mobile positron "cameras" and positron emitting "tags" are discussed with particular reference to research in Birmingham.

PET is illustrated with reference to an extrusion experiment, where images in tomographic form were produced every 30s with a resolution (FWHM) of 8mm. Using the same camera imaging algorithms permit single particle location every 0.1s to within 3mm. Particle trajectories in powder mixers are presented, from which quantitative data towards the optimization of mixer operation and design have been obtained.

1. INTRODUCTION

Positron emission tomography (PET) is well established as a medical imaging technique for observing the evolution of a bolus of metabolic fluid which has been labelled with an appropriate positron-emitting radionuclide. Each positron formed rapidly annihilates with an electron, giving rise to a pair of 511 keV γ-rays which are emitted almost exactly back-to-back, so that subsequent location of both γ-rays defines a line in space close to which the original positron emission must have occurred. By viewing the region containing activity from all sides and detecting a large number of pairs of γ-rays, the spatial distribution of the radionuclide can be reconstructed using the standard tomographic approach. Medical PET scanners usually employ one or more rings of scintillator detectors and construct the 3D image as a stack of independent 2D slices, although there is currently interest in fully-3D detector systems.

The same technique can be applied to non-medical flow studies. An important property of the 511 keV γ-rays is that they can penetrate considerable thickness of material, so that the fluid of interest may be successfully imaged from outside its casing. The γ-ray intensity is attenuated by a factor $1/e$ in traversing approximately 45mm Al or 15mm Fe, implying the possibility of imaging through a 25mm steel casing. Where such attenuating material is distributed inhomogeneously through the field of view it is necessary to make appropriate corrections to the measured data, but in an engineering context this is straightforward since the geometry of the plant is usually accurately known; if not then attenuation factors can be measured experimentally, without the concern for the effect of additional radiation dose to the subject which is a vital consideration in medical PET (the dose to the operator can be kept small, as in medical PET).

A wide range of positron-emitting radionuclides can be produced using a cyclotron. Whereas in medical PET, where biochemical pathways are being studied, the exact chemical form of the radiolabel is critical, in process engineering the intention is generally to use the positron emitter as an inert tracer, and the choice of radionuclide is often based primarily on the need for an appropriate half life: long enough to survive the process being studied but not so long that a problem arises from radioactive contamination of plant.

The Birmingham positron camera was installed in 1984 for the purpose originally of studying lubrication in engines and gearboxes. It remains the only PET facility devoted to non-medical imaging, and, in conjunction with the two cyclotrons belonging to the University of Birmingham, has been used for a wide range of engineering studies, some of which are mentioned below.

The camera is now used in two distinct modes, which are separately described in Sections 3 and 4 below. Conventional tomography requires the collection of large volumes of data, so that acquisition of an image takes typically several minutes. On the other hand, if it is known that only a single positron-emitting particle is present within the field of view, its position can be accurately determined from a small number of detected events. Such a particle can thus be used as a flow tracer and can be located many times per second, providing a direct measure of the velocity field within a flow system.

2. THE BIRMINGHAM POSITRON CAMERA

The camera, which was designed and constructed at the Rutherford Appleton Laboratory, has been fully described elsewhere (Hawkesworth *et al* 1986, Hawkesworth *et al* 1991), and will only be briefly summarised here.

Two position-sensitive detectors, each with an active area of 600x300 mm^2, mounted on either side of the field of view, are used to detect the pairs of coincident annihilation photons. Each detector consists of a multiwire proportional chamber, containing a stack of thin lead cathodes with intervening planes of anode wires (held at a potential of 3.5kV relative to the cathodes), and filled with a mixture of isobutane and freon at atmospheric pressure. An incident γ-ray can interact by photoelectric absorption or Compton scattering in one of the lead cathodes and release an electron into the gas, thereby triggering an avalanche of ionisation around the adjacent anode, which can be detected via the charges induced on this anode and its two neighbouring cathodes. The lead cathodes are divided into parallel strips, aligned orthogonally on successive cathodes, so that the (x,y) position of the interaction within the anode plane can be determined.

Only coincident events in which γ-rays are detected in both detectors within the resolving time of the system (approximately 15ns) are accepted, and are stored event-by-event on disk using a VAX4000/200 computer. For each such event, the coordinates of detection of both γ-rays are recorded, together with the time of detection.

The probability of detecting a 511 keV γ-ray which passes through one of the detectors is only about 7%, giving an overall probability of detecting a pair of such γ-rays of 0.5%. For every valid coincident event, many more γ-rays are detected which are not coincident, and these load the electronics, so that the maximum useful data rate is around 3000 coincident events per second.

The separation of the two detectors is adjusted to suit the particular application, and the geometrical efficiency varies accordingly; it also varies across the field of view, being highest at the centre. When a small system is being studied, a separation of 300mm is usually adopted, giving a field of view 600x300x300mm^3, as shown in Fig.1. For points close to the centre of this field of view the stationary pair of large area detectors covers a sufficiently wide range of angular views that tomographic reconstruction is possible, although the resolution of the resulting images is notably poorer in the z-direction (the axis linking the two detectors) than in the other two directions. This geometry also provides the basis for the particle tracking studies. For imaging larger systems, detector separations up to 600mm are routinely used, and in this case full 3D tomographic reconstruction can only be achieved by rotating the pair of detectors through 180° about a central axis.

The camera was designed to be transportable and sufficiently rugged to operate in an industrial environment. Indeed in its early years it was used successfully for imaging the lubricant distribution within an aero engine operating at full power on a test rig. Generally, however, measurements are made at Birmingham on small-scale test rigs.

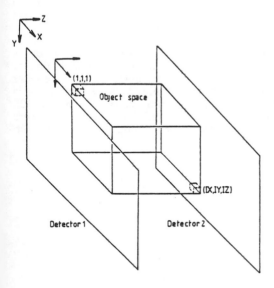

Fig. 1. Schematic view of the detector geometry and coordinate system.

3. TOMOGRAPHIC STUDIES

The process of forming a tomographic image basically involves measuring positron annihilation γ-rays over a wide range of angles, backprojecting each detected event uniformly along the γ-ray path (with appropriate correction for attenuation by material on the path, if any) into an object space comprising a 3D array of cubical voxels (Fig.1), and finally deconvolving from the resulting backprojected image the image of a point source measured under the same conditions, the "point spread function" (PSF). Implicit in this approach is the assumption that the PSF is invariant over the field of view. In fact this is never the case, since a much wider range of emitted γ-ray directions can be detected for a point at the centre of the field of view than for one near the edge. However, by arbitrarily restricting the γ-ray paths used to those subtending less than some limiting angle with the normal linking the two detectors, uniform response can be achieved over a central portion of the field of view, albeit by throwing away a significant fraction of the original data. The tighter this "angle limit", the larger the field of view over which uniform response is achieved, at the expense of accepting less and less of the data, and reducing the stereoscopic view of the detectors, so that the resulting images have good resolution in the x and y directions but much poorer resolution in the z direction.

For example, with a detector separation of 300mm, by restricting the accepted γ-rays to those subtending an angle of less than $25°$ to the normal, it is possible to achieve uniform response over approximately one quarter of the volume of the full field of view, with a PSF having a FWHM resolution of approximately 8mm in the x and y directions and 25mm in the z direction.

To achieve 3D reconstruction with better resolution in the z direction, it is necessary to rotate the detectors about the field of view. In this case the requirement to impose angle limits can be removed in the radial direction since, for each point within the central region of the field of view, all radial angles of emission are sampled equally as the detectors are rotated continuously through 180°, and a simple radial normalisation can be applied to compensate for the residual radial variation in detection efficiency (Clack *et al* 1984). It is still necessary, however, to apply an angle limit in the axial direction. A typical imaging situation uses a detector separation of 600mm, rotation about the central x-axis, and an axial (x) angle limit of 15°; the resulting PSF is invariant over a field of view consisting of a cylinder, 280mm in diameter and 350mm long (plus an additional conical region at each end) and has a FWHM resolution of 8mm in the axial direction and 12mm in the radial direction.

As an indication of the power of the tomographic technique, Figs 2 and 3 show results obtained from measurements made in the geometry just decribed on a system consisting of line sources of ^{22}Na: two lines 100mm long oriented in a vertical plane and forming the letter "V" and five lines 50mm long arranged to form a horizontal "H". Fig. 2 shows four views of the image obtained after recording 10^7 events, backprojected into an array of 128x128x128 voxels, each 2.5x2.5x2.5mm^3, after deconvolution of the measured PSF. These data were actually recorded as 20 distinct views, with the detectors rotated through 9° between each view.

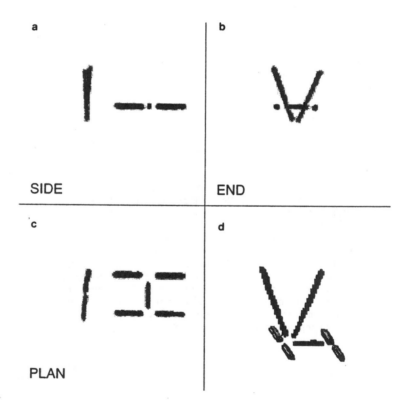

Fig. 2.   Four views of the 3D image of seven line sources (10^7 events) in 128x128x128
2.5x2.5x2.5mm^3 voxels: (a)-(c) are projected views showing (grey scale) the
maximum voxel contents in each column of 128 voxels; (d) is a 3D view of
those voxels having contents higher than 50% of the maximum.

Fig. 3 shows just the single horizontal tomograph, 2.5mm wide, containing the letter "H". Profiles in the axial and radial directions are shown for the full image constructed from 10^7 events; the FWHM resolution is seen to be approximately 8mm in each coordinate. The corresponding radial profile is also shown for two other images, obtained using just 10^6 and 2×10^5 events respectively. It is apparent that as less and less data is used the images become more and more noisy, making it necessary to impose additional smoothing in order to see the genuine features. It can be seen that, even for a relatively simple system such as this one, it is necessary to detect something of the order of 10^5 events in order to obtain an acceptable tomographic image.

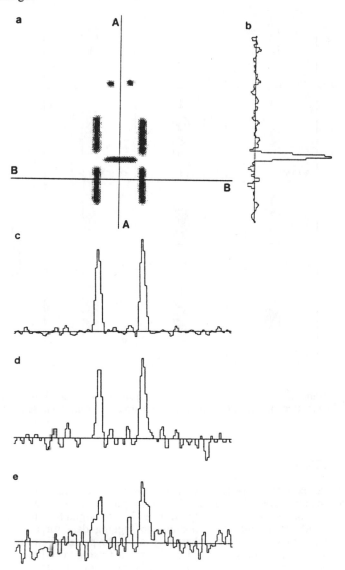

Fig. 3. (a) Single horizontal tomograph (2.5mm thick) from the image shown in Fig. 2
         (b) Axial profile across this tomograph between points AA
         (c) Radial profile between points BB
         (d) As (c), but constructed using only 10^6 events
         (e) As (c), but constructed using only 2×10^5 events

As an example of a real application in process tomography, Fig. 4 shows a sequence of vertical tomographs through the centre of a mould into which radiolabelled dough was hydraulically extruded. Each image corresponds to 60 secs data. The PET images show the formation of a blockage halfway down the mould after the initial rod of dough hit the bottom and became kinked, seriously hindering subsequent filling of the bottom of the mould.

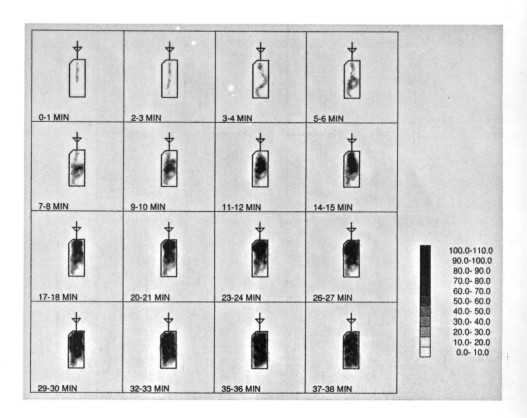

Fig. 4. Centre-plane vertical tomographs selected from a sequence showing extrusion of ^{68}Ga-labelled dough into a mould; each image comprises 60s data.

4. PARTICLE TRACKING

The initial impetus to explore the possibility of tracking a single particle came from the need to study processes which develop on timescales much shorter than a minute. As explained above, reconstruction of even a relatively simple 3D tomographic image requires the measurement of around 10^5 events, corresponding to logging data for at least 30s. It was realised that if it was known *a priori* that only a single positron emitting particle was present in the field of view, its location could be determined using very little data (hence in a very short time), since in principle all of the measured γ-ray paths should meet at its position. In the absence of undesirable experimental effects, therefore, measurement of just two events should be sufficient to locate the particle by "triangulation". In practice, of course, a significant fraction of the detected coincident events are "corrupt" and must be discarded, but whereas the paths of the "valid" events meet (to a good approximation) at a point, these "corrupt" events are broadcast randomly, so that if a sufficient number of events are compared it is possible to discriminate with reasonable success against the "corrupt" ones. As shown below, a sample of 80 events is found to be appropriate in many circumstances, and at a logging rate of 2500 events/s this means that the location of the particle can be determined approximately 30 times per second. Provided, therefore, that it is possible to introduce a positron-emitting particle whose motion faithfully follows that of its surrounding fluid, the particle tracking technique can be used to study high speed fluid motion.

Before applying the technique to systems of interest, it was necessary to develop and validate the location algorithms by tracking a particle under known conditions. The algorithm proceeds roughly as follows: given an initial sample of N detected coincidence events, the point in 3D space closest to which all these N γ-ray paths pass is found; then those paths which pass furthest from this point are rejected as "corrupt", and the process is repeated for the remaining paths; the algorithm iterates until only a fixed fraction f of the original N paths remain, whereupon these remaining paths are assumed to be "valid" and the point closest to which they all pass is taken as the location of the particle. The reliability of this algorithm was first investigated by using it repeatedly to locate a stationary particle (a 100 μCi ^{22}Na source) and establishing the scatter in the resulting values. For a wide range of values of N, the most consistent location was found to be achieved with a value of f of approximately 0.15, which corresponds to rejecting approximately 85% of the measured events.

It is interesting to compare this result with the expected contribution of "corrupt" events. These arise from two sources: (i) detection of events which do not in fact correspond to a pair of annihilation photons from a single positron annihilation, and (ii) events in which one or other of a genuine pair of annihilation photons has been scattered (either by scattering material within the field of view, or in the front part of the camera itself) prior to detection, so that its coordinates are shifted. Together, these two types of process are estimated to be responsible for approximately 60% of all detected coincident events from the ^{22}Na source. Presumably, the fact that optimum location is achieved when 85% of events are rejected indicates that the algorithm cannot perfectly discriminate between "valid" and "corrupt" events, and inevitably discards some valid events.

It was also found that, using a detector separation of 300mm, accurate location could be achieved over most of the field of view. Inevitably the accuracy becomes significantly poorer as the source approaches the extremes in the x or y directions, since the range of angles over which coincident pairs of γ-rays can be detected becomes too limited to provide good "triangulation".

For a stationary particle the precision of location can be arbitrarily improved by using larger and larger values of N, the number of events in the initial sample, which corresponds to measuring over a longer interval. For a moving particle this is no longer the case, since as the time interval increases movement of the particle during the period of measurement becomes significant, and, in general, at a given speed there is found to be an optimum value of N, which decreases with speed. Measurements were made on a particle fixed at a radius of 95mm on a turntable rotating at constant speed in the centre of the field of view, and the sequence of locations was determined using various parameter values in the tracking algorithm. Note that the time at which each event is detected is recorded (in tenths of a millisecond) so that after the algorithm has reduced the initial sample of N events to one containing only fN events, the time corresponding to the resulting location is just given by the average of these fN recorded times. Thus each location in fact comprises four values (x,y,z,t).

The precision of location in these turntable studies was determined by finding the scatter of the resulting locations about the known sinusoidal equation of motion of the particle (where in fact the exact parameters, such as the angular velocity and the starting coordinates, of this equation of motion were established by least-squares fitting to the sequence of locations). The resulting 3D location error, $\Delta = (\Delta_x^2 + \Delta_y^2 + \Delta_z^2)^{0.5}$, (where Δ_x represents the root mean square error in the x-direction, etc.) is shown as a function of speed in Fig. 5a for two orientations of the turntable. As already mentioned, the optimum value of the sample size varies with speed, and the results shown correspond to values of N ranging from 400 at low speed to 40 at the highest speeds. A dramatic difference is apparent between the results achieved with the two different orientations of the turntable, which is principally attributed to unreliable location when the source nears the edge of the field of view, as it does when the turntable is vertical (in the y-direction the source then moves to within 55mm of the edge). In all cases, as expected from the detection geometry, the error in the z direction dominates the value of Δ , being typically a factor of 3 larger than the errors in the other two directions.

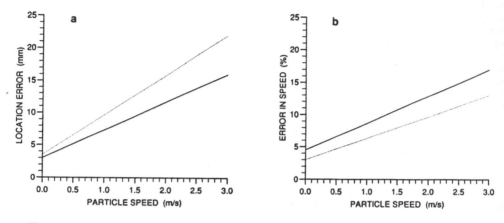

Fig. 5. Approximate r.m.s. error in (a) location, and (b) speed determination from tracking 100μCi ^{22}Na particle fixed at a radius of 95mm on a horizontal turntable (solid curve) and a vertical turntable (dashed line), as a function of particle speed.

Of equal interest is the precision in determining the instantaneous velocity of the particle. From a sequence of locations, the velocity can be obtained simply as the distance moved between successive locations divided by the difference in time. In fact it has been found more reliable to average over three successive points, so that the velocity $v_i = (v_{xi}, v_{yi}, v_{zi})$ associated with location i is given by

$$v_{xi} = \frac{(x_i - x_{i-1})}{2(t_i - t_{i-1})} + \frac{(x_{i+1} - x_i)}{2(t_{i+1} - t_i)} \quad , \qquad \text{etc.}$$

For the turntable studies, since the particle was moving at constant speed, it was most straightforward to analyse the velocity measurements in terms of the r.m.s. deviation of the measured speed, $v = \sqrt{v_x^2 + v_y^2 + v_z^2}$, from the true particle speed. The results are shown in Fig. 5b. Whereas in terms of precision in location the horizontal turntable results were superior to those from the vertical turntable, in speed determination the situation is entirely reversed. This arises from the fact that the particle location is always determined much more accurately in the x and y directions than in the z direction; in the case of the vertical turntable (rotating in the x/y plane) the poorly-determined z-coordinate has little effect on the overall speed determination.

It is clear that no simple single figure can be quoted for the accuracy of location or velocity determination which can be achieved by the tracking technique, since these depend not only on the position of the particle within the field of view but also on its speed, direction of motion, and acceleration. The curves shown in Fig. 5 provide a reasonable indication of what can be achieved for typical motion provided the particle does not approach the extremes of the field of view in the x or y directions. The situation can be broadly summarised as follows: at slow speeds (less than 0.1m/s) the particle can be located to an accuracy of better than 3mm in 3D, and its speed determined to within 5%, once every 0.2s; at a speed of 1m/s it can be located to within about 8mm and its speed measured to within 10% once every 0.04s. These results apply to a 100 μCi ^{22}Na source. For sources of different activity similar results are achieved, but the dependence on speed scales with the source strength, so that a 50 μCi ^{22}Na source travelling at a speed of 1m/s would be located with the same accuracy as a 100 μCi ^{22}Na source travelling at 2m/s. Because of the limit to the logging rate of the camera, it is not practical to track sources much stronger than 100 μCi.

When the active particle is surrounded by material, so that the emergent γ-rays suffer absorption and scattering, the accuracy of location is somewhat degraded, but not seriously provided the effect of absorption is compensated for by using a correspondingly stronger source.

To make the technique useful, it remains to develop positron-emitting particles which faithfully follow the flow streams within the system of interest. The simplest way to produce a positron-labelled particle is to encapsulate a small quantity of ^{22}Na, which has a half-life of 2.6 years, within, for example, a glass bead. However, it is difficult to produce particles smaller than several mm diameter in this way, and the density of the resulting particles is generally higher than desired. Furthermore, ^{22}Na is not an ideal radiolabel for two reasons. Firstly, its very long half life means that it is necessary to recover the particle at the end of the study to avoid problems with radioactive contamination of plant. Secondly, its decay mode involves the emission of a γ-ray of energy 1.27 MeV in addition to the pair of annihilation photons, and the Birmingham camera is unable to distinguish these γ-rays, which accordingly contribute to the detected "corrupt" coincidence events. In fact, more than one third of the detected "corrupt" events are attributable to this γ-ray, so that a significant improvement in location is anticipated if a pure positron-emitting radionuclide (without other γ-rays) could be used. Such a nuclide is ^{18}F, which has a half-life of 110 minutes and is produced by cyclotron irradiation of oxygen. One method for producing small particles containing ^{18}F is therefore to irradiate pellets of silica, and this technique has recently been developed at Birmingham, with 2mm diameter silica pellets.

As an illustration of the power of this tracking technique, Figs 7-9 show early results obtained tracking an 8mm steel capsule containing ^{22}Na in a small Lodige ploughshare mixer (Fig 6) partially filled with a powder of average grain size approximately 1mm. The mixer consists of a horizontal cylindrical chamber, 190 mm in diameter, with a central horizontal shaft fitted with two ploughshare blades which effectively divide the volume into three sections. Measurements were carried out with fill fractions ranging from 10% to 70% of the total mixer volume. Figure 7 shows the variation of the axial (x) location of the particle with time, over a 300 second period, for two different fill levels. At low fill, movement between the three sections of the mixer occurs irregularly. At high fill, on the other hand, the particle moves more continuously.

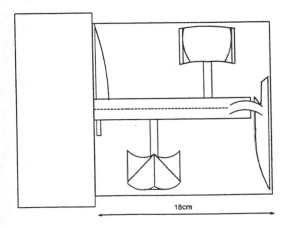

Fig. 6. Schematic diagram of the small Lodige powder mixer.

18cm

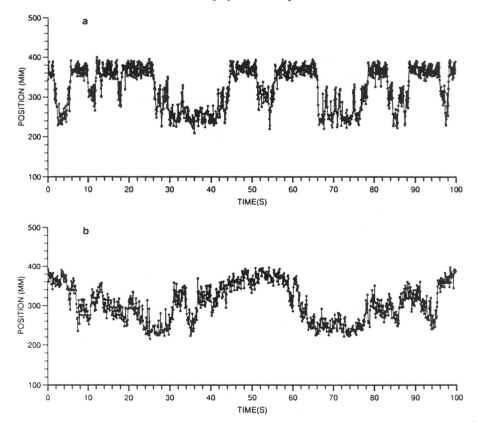

Fig. 7. Examples of tracking data obtained from the mixer: variation of axial location
over a period of 100s with (a) 16% fill, and (b) 70% fill.

In a closed system such as this, where the particle remains within the field of view for a long period, it is possible, in addition to analysing its path, to average the results over an extended period to obtain information on the fraction of the time the particle spends in each region and its average velocity at each point. For each fill level, the particle was tracked for a period of 1000 seconds, and the resulting set of locations provided the results presented in Figs 8 and 9. Fig. 8 shows the fraction of time spent in different radial regions, for the same two levels of fill shown in Fig 7: each location (x_i, y_i, z_i, t_i) is assigned to a particular 10mm square bin in the radial (y/z) plane, and it is assumed that the particle occupied this bin for a period $(t_{i+1} - t_{i-1})/2$ before moving to the bin corresponding to the next location. Note that in this way the data is automatically compensated for variations in detection efficiency (due to changing solid angle and possible variations in γ-ray absorption) as the particle explores different regions of the field of view - when the particle enters a region of lower detection efficiency the located points will be spaced further apart in time, but each will carry correspondingly greater weight when the entire set of locations is averaged. Although in these measurements the tracer particle was considerably larger than the powder and did not necessarily follow the bulk motion at all times, the distributions shown in Fig 8 are very similar to the expected bulk distribution. Similarly Fig 9 shows the average velocity in the y/z plane found within each 10mm square bin. It is doubtful whether any other technique can provide this type of information.

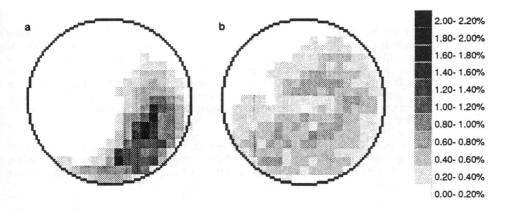

Fig. 8. Average occupancies in the radial plane of the mixer, integrated over 1000s: (a) 16% fill, and (b) 70% fill.

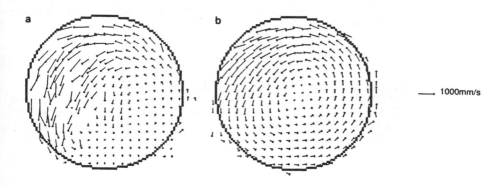

Fig. 9. Average y/z-velocity at each point in the radial plane of the mixer, integrated over 1000s: (a) 16% fill, and (b) 70% fill.

It should be noted that although Figs 8 and 9 show the variation in two-dimensions, the data are fully three-dimensional, so that, for example, distributions such as those shown could be separately presented for each axial location within the mixer. Furthermore, in addition to determining the average velocity at each point it is also possible to determine the spread of velocities and many other quantities, so that the method chosen for presenting the data is likely to depend very much on the particular application.

5. SUMMARY

The capabilities of the Birmingham positron camera for studies in process engineering have been briefly described. Conventional 3D tomographic imaging with a FWHM resolution of around 8mm is possible over a cylindrical field of view approximately 350mm long by 300mm in diameter, but generally requires several minutes to acquire sufficient data to form each image. A single positron-emitting particle can be located several times per second, to an accuracy of 3mm (in 3D) at low speeds and an accuracy of around 8mm at 1m/s; the corresponding accuracy in determining the particle's velocity ranges from around 5% at low speed to 10% at 1m/s.

In a closed system in which the labelled particle moves continuously around the field of view, provided its motion is representative of that of the surrounding fluid, the set of particle locations measured over an extended period can also be used to provide a tomographic image of the fluid. It is interesting to note that this may actually offer a more powerful way of observing the bulk distribution than conventional tomographic imaging, since in the latter technique the "corrupt" events distort the image in a way which can only partially be corrected after backprojection, whereas in the former "corrupt" events are largely discarded by the tracking algorithm.

ACKNOWLEDGEMENTS

The authors gratefully acknowledge the part played in this work by Dr P Fowles, C J Broadbent, T D Fryer and P McNeil, and financial support from the Science and Engineering Research Council, including support through its Specially Promoted Programme in Particulate Technology, and from Unilever Research.

REFERENCES

Clack R, Townsend D and Jeavons A 1984 *Phys. Med. Biol.* 29 1421
Hawkesworth M R, O'Dwyer M A, Walker J, Fowles P, Heritage J, Stewart P A E, Witcomb R C, Bateman J E, Connolly J F and Stephenson R 1986 *Nucl. Inst. and Meth.* A253 145
Hawkesworth M R, Parker D J, Fowles P, Crilly, J F, Jefferies N L and Jonkers G 1991 *Nucl. Instr. and Meth.* A310 423

Advances in and Prospects for the Use of Electrical Impedance Tomography for Modelling and Scale—up of Liquid/liquid and Solid/liquid Processes.

O M Ilyas, R A Williams, R Mann, P Ying and A M El—Hamouz
Department of Chemical Engineering, University of Manchester Institute of Science & Technology, P O Box 88, Manchester M60 1QD, U.K.

F J Dickin
Department of Electrical and Electronic Engineering, University of Manchester Institute of Science & Technology, P O Box 88, Manchester M60 1QD, U.K.

R B Edwards
Unilever Research Port Sunlight Laboratory, Quarry Road East, Bebington, Wirral L63 3JW, U.K.

A Rushton
British Nuclear Fuels plc, Springfields Works, Salwick, Preston PR4 0XJ, U.K.

ABSTRACT
Experimental results derived from a study of liquid/liquid mixing in a 0.29 m diameter baffled stirred tank using pseudo 3—dimensional electrical impedance tomography are presented and compared with complementary information derived from conventional visual interrogation (using dye tracers and video analysis) and predictive computational network mixing models. The work demonstrates the potential utility of electrical tomographic techniques in being able to provide hitherto inaccessible experimental data for design purposes. Future prospects for a number of important process engineering applications of the methodology are highlighted pertaining to liquid/liquid and solid/liquid mixtures.

1. Introduction

The design of process equipment for the purposes of dispersing and mixing components in similar or dissimilar phases represents a major and important step in many chemical and biological processes. In some instances the mixing process itself may also induce or involve a change of phase (*e.g.* precipitation and crystallisation).

The problem faced by process engineers attempting to design mixing or homogenisation systems for various types of mixtures is to optimise (a) the geometry of the equipment (b) the manner in which the process is performed (*e.g.* batch, continuous operation, how feed and products streams are added and removed from the reactor, respectively) (c) the ease of controlling and monitoring the process to avoid malfunction (*e.g.* to allow for maximum flexibility in the process throughput, or changes in the type of feed stream). Traditionally this situation has been approached with recourse to previous experience coupled with experimental investigation at a laboratory and then pilot–plant scale, since predictions from *first principles* are difficult due to the complex hydrodynamics encountered in most types of mixing processes.

Recently, the availability of powerful computational resources has allowed, to a limited degree, some direct prediction of mixing kinetics and behaviour using computational fluid dynamics calculations. For example, subject to certain limiting conditions, the mixing behaviour in standard stirred tanks coupled with a reaction kinetics model can be employed to predict the dynamic response in 2–dimensions in an axial direction. More sophisticated models also claim to produce 3–dimensional profiles, which are a useful guide for process design but are often difficult to validate experimentally without using invasive instrumentation. It is in this context that tomography offers the opportunity to radically transform the confidence of the design engineer in producing robust models for mixing phenomena and hence reliable simulations. Furthermore, tomographic experimentation has the potential of yielding results of direct use in the interpretation and control of process behaviour.

In this contribution, a particular case study will be described which exemplifies the use of electrical tomography for the interrogation of complex phenomena. The case study concerns the mixing of two miscible aqueous liquids, and exploits differences in the electrical conductivity of the two media.

2 Liquid Mixing Experiments

2.1 Imaging instrumentation

A medical electrical impedance instrument (IBEES Ltd, Sheffield) was adapted for use on a process vessel, to yield images showing the *relative changes* in electrical conductivity at various cross–sections of a mixing vessel. The system uses 16–electrodes and a fast back–projection algorithm to reconstruct measured data, as described in detail by Barber and Brown (1984). The images produced are semi–quantitative in the sense that the regions visualised as having different conductivities represent regions of relative change (scaled and normalised by the user and presented on an arbitrary colour scale) rather than quantitative values of the absolute conductivity. The 80x80 cubic pixels produced on the screen image represent a slightly higher spatial resolution than is justified in the strictest sense according to the reconstruction method employed. This had been achieved by interpolating between raw reconstructed zones (32x32 pixels) resulting in smoothing of the conductivity profiles.

The measurements presented in this work have been obtained by collecting measurement signals averaged over a period of 79 ms, typically at a frequency of one such measurement every 1 second. Experimental measurements were stored for reconstruction off–line, each image requiring about 2 seconds to render to the screen. The measurements were made using the adjacent electrode technique (Dickin et al., 1991) whereby one electrode pair is used to inject a small (5 mA) alternating current (50 kHz) whilst monitoring the resultant voltage at an adjacent electrode pair; this procedure being repeated for all electrode pair combinations. Measurements were made at four imaging planes, although it was not possible to perform data collection simultaneously. This necessitated that each test condition (Section 2.3) had to be repeated four times in order to collect measurements at each cross–section.

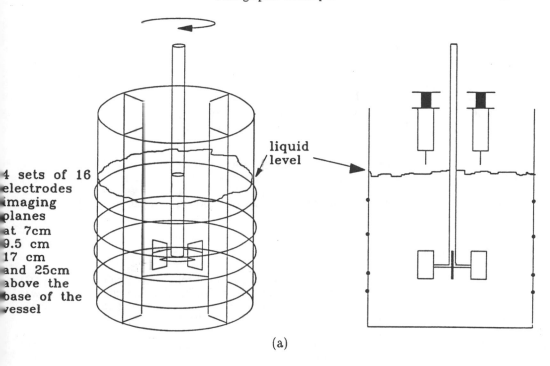

4 sets of 16
electrodes
imaging
planes
at 7cm
9.5 cm
17 cm
and 25cm
above the
base of the
vessel

liquid
level

(a)

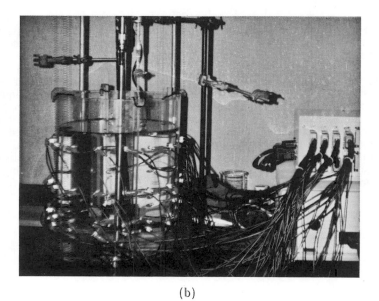

(b)

Figure 1: Experimental arrangement for interrogating batch mixing (a) showing location of image planes, baffles, stirrer and method of secondary liquid addition via four syringes (b) photograph of the axisymmetric instrumented tank, with a burette in position for asymmetric addition of secondary liquid.

2.2 Mixing vessel

Experiments were performed using a Perspex mixing tank 290 mm in diameter equipped with baffles and with agitation provided by a variable–speed six–bladed Rushton turbine impeller. The turbine was constructed from mild steel and mounted on an aluminium shaft, operating in the range of 0–200 rpm. The geometry of the tank was arranged so that it conformed to the standardised dimensions required to allow prediction of scale–up characteristics (Harnby et al., 1992). Sets of 16 electrodes were installed at four places across the vessel — two planes were in the vicinity of the impeller itself and the other two above the impeller, Fig. 1(a,b).

Mixing of miscible aqueous liquids was investigated by introducing the secondary liquid either *via* a burette or from a farm of syringes mounted just above the level of the primary liquid in the mixing tank, as shown in Fig. 1(a). For some tests the secondary liquid was added close to the impeller itself *via* a long narrow–bore tube adjacent to the impeller shaft.

2.3 Experimental procedures

The tank was filled with a primary liquid (0.1 wt. % NaCl solution, 1.9 mS cm^{-1} at 18 °C) to which an aliquot of the secondary solution (1 wt. % NaCl, 18.22 mS cm^{-1} at 18°C) was added. The volume of the aliquot(s) varied between 8–22 ml according to the particular experiment. Principally, two types of secondary liquid addition were employed.

(i) axisymmetric addition, in which the secondary liquid was introduced from four syringes mounted above the liquid level in the tank. This represents a condition in which the more concentrated liquid is added to the tank in a symmetric fashion.

(ii) asymmetric addition, in which the secondary liquid is added *via* one syringe, or from a burette, positioned midway across the radius of the tank. This represents an asymmetric method of addition.

In general the secondary liquid was added as a pulse over a short time interval (< 2s), although experiments could equally–well be performed whilst adding the secondary liquid over longer periods (Ilyas, 1992).

Experiments were performed to examine the influence of agitation rate (in terms of the rpm of the stirrer) and the symmetry of the addition of the secondary liquid. Parallel experiments were performed using injections of a Nigrosine dye–tracer, in place of the secondary liquid, and observing the resultant dispersion of the dye using a video camera. This provides complementary two–dimensional (vertical) information based on *external* observation of the tank for comparison with the two dimensional (horizontal) information derived from the *internal* observations facilitated by electrical impedance imaging. Theoretical simulations of the same experiments were also performed using a network simulation model, described below.

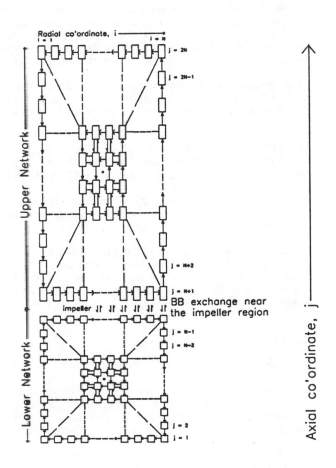

Figure 2: Simulation of mixing behaviour using a 2–d network of zones model for an impeller at one–third clearance.

2.4 Theoretical analysis of mixing behaviour

In the work reported here experiments have been conducted using an impeller at a clearance above the base of C = H/3 for a standard geometry tank with H = T. It is thus necessary to modify the former 'standard' single impeller. However, unlike previous work using the model at one–third clearance (Mann and El–Hamouz, 1991), instead of having an NxN network below the impeller and an Nx2N arrangement above the impeller (where all the cells are of equal volume), this development has retained the simpler (NxN)+(NxN) algorithm, but reduced the volume of the cells below the impeller by 2/3 and correspondingly increased the volume of the cells above the impeller by the factor 4/3.

Figure 2 shows the schematic arrangement of the zones. Note the ones above the impeller have been 'stretched' to accommodate the adjustment in zone volumes. To indicate the general N x N network structure, the outer loops of zones in this figure are shown partially complete.

The impeller is located between j = N and j = N+1. The focus of the lower circulation loops is between i = N/2 and i = N/2 + 1 and j = N/2 and j = N/2 + 1. The upper loop focus is then between i = N/2 and i = N/2 + 1 and j = (3/2)N and j = (3/2)N + 1.

For the present case, N has been chosen to be 20, which gives an overall total of 800 zones. This number represents a good compromise between having a reasonably fine spatial discrimination, without excessive computing time.

Each cell undergoes an equal and opposite exchange flow with adjacent cells in the lateral inner and outer flow loops which imitates the effect of turbulent exchange between parallel flowing streams of fluid which circulate by the action of the impeller. A turbulent exchange flow parameter of $\beta = 0.2$ provides accurate simulations of the experimental dispersion of inert and reactive tracers.

3 Experimental Results

3.1 Effect of agitation on mixing kinetics

Figure 3, shows a photograph of a time sequence of images for measurements performed at one cross–section (17 cm above the base of the tank), for asymmetric addition of the secondary liquid for three different impeller speeds. The major features of interest can be seen from these images (originally in colour but reproduced here in mono–tone).

Considering the sequence for 50 rpm, the first images (time = −1 s) is a 'reference' image obtained with the tank containing the primary liquid and whilst agitating the liquid. The second image (time = 0) corresponds with the time when the secondary liquid has been added, hence large changes in conductivity are perceptible from the image (the region of highest conductivity is the white core surrounded by a darker area). With continued mixing this high conductivity zone is dispersed until after 19 s no further statistical changes in the image can be deduced. Nevertheless having achieved a homogeneous mixture some artifacts associated with the conducting central impeller and wall conduction are seen on the final image.

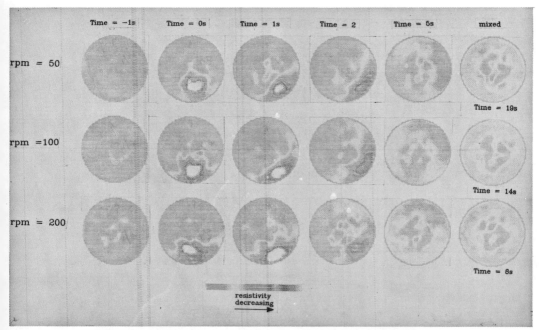

Figure 3: Effect of impeller speed on mixing following asymmetric addition of a secondary liquid (at time =0), visualised at a cross−section 17 cm above base of vessel.

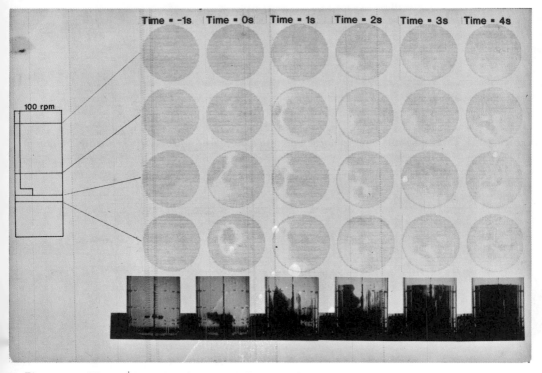

Figure 5: Three dimensional tomographic visualisation of asymmetric mixing compared with stills taken from a video−dye tracer mixing experiment.

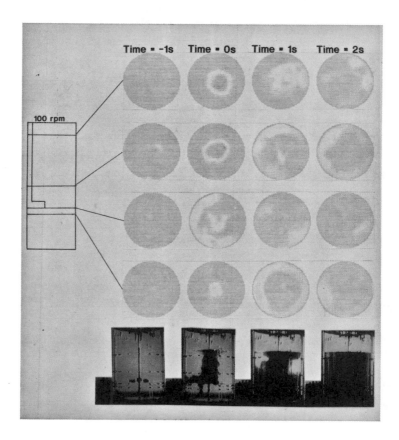

Figure 4: Three−dimensional tomographic visualisation of axisymmetric mixing compared with stills taken from a video dye−tracer experiment.

For tests performed at higher mixing speeds, some 'noise' is detected within the reference image (obtained with the primary liquid and stirred at the appropriate rate). On addition of the aliquot of concentrated solution, it is dispersed rather more effectively, and the corresponding times to achieve mixing to a homogeneous state were 14 s and 8 s for impeller speeds of 100 rpm and 200 rpm, respectively.

Hence, the tomographic method offers a convenient way to assess the mixing times required to achieve a uniform distribution of the secondary liquid. A comparison of data measured with those derived from theoretical considerations will be discussed in Section 3.3.

3.2 Axisymmetric and asymmetric mixing

Axisymmetric
Figure 4 compares cross–sectional images from electrical tomography with visual images obtained from external observation using a dye–tracer and captured on video for mixing at 100 rpm. Experimental measurements were made at the four image cross–sections (Figure 1(a)) by the axisymmetric addition of a second liquid. Video stills cropped from the video record are produced beneath the corresponding impedance image. The video still close to time t=0 (the time when the dye was injected) exhibits some asymmetry at the base of the plume to the left–hand side (the impeller is rotating in a clockwise direction). This feature is detected by the second image plane up from the base of the tank. Further similar asymmetric features are perceivable from the impedance image at time t = 1 s, *e.g.* on the third plane up from the base – the exact cross–sectional co–ordinates (x,y) locating such features could not be discerned from external video observations alone.

Asymmetric
In the sequences shown in Figure 5, the secondary liquid (and dye tracer) was added at one location just above the turbine region. On addition it is dispersed to the left–hand side (driven by the clockwise motion of the turbine at t = 1 s and then upwards (t = 2 s) also being broken up by the baffles. By adding the liquid close to the impeller, the mixing kinetics are very much faster than adding the liquid just below the level of primary liquid surface (Figure 3). As in the previous case the impedance tomograms allow detailed structure of the mixing characteristics to be followed, in a manner than could not otherwise be seen.

3.3 Comparison of mixing models with experimental images

Not only is electrical impedance tomography a non–intrusive experimental technique it also delivers a vast amount of information with respect to position and time in the mixing vessel. This sort of information is comparable to the type of data that is produced by predictive mixing models, and an example of such a model is the *networks of back–mixed zones* (Section 2.4). The network of zones model was used in a preliminary study to predict the mixing times for various impeller speeds (similar conditions and geometry to the experiments described in Section 3.1). The results obtained from the model were in excellent agreement with the electrical impedance images. For example the model predicted a mixing time of 13.8 s for an impeller speed of 100 rpm (Figure 6), while tomography gave a mixing time of 14 s (Figure 3).

This model comparison work has been extended to compare the concentration profiles predicted by the model with those obtained experimentally using electrical impedance tomography, and this work will be reported at a later date (Ilyas et al, 1992). It is envisaged that one of the potential applications for this technique is to help validate and improve modelling of mixing phenomena and hence optimise design of mixing equipment.

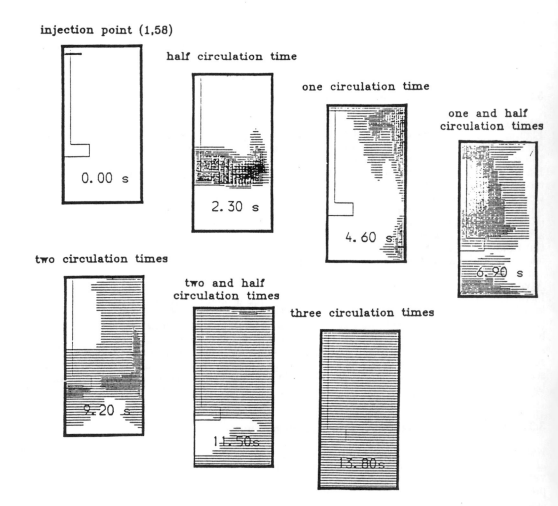

Figure 6:   Theoretical network mixing model for experimental conditions corresponding to axisymmetric mixing experiment at 100 rpm (Figure 3), which predicts a mixing time of 13.8s is required to produce a homogeneous mixture. Each diagram corresponds to a vertical slice through one half of the vessel (with the turbine on the left–hand–side). Circulation time corresponds to the period of time required for the turbine to 'turn–over' a volume of fluid equal to the volume of the vessel.

For instance, Figure 7 shows relative concentration profiles with time derived from the impedance images in Figure 4 along a line across the diameter of the tank at the top electrode sensor plane (25 cm above the base of the vessel).

Figure 7 has been constructed from the normalised pixel data files to produce a relatively crude scale (1–5) of the relative concentration with respect to the reference image (t=−1s). The symmetric addition of the secondary liquid is easily distinguished (t=0 s) and its dispersion with time (t=1, 2 s ..). Such procedures can be repeated for any line across a diameter through the cross–section as a function of time. Hence it is possible to construct relative concentration maps at multiple–planes in the mixing tank and to examine how they change with mixing time and mixing rate.

4 The Need for Quantitative Images and Intelligent Image Interpretation

4.1 Image quality versus dynamic response capability

From the perspective of a process design engineer it is imperative that any imaging device can produce information on a timescale and spatial dimension that is congruent with the process itself. For example, to observe mixing phenomena that are occurring over short periods of time in a small zone in the mixing vessel. Inevitably it would appear that some trade–off exists between the quality of the images that can be obtained (spatial resolution, sensitivity to conductivity changes, non–linearities in the sensing capability within a given cross–section) and the measurement time required to collect and average signals. Whilst there are applications for impedance tomography where the measurement (or "aperture") times could be quite long (a few seconds) if the process was in a steady–state condition, such a luxury cannot be afforded in the interrogation of mixing processes. In mixing, measurement times must be small, ideally in the range 0.1 − 50 ms. The frequency at which these measurements have to be repeated will vary according to the nature of the mixing process, but a value of 1 Hz is likely to be the lowest frequency acceptable and 100 Hz would be highly desirable. This specification, therefore, sets a target for those engaged in instrument design. Typically a baseline spatial resolution of 5% is sought, but the criterion of sensitivity is still not defined adequately. For laboratory purposes, the conductivity tracers employed in tests can be selected to suit the sensitivity of the instrumentation available, although for the more general purpose applications of impedance tomography there is a great need to define and quantify the performance of a given imaging system. This represents an urgent need which the process tomography community will have to address in the near future.

This discussion has, deliberately, not yet embraced the problem of image reconstruction. It is evident that the process–driven need to acquire information *via* short measurement 'snapshots' and to repeat this at a high frequency will impose a considerable information handling and computational burden. However, whilst this is a challenging problem, it should be borne in mind that the requirement to render such images in real–time is of very much lower priority than to succeed in producing the highest quality images possible. The implication being that the process engineering community will first need to be convinced that the technology is fundamentally sound and can assist in practical design problems, and the next stage is to speed up computational bottlenecks; it could be argued that the latter is largely a matter of financial resources.

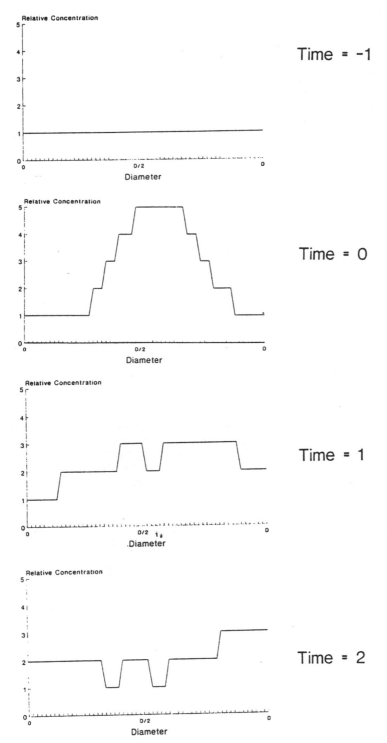

Figure 7: Relative concentration profiles across the mid—horizontal diameter of top imaging plane of Figure 4. as a function of time, computed from the pixel data.

4.2 Image interpretation

Obtaining a good quality image represents the first stage of information input to the process engineer. The ultimate goal is quantitative (numerical) interpretation of an image or, more likely, many hundreds of images corresponding to different spatial and temporal conditions. In most circumstances a visual diagnosis based on glancing at the images will be insufficient, except perhaps to diagnose gross malfunction of a process. This represents a major and fundamental difference between the general philosophy of medical tomography and that of process tomography. A second important distinction is that the images should ideally convey quantitative information rather than relative changes. For example, the work presented in this paper is based on subtracting measurements from a reference image. This has certain instrumental and algorithmic advantages but does not yield information in terms of measurable parameters, such as absolute electrical conductivities. Ultimately absolute measurements will be required, but this imposes quite severe demands on the models used to reconstruct the images and the manner in which the process is probed to extract the resistivity profile. These aspects are discussed in further detail elsewhere in this volume.

Hence assuming pixel–by–pixel data sets were available giving absolute conductivities in one or more cross–sections of a mixing vessel as a function of time, the image sets can be selected, plotted and re–analysed in the form required by the process engineer. For example, following the change in conductivity in a particular pixel with time, or in a vertical slice through the vessel. This represents the ultimate goal for impedance imaging of mixing processes, and carries with it the inherent implication that it will be possible to acquire and solve measurement information in 3–dimensions. This goal is not yet within our grasp, since the problem of solving interacting electrical field equations in a quantitative manner is by no means a trivial task.

4.3 Extension to solid–liquid systems

In principle, the same techniques can be applied to solid–liquid mixtures in order to discern the phase ratio or concentration profiles of solids in an aqueous–based continuum. Such systems are more difficult to work with and to calibrate, particularly if the solid phase exhibits any solubility in the continuous phase (Sinclair and Holdich, 1992) which will alter the conductivity of the liquid with time. The instrumentation system may also have to cope with additional 'noise' induced by solid particles impinging on the sensor electrodes. Nevertheless work is in progress to test impedance systems for interrogating cyclonic separators and hydraulic conveying processes.

5 Conclusions

This paper has demonstrated, for the first time, how the component concentration profiles derived using electrical impedance tomography can be compared with those obtained from dye tracer experiments and from a theoretical mixing model. The results are sufficiently encouraging to suggest that electrical impedance tomography is likely to have a number of important applications in process engineering, in particular, in the design of efficient process reactors and the manner in which they should be operated. Before the full potential of this technique can be realised it will be necessary to derive instrumentation that can produce quantitative information in terms of absolute conductivities and to acquire the information over 0.1–50 ms up to 100 times per second. The ultimate goal would be to perform such measurements at multiple–image planes simultaneously to produce a true 3–dimensional representation of mixing processes as a function of time.

Acknowledgements

This work was performed with the support of British Nuclear Fuels plc and Unilever Research in association with additional facilities provided by a European Coal and Steel Community Contract 7220/EA/829 and the Science and Engineering Research Council. The authors express their thanks to all the respective industrial partners involved.

References

Barber, D.C., and Brown, B.H., 1984, *J.Phys.E: Sci. Instrum.*, 17, 723–733.

Dickin, F.J., Williams, R.A., and Beck, M.S., (1991) "*Interrogation of multi–component mixtures in Process Vessels Using Electrical Impedance Tomography (EIT), I:Principles and process engineering applications*", submitted to *Chem. Eng. Sci.*

Harnby, N., Edwards, M.F., Nienow, A.W., 1992, *Mixing In The Process Industries*, 2nd Ed. (Oxford: Butterworth–Heinemann).

Holdich, R.G. and Sinclair, I., 1992 "*Measurement of slurry solids content by electrical conductivity*", *Powder Technol.* (in press).

Ilyas, O.M., 1992 "*Interrogation of Liquid/Liquid and Solid/Liquid Processes Using Electrical Impedance Tomography*", M.Sc. Thesis, University of Manchester Institute of Science & Technology.

Ilyas, O.M., Williams, R.A., Mann, R., Ying, P., Dickin, F.J., Edwards, R.B. and Rushton, A., 1992, to be submitted for publication.

Mann, R. and El–Hamouz, A.M., 1991, "*Effect of Macromixing on a competitive/consecutive reaction in a semi–batch stirred reactor*", Proc. 7th Europ. Conf. on Mixing, Brugges, 1.

Use of Tomographic Technology for Fluid–Based Conveying Processes

S L McKee, T Dyakowski and R A Williams

Department of Chemical Engineering, University of Manchester Institute of Science & Technology, P.O. Box 88, Manchester, M60 1QD, U.K.

ABSTRACT

This paper focuses attention upon instrumentation that is capable of interrogating the behaviours encountered in solid/liquid and solid/gas conveying. A critical review of relevant sensor technologies for measurements with dense phase and light phase mixtures is presented. It is demonstrated that dielectric and resistivity sensors appear to offer particular advantages and can be used to provide 2–dimensional images which can be used in enhancing the modeling of conveying processes. The principles, uses and limitations of such systems, are illustrated.

1 Introduction

The reliance of process engineers upon past experience in the design of process plant is well established. Some modeling techniques can be employed to describe a process, often inherently assuming conditions which, in reality, can deviate considerably from the true performance of a process vessel. However, the ability to interrogate the contents of such vessels, by imaging the interior, is provided by application of various tomographic techniques. Possible tomographic sensing methods include optical, radiation–based, ultrasound and electrical (resistive and capacitance) techniques. The potential simplicity of the electrically–based tomographic sensing methods lends the technique to an immediate and wider range of industrial examples than, for example, radiation–based tomography. For this reason, the prime focus of attention will be upon the use of capacitance and resistive sensors to investigate gas/solid and solid/liquid systems. The latter sensors are classified as being soft field, that is the sensing field is influenced by the physical nature of a mixture/flow being imaged. In contrast, with hard field sensors, as utilized in radiation based tomography, the sensing field is independent of the nature of the subject under interrogation and the spatial definition of the sensing zone is better delineated.

2 Principles of transportation processes

2.1 Hydraulic and pneumatic operations

Hydraulic and pneumatic conveying can be employed to transport solids over long distances, sometimes several hundred kilometres, which may offer a less expensive method than conventional transportation by road or rail. Conveying processes can also prove a more economic method of disposal, as for example in the hydraulic transport of sewage sludge, suggested by Raynes & Larson (1971), to aid in the reclamation of land, as opposed to the normal procedure of incineration. Further, the use of a pipeline designated for the conveying of a specific substance, such as a pharmaceutical, will negate the possibility of any extraneous contamination.

Considering the case of solid/liquid transportation, a range of flow regimes can occur, subject to process parameters such as phase volume fraction of solids, flow velocity, hydraulic pressure gradient and the physical properties of both the solid and the suspending liquid. The particle size of solids also has a significant effect upon the resultant flow regime produced. Generally, a slurry is identified as being either *homogeneous* or *heterogeneous*. In the former, a high concentration of fine solids is suspended, while the latter is characterized by an asymmetric distribution of solids in the suspending liquid, with particles readily demonstrating a tendancy to settle and form either a moving or a stationary bed of particles on the base of a horizontal pipeline. The velocity at which such a situation can arise is referred to as the critical deposition velocity, u_{crit}, and represents a fundamental parameter in the design of slurry pipelines. The variation of pressure drop on mean slurry velocity is illustrated in Figure 1, with the minimum on the curve corresponding to the critical deposition velocity. Another phenomenon characteristic of a heterogeneous slurry is saltation, in which the suspension of particles due to turbulence, is surpassed by gravitational force and particles are subsequently suspended and deposited periodically on the surface of a moving or stationary bed. A frequently used correlation in the classification of flow regimes is that proposed by Newitt *et al* (1955), involving mean slurry velocity, u, and mean particle diameter, d_p. Typical ranges for significant parameters encountered in hydraulic conveying are also highlighted on Figure 1, namely, the phase volume fraction of solids, ϕ, the ratio of solids density, ρ_s, and the fluid density, ρ_f. Characteristic pipe diameters for both pneumatic and hydraulic conveying can be considered to lie in the range 50 mm to 2 m.

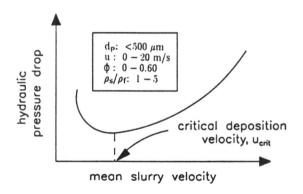

Figure 1 Variation of pressure drop with mean slurry velocity
for hydraulic conveying in a horizontal pipe

In horizontal pneumatic conveying, the flow regimes encountered are largely dependent upon the suspending gas velocity. As the velocity is reduced the trend is for the distribution of solid particles to become progressively less uniform. Eventually, a moving bed of particles can form coupled with a saltation effect similar to that described above. At sufficiently low velocity, the particle bed can build up to result in a blockage of the conveying line. Clearly, the flow velocity is significant and, as in the design of pipelines for hydraulic conveying, both the flow velocity and pipeline pressure drop represent essential design parameters. Figure 2 illustrates the change in pressure drop with superficial gas velocity, defined as the volumetric gas flowrate divided by the cross sectional area of the pipe. The diagram also suggests a suitable range for the loading factor, LF, defined as the ratio of the mass flow of particles to the mass flow of gas. Figure 3 shows images obtained, by the authors, using a capacitance tomography instrument for different flow behaviours encountered in horizontal pneumatic conveying.

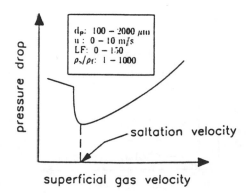

Figure 2 Variation of pressure drop with gas velocity
for horizontal pneumatic conveying

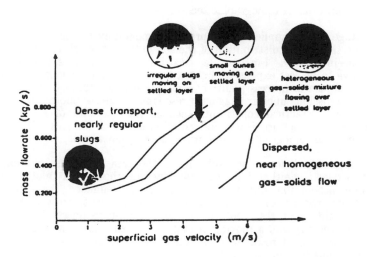

Figure 3 Variation of mass flowrate with superficial gas velocity
for horizontal pnuematic conveying

In vertical pneumatic conveying, the choking velocity is a significant parameter representing a gas velocity so low that a sequence of 'slugs' result. Generally, as the superficial gas velocity is decreased, a transition from dilute–phase to dense–phase will be observed. Pneumatic transport with low air velocity allows pressure drop to be minimized and as a consequence to reduce the amount of energy provided to the compressor. For vertical pneumatic transport, the relationship between pressure drop and superficial gas velocity is illustrated in Figure 4.

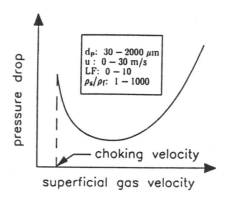

Figure 4 Variation of pressure drop with gas velocity
for vertical pneumatic conveying

2.2 Potential applications of tomographic techniques

A prime advantage in the application of process tomography to such systems, is the ability to explore the spatial distribution of the contents of a vessel, in an intrinsically safe manner, non—invasively. Further, electrical tomography is an attractive method since it may prove to be less expensive, have a better dynamic response and be more portable for routine use in process plant than radiation based tomographic techniques such as positron emission, nuclear magnetic resonance, gamma photon emission and X—ray tomography. Practical constraints such as the diameter of a large process vessel, will render the direct application of radiation—based techniques difficult and in this instance, electrical tomography would prove more advantageous.

Other process applications for tomography lie in the area of process control, in the detection of blockages in either full—scale pipelines or those of a pilot plant — to identify possible production difficulties would greatly enhance the efficiency of operation. The flow regimes discussed previously could be identified with ease and so further act as an aid to process control. In the case where flow velocity is below critical deposition velocity and a moving or stationary bed results, access to real time images would allow a rapid response to be taken, thereby allowing the operation to continue without being further impaired.

The accurate determination of flow velocity, used in basic design equations for the design of both pipelines and pump power requirements, will enable a process engineer to refine the design of such equipment cost—effectively. Process tomography should also enhance an understanding of particle dynamics for both steady and unsteady flow and further, assist in the validation of fundamental design equations through accurate determination of parameters such as phase mass flowrate and flow velocity. The spatial variation of solids concentration and velocity should be readily determined, along with concentration profiles as a function of concentration, particle size distribution and flow velocity.

3 Current status of suitable tomographic technology

The application of tomographic techniques to the process industry can still be regarded as being in its infancy, in contrast to the extensive uses found in the medical field. However, to date tomography has assisted in understanding the mechanics of various processes ranging from liquid distribution in a trickle bed reactor (Lutran *et al*, 1991) to fluidization in a gas–fluidized bed (MacCuaig *et al*, 1985). Among the techniques which have been utilized are gamma–ray, X–ray and electrical tomography. This section will highlight some recent studies concerned with flow, which reflect the potential applications of tomography.

With reference to capacitance and resistance tomography, both methods essentially rely upon the use of electrodes placed around the periphery of a process vessel or pipe, the electrodes in the capacitance unit being much larger than those used in resistance tomography. In contrast to capacitance tomography, the electrodes used in resistance tomography do penetrate the pipe wall in order to establish electrical contact with the process mixture. Capacitance tomography can be used to interrogate electrically insulating fluids, while resistance tomography is associated with conducting fluids. Figure 5 illustrates the basic components of a process tomography system. Each tomographic arrangement comprises two units of hardware, the electrodes and a data acquisition system, and one unit of software, the image reconstruction and image interpretation system. The capacitance tomography system measures the sensitivity distribution between electrode pairs and through the use of a suitable reconstruction algorithm, the dielectric distribution is determined. Measurements between all possible combinations are made and the information is utilized by the image reconstruction system, via the data acquisition system, to reconstruct a 2–D image of the dielectric distribution within a vessel. In electrical resistive tomography, one sensor excitation approach that may employed, is to inject alternating current into an electrode pair, while the potential at all other electrodes is measured. As in capacitance tomography, the data acquisition system supplies the image reconstruction system with all the information necessary, but in this case an image of the electrical resistivity profile is produced. The final and important stage is to interpret the images and so extract *quantitative* information pertaining to the process under investigation. For instance, as indicated in Figure 5, the component concentration at a given location [c(x,y)] as a function of time. Without a quantitative image interpretation facility, any wholly qualitative visual image is of limited use to the process engineer.

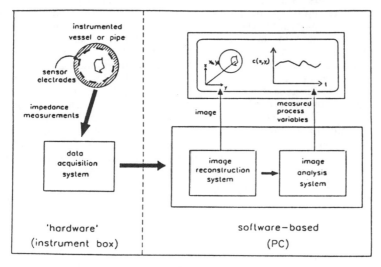

Figure 5 Basic components of a process tomographic instrument

3.1 Static flow

Capacitance tomography has successfully facilitated imaging solid/gas conveying. An early publication by Huang *et al* (1989) discussed the experimental application of this technique to the imaging of two component flow. Eight brass electrodes were mounted in the same plane around the periphery of a three–inch diameter Perspex pipe and, after selecting a pair of electrodes, one was charged and discharged continuously, while the other was earthed. Measurements of capacitance between all possible combinations of electrodes, generating a total of 28 independent measurements, then enabled a linear backprojection algorithm to replicate the dielectric distribution. Such was the procedure applied in the static imaging of various simulated flow regimes of sand in a pipe, from annular to core flow. However, this early study recognised the limitations of this unit in the form of low resolution and slow image speed. Further, image distortion was found to occur due to the assumptions that the influence of the sensitivity distribution of the sensors upon the dielectric distribution was negligible and also that changes in measured capacitance arose due to a uniform dielectric change over the entire cross section of the pipe. Subsequently, it was deemed necessary to improve the reconstruction algorithm. In this study, the data collection time for 28 measurements was 5 ms, while the reconstruction time was 5 s. An improvement on these figures was reported by Salkeld *et al* (1990) to 2.5 ms and 48 ms respectively. This was achieved by employing T414 transputers, but the spatial resolution of the images obtained was still impaired by the limited number of measurements which could be made. To overcome these difficulties, current work at UMIST involves the use of 12 electrodes and consequently 66 measurements of capacitance. A 20 x 20 pixel grid array is being used, as opposed to the 64 grid array employed in the study of Salkeld *et al* (1990). Images can be obtained at a rate of 40 frames per second by the use of five T800 transputers. These modifications have subsequently shown an improvement in the spatial resolution of the images obtained.

3.2 Flow in fluidized beds

Investigation of the solids concentration in a circulating fluid bed was conducted by Azzi *et al* (1991) using gamma radiation, with the aid of a suitable source and detector. The industrial unit studied was a gas–oil fluidized catalytic cracking vessel, with particular attention focused upon the distribution of catalyst within a riser pipe. Ultimately, with the aid of a suitable reconstruction algorithm, local density measurements were replicated in the form of density maps. However, the resolution of such images was impaired by the limited number of measurements which could be made. An improvement in the resolution of the technique has enabled Martin *et al* (1992) to produce better quality images, as illustrated in Figure 6, which shows the density map of a catalyst in an industrial riser, for a superficial gas velocity of 25 m/s. Extensive work on gas fluidization by Halow (1992) at the Morgantown Energy Centre, USA, employed capacitance tomography in analysing fluidized beds. The imaging system comprised four sets of 32 electrodes positioned at various depths along the height of the bed. The images obtained revealed hitherto inaccessible information on the process of void coalescence and on void shapes. Plots of the average void fraction versus time also facilitated determining characteristics of the resultant bubbles, such as bubble rise velocity and bubble length. A notable achievement in this work was the direct observation of bubble coalescence phenomena. An image of the cross–section of a void, with the lighter regions representing areas of low solids volume fraction and the darker regions representing areas of high void fraction, is illustrated in Figure 7.

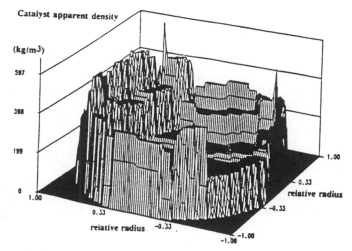

Figure 6 Density map of catalyst in an industrial riser unit visualized
using γ–ray tomography
[from Martin *et al* (1992)]

A study of the mechanics of fluidization in the jet region of a gas–fluidized bed, was
addressed by MacCuaig *et al* (1985) and Seville *et al* (1986) by the use of gamma–ray
tomography. The former study looked at a fluidized bed, having a diameter of 51 mm
and an average bed height of 60 mm. Compressed air fluidized a bed of either ballotini
or quartz sand, using a minimum fluidization velocity of 5 cm/s and 11.4 cm/s,
respectively. The experiments were found to successfully yield density profiles, but the
physical size of the apparatus limited its application to only small scale investigations.
A larger fluidized bed was studied by Seville *et al* (1986), having a diameter of 14.6 cm
and a bed height of 15 cm. In this instance, the minimum fluidization velocity
achieved was 9.2 cm/s. The images obtained, facilitated a comparison with various
proposed correlations related to the height of the jet.

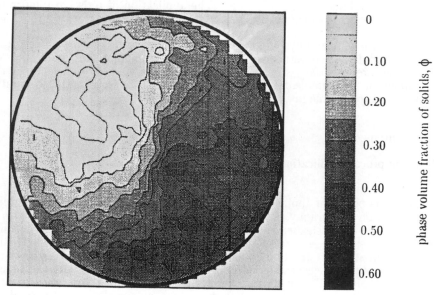

Figure 7 Cross–sectional image of a large gas bubble visualized
using capacitance tomography
[from Halow (1992)]

3.3 High and low velocity flows

Tomographic interrogation of pneumatic conveying in both vertical and horizontal pipelines, for light and dense phase respectively, was reported by Plaskowski *et al* (1991) and for dense phase by Williams *et al* (1992). In the former, rape seed was transported in a glass flow rig and the tomographic arrangement employed was essentially similar to that of Huang *et al* (1989). Air velocities ranged from 20 m/s, for the light phase transportation, to 5 m/s for the dense phase. Solids velocity was measured using two capacitance transducers as part of a cross correlation system. Quality images were achieved of stratified flows, but at high velocity and low volume concentration of solids, distinct images were unable to be obtained. The errors with the technique were the frequently cited assumptions related to the sensitivity distribution between electrodes and those inherent in the reconstruction algorithm. Williams *et al* (1992) also highlighted the use of an eight electrode capacitance system to investigate the conveying of a dense phase. In this instance, the air velocity employed resulted in the formation of particulate slugs within the pipeline with a good correlation between reconstructed images and those obtained by external visual observation.

In summary, the current limitations of capacitance tomography include resolution and image speed. Improvements with respect to both of these will be achieved by advancing the reconstruction algorithm, which will be discussed later.

3.4 Solid/liquid flow

It has been suggested that both *component* mass flowrates and velocities in solid/liquid flow can be obtained by the use of resistance tomography (Dickin *et al*, 1991). In hydraulic conveying the distribution of solids is frequently non–uniform and the velocities can vary considerably. To obtain the volumetric flowrate, the velocity profile has to be determined and to this end, a cross correlation system could, in principle, be employed to compare images obtained at two different locations along a horizontal pipe. Mass flowrates then result from knowledge of the component velocity, density and phase volume fraction of solids. The application of resistive tomography to solid/liquid processes is discussed by Ilyas *et al* (1992), elsewhere in this publication.

Although resistance tomography differs from capacitance tomography with respect to measurements and details concerned with the reconstruction algorithm, the limitations of the techniques are essentially similar, in the form of poor spatial resolution, due to a limited number of measurements, and the requirement for substantial computing resources to enable real–time image reconstruction.

4 Future requirements

4.1 Advancing process applications

A summary of the potential applications of process tomography is provided in Table 1. Without the use of tomography, a broad spectrum of instruments would have to be employed to obtain the measurements highlighted. As an example, one approach to measuring solids velocity, in vertical pneumatic conveying, is to use electrodynamic transducers (Williams *et al.* 1991). During the transport of gas/solid flows, electrostatic charge can be generated due to particle/particle collisions and collisions of particles with the pipe wall. and to this end a cross–correlation system, incorporating two separated sensors, was employed to determine the average velocity of the solids.

In the example cited (Xie *et al*, 1989), the two detecting electrodes used were separated by a distance of 50 mm on the exterior of a vertical Perspex pipe to interrogate the flow, of polypropylene plastic granules at varying mass flowrates. The main error in measured velocity was attributed to errors with respect to transit–time measurement. This itself is an inherent property of the cross–correlation technique, the standard deviation of such measurements being largely influenced by the properties of the solids. Despite this, the errors associated with transit–time measurement were low, being in the range 0.2% to 0.6 %. Similar methodology was employed to determine mass flowrate of solids falling under gravity via the measurement of solids concentration, involving a combination of electrodynamic and capacitance transducers. As in the preceeding example, the electrodynamic transducers enabled stream velocity to be determined. Two different configurations were used, with respect to electrode dimensions and position, but each comprising an electrode pair surrounded by a screen. Measurements obtained with flows of sand were found subject to errors. Principally, the errors were attributed to the non–uniform sensitivity field distributed over the entire pipe cross–section and, more fundamentally, measurements associated with the capacitance transducers such as the influence upon resultant measurements by electrostatic charge, arising from particle collisions. Such impairments limit the application of this arrangement to systems in which particle recirculation is absent from the flow. These restrictions on information derived from averaging signals from transducer pairs traversing the pipe, are not encountered in the application of process tomography.

Purpose	Measurements
Equipment design	Component distribution
Process modeling	Quantitative concentration gradients
Process control	Dynamic changes
Process monitoring:	Flow regime identification
	Velocity measurements
	Mass flowrate measurements
	Component flow measurements
	Component velocity and mass flowrate measurements

Table 1 Potential applications of process tomography
and associated measurements

There are a number of parameters of prime concern in establishing the specification of a process tomographic instrument. As an illustrative example, Table 2 provides a synopsis of the typical specifications for an electrical resistive instrument.

Parameter	Specification
Number of electrodes	32
Frame acquisition time	40 ms
Reconstruction time	24 s
Spatial resolution	12%
Imaging rate	100 frames/s
Sensitivity	?

Table 2 Specification of a typical resistive tomographic instrument

Figure 8 provides a general summary of two aspects of prime concern; variation of flow regimes with carrier fluid velocity and spatial resolution of the tomographic image. Existing resistive tomographic techniques can achieve a spatial resolution of 12% or greater, for both homogeneous and heterogeneous flow.   The diagram also highlights the regions which can be employed by either hard or soft field sensors.   The shaded region represents currently unexplored territory and as sensitivity and spatial resolution improve, the limiting boundaries for both homogeneous and heterogeneous flow will be pushed—back.

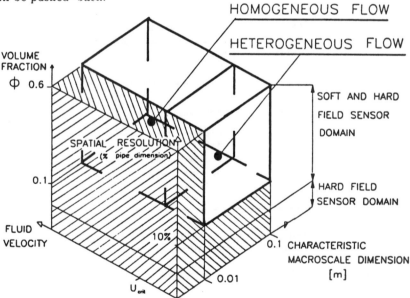

Figure 8 Limits of tomography defined by spatial resolution and geometrical dimension

One of the key parameters in Table 2, is the imaging rate and this dictates the ability of the technique to interrogate fluid systems in both micro— and macro—time scales. An important parameter which can be used to characterize particle motion is relaxation time (Hestroni, 1989), representing the time taken for a particle to accelerate to 63% of the carrier fluid velocity, for Stokes interaction only, between fluid and particles. As an example, the relaxation time for particles having a diameter of 250 mm, is about 10 ms. Subsequently, this imaging rate of 100 frames/s, enables particle motion, under turbulence, to be followed on a micro—scale basis. With respect to flow regimes, characteristic time scale for changing from one flow pattern to the another, is of the order of 100 ms. Thus the tomographic technique can be used to witness flow transition from one pattern to another.

4.2 Limitations and improvements in electrical tomography

Referring to Figure 5, it should be noted that tomography involves the solution of both a forward and an inverse problem, to result in the production of an image. The forward problem of resistivity tomography is influenced by such phenomena as spatial variation of current density and physical processes in the vicinity of electrodes. Currently, knowledge of such physical phenomena is limited. Also it is well established that noise, associated with the data acquisition system, can affect the intensity of the measured impedance signal, and it is these physical constraints which limit the dimensions of the electrodes.

The inverse problem for resistive tomography is concerned with obtaining an image of the resistivity distribution, while the inverse problem for capacitance tomography aims at producing an image of the dielectric distribution. The reconstruction algorithm is a function of electric field properties, for both hard and soft field sensors. Ultimately, significant improvements in spatial resolution and image quality lie in the development of a reconstruction algorithm which recognizes the non—linearity of the sensing field. Simply increasing the number of electrodes does improve both image quality and resolution, but at a cost to the procurement of images in real time, required for on—line process control, since the reconstruction of images requires longer computation time. Future efforts should concentrate upon advancing the reconstruction algorithm and interpretating images to obtain quantitative data which can be used by the process engineer to effectively design process equipment.

Awknowledgements

The authors would like to thank the SERC, for the provision of a studentship for SLM, and the Particle Science & Technology group at E.I. du Pont de Nemours & Co., USA, for their support of this work.

References

Azzi, M., Turlier, P., Bernard, J.R., and Garnero, L. (1991) "Mapping solid concentration in a circulating fluid bed using gammametry", Powder Technol., 67, p27.

Dickin, F.J., Williams, R.A., and Beck, M.S. (1991) "Interrogation of multi—component mixtures in process vessels using EIT. 1. Principles and process engineering applications", Chem. Eng. Sci., (submitted).

Halow, J.S. (1992) "Application of capacitance imaging to fluidized beds", U.S. Dept. of Energy, Morgantown, WV, in "Process Tomography — Principles, Techniques & Applications", (to be published by Butterworth — Heinemann).

Hestroni, G. (1989) "Particles—turbulence interaction", Int. J. Multiphase Flow, **15**, p735.

Huang, S.M., Plaskowski, A.B., Xie, C.G., and Beck, M.S. (1989) "Tomographic imaging of two—component flow using capacitance sensors", J. Phys. E : Sci Instrum., **22**, p173.

Ilyas, O.M., Dickin, F.J., Mann, R., Williams, R.A., Ying, P., Edwards, R.B., and Rushton, A. (1992) "Advances in and prospects for the use of electrical impedance tomography for modelling and scale—up of liquid/liquid and solid/liquid processes", (in this volume).

Lutran, P.G., Ng, Ka M., and Delikat, E.P. (1991) "Liquid in trickle beds. An experimental study using computer — assisted tomography", Ind. Eng. Chem. Res., **30**, 6, p1270.

MacCuaig, N., Seville, J.P.K., Gilboy, W.B., and Clift, R. (1985) "Application of gamma—ray tomography to gas fluidized beds", Appl. Optics, **24**, 23, p4083.

Martin, M.P., Turlier, P., Bernard, J.R., & Wild, G. (1992) "Gas and solid behavior in cracking circulating fluidized beds", Powder Technol. (to be published).

Newitt, D.M., Richardson, J.F., Abbott, M., and Turtle, R.R. (1955) "Hydraulic conveying of solids in horizontal pipelines", Trans. Inst. Chem. Eng., **33**, p93.

Plaskowski, A., Bukalski, P., Habdas, T., and Solimowski, J. (1991) "Tomographic imaging of process equipment — application to pneumatic transport of solid material", Proc. 5th Conf: "Sensors & their Applications", Edinburgh, in Grattan, K.T.V. (Ed) "Sensors : Technology, Systems & Applications", Adam Hilger (Bristol) p215.

Raynes, B.C., and Larson, H.F. (1971) "Economic transport of digested sludge slurries", in Zandi, I. (Ed) "Advances in Solid—Liquid Flow in Pipes and its Applications", 1st Edn, Pergamon Press (Oxford), p211.

Salkeld, J.A., Hunt, A., Thorn, R., Dickin, F.J., Williams, R.A., Conway, W.F., and Beck, M.S. (1990) "Tomographic imaging of phase boundaries in multi—component processes", in Williams R.A. and de Jeager, N.C. (Eds) "Advances in Measurement & Control of Colloidal Processes", Butterworth—Heinemann, (Oxford) p 95.

Seville, J.P.K., Morgan, J.E.P., and Clift, R. (1986) "Tomographic determination of the voidage structure of gas fluidized beds in the jet region", in Oestergaard, K and Sorensen, A. (Eds) "Process Fluidization V : Engineering Foundation Conference", Eng. Found. (New York), p87.

Williams, R.A., Dickin, F.J., Dyakowski, T., Ilyas, O.M., Abdullah, Z., and Beck, M.S. (1992) "Looking into mineral process plant?", Minerals Eng., **5**, 8, (in press).

Williams, R.A., Xie, C.G., Dickin, F.J., Simons, S.J.R., and Beck, M.S. (1991) "Multi—phase flow measurements in powder processing", Powder Technol., **66**, p203.

Xie, C.G., Stott, A.L., Huang, S.M., Plaskowski, A., and Beck, M.S. (1989) "Mass—flow measurement of solids using electrodynamic and capacitance transducers", J.Phys. E: Sci. Instrum., **22**, p 712.

A Prototype Distributed Pressure Sensor Utilising Electrical Impedance Tomography; Initial Results

I Basarab-Horwath, M Faraj
School of Engineering Information Technology
Sheffield City Polytechnic
Sheffield
S1 1WB

Abstract

A prototype pressure sensor has been constructed to measure distributed planar pressure. The transduction element is a conductive elastomer sheet; the applied pressure produces resistance changes in the sensor element. These changes can be measured using tomographic techniques. Initial results for different loads and elastomers are described and discussed.

The main objective of the work described in this paper is to develop a sensor to measure distributed pressures. The distributed pressures are applied to a planar conductive elastomeric material; these produce a graded response in the deformable sensor element.   The space-distributed changes in dimension due to the applied load result in local changes in resistance; these can be measured using electrical impedance tomography. Such a sensor would be used to obtain tactile information.

Tactile sensing provides information about the state of contact between the sensor element and object or load and the magnitude and distribution of that contact. There is an obvious application in robot gripping. Tactile sensing normally refers to skin-like properties; that is, properties with which areas of force sensitive surfaces are capable of reporting graded signals and parallel patterns of touching (1, 2, 3). Tactile sensors are based on direct measurement force transducers - these force transducers are arranged in a two-dimensional area and measure the mechanical deformation produced by the applied force acting on each transducer. Tacile sensors have been constructed using a wide variety of technologies, eg resistive, capacitive, optical and inductive methods. These are well documented in the literature (1, 2, 3). There are advantages and disadvantages with each technology. However, the basic concept has been to produce an array of tactels and to interrogate each tactel to determine the applied load. In the sensor described in this paper, there are no individual tactels; instead the whole 'array' is interrogated

The sensor element is a conductive elastomer. The elastomeric materials used in this reported experimental work were obtained as samples from an industrial company manufacturing rubber products. They are designed to be used in sensor applications; force/resistance curves are shown in Figure 1. It can be seen that there are two distinct types of material; one type gives a graded response while the other type has a switching characteristic. Results from both types of material are reported in this paper.

The main problem encountered in the construction of the transduction element was in the formation of good, reliable electrical connections to the elastomer sheet. These connections had to be such that the elastomer sheet could be removed and replaced with other elastomer sheets. It has been found from previous unpublished work, by Basarab-Horwath et al, that gluing electrodes to the polymer surface does not produce a reliable connection. For this prototype device, it was decided to use a pressure type connection whereby brass screws with flat ends were vertically screwed down to make a firm contact with the surface of the conductive elastomer. Care has to be taken to limit this pressure so as not to damage the surface of the material. It is difficult to obtain the same contact pressure for each electrode.

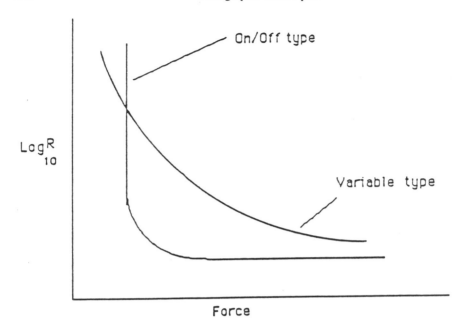

Figure 1: Force-resistance curves for the elastomer

Connection to each electrode is made via wires soldered to each electrode. The test rig is constructed so as to allow the elastomer sheet to be changed easily and simply. Figure 2 shows the electrode contact points around the periphery of the material sample.

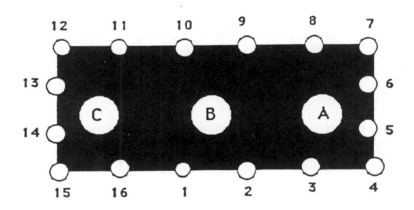

Figure 2: Diagram of the electrode configuration for the elastomer sheet

A block diagram of the data acquisition system is shown in Figure 3. A current source is connected to 2 adjacent electrodes and the resulting differential voltages on the periphery of the sheet are fed into an RMS to DC converter and then into a PC using a 12 bit ADC. The current source is set to a fixed optimum frequency, determined by the material.

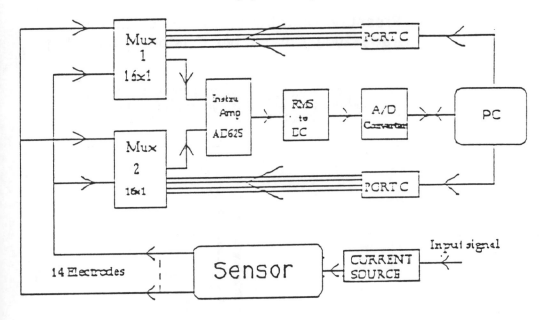

Figure 3: Block diagram of the data-collection system

All the data acquisition software was written in BASIC. In the prototype sensor reported here, the object was to validate the general approach rather than to aim for rapid data acquisition. Noise reduction in the measured voltage signals was carried out within the software using averaging techniques

Typical results for two materials tested are shown in Figure 4, 5, 6 and 7. The two materials are labelled Grade 2000 and Grade 3000 and the results shown for each material are for a load of 200 g and 1 kg; the load being distributed evenly over a 13 mm diameter area. Grade 2000 exhibits a variable resistance/load characteristic; Grade 3000 has a switching or on-off characteristic. Each load was applied in turn to three distinct previously defined locations on the elastomer sheet. These locations are shown in Figure 2.

The results show that there is a measurably difference in the output with changes in applied load. They are the boundary voltage readings when the current source is connected between electrodes 9 and 10. The resulting current distribution means that the sensor will have greatest sensitivity near to this electrode pair and in fact this can be seen in Figures 4 to 7. Smaller changes can be observed in the differential voltage between the other pairs of electrodes. These are initial results and are encouraging in that the data-collection system is not optimised and also the present sensor construction is crude. However, the results do show that it is possible to obtain repeatable results from a conductive elastomer sheet using electrical impedance tomographic techniques.

References

1   L D Harman, Automated tactile sensors. Int J Robotics Res, 1, 2, 2-32, 1982

2   Ruocco S R, Robot sensors and transducer, Halstead Press and OUP.ISBN 0-335-15408-5

3   J G Webster, Tactile sensors for robotics and medicine, John Wiley and Sons, 1988.

Pressure Distribution Representation for Grade 2000 Conductive Elastomer for 200g Load

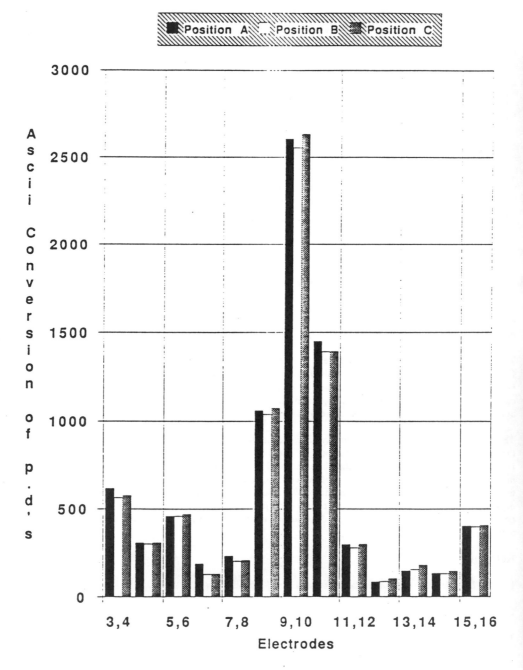

Figure 4

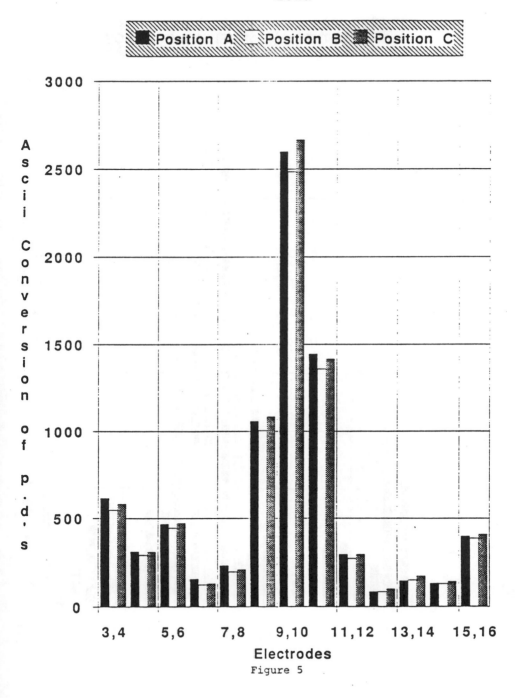

Figure 5

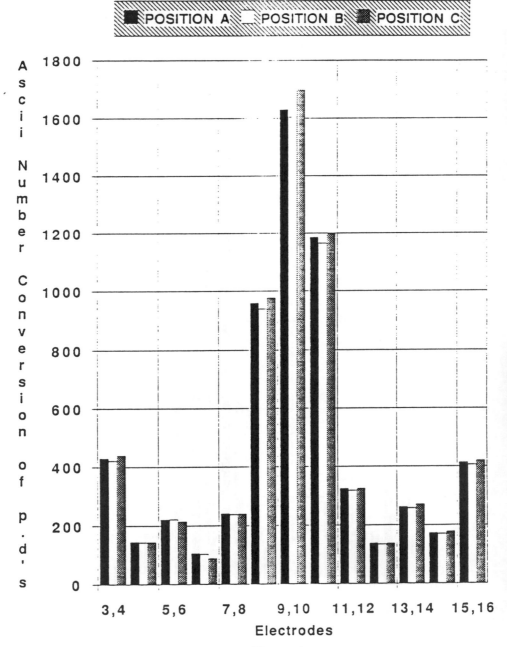

Figure 6

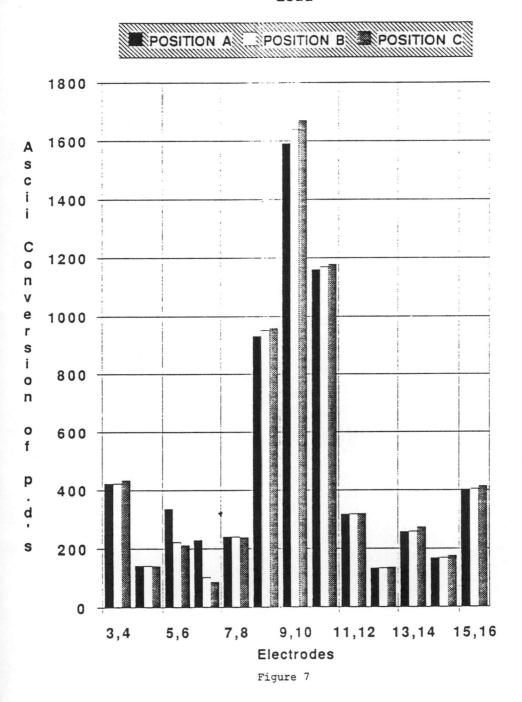

Figure 7

Efficient reconstruction with few data in industrial tomography.

L. Desbat*, P. Turlier°

*Observatoire de Grenoble, CERMO BP 53 x, F-38041 Grenoble
°Centre de Recherche Elf Solaize, BP 22, F-69360 Saint Symphorien d'Ozon.

ABSTRACT: Recent works on algebraic reconstruction from interlaced schemes allow us to apply these geometries in industrial tomography with few data. In this paper, we propose a modified version of the Klaverkamp's algorithm to solve the direct algebraic problem from interlaced data. We show that the reconstructions from interlaced geometries (i.e with twice less data) are as good as those obtained in the corresponding standard geometry. Reconstructions from a real experiment are given.

1 INTRODUCTION

Tomography is used by the Elf company for mapping the solid catalyst concentration in a cross section of a circulating fluid bed reactor for gas oil cracking. It is also used as a diagnostic tool for detecting choked pipes or flow problems. The crucial point we are dealing with is the little amount of data. Whereas the number of data in the medicine field is usually in the range of 10^5-10^6, we have to produce a reconstruction from between 20 and 300 data. In this domain of very few data the algebraic reconstruction methods seem to yield the best results (Girard 1987, Natterer 1980).

1.1 Analytic approach

This approach is based on known analytic expressions for the inverse of the Radon transform:

$$\mathcal{R}f(\theta,s) = \int_{(x,\theta)=s} f(x)dx, \qquad (1)$$

where x is a point of the support (supposed to be the unit disk in the rest of this paper) of the unknown function f, θ is the unit vector $(\cos\phi, \sin\phi)$, $s \in \mathbb{R}$. Because of the necessary finite number of data, the inversion formula has to be discretized. The mathematical properties of the Radon transform lead to different inversion formulae using filtering and Fourier transforms. The well known filtered back-projection algorithm produces very efficiently good reconstructions when dealing with 10^5-10^6 data, but it is not so well suited for few data.

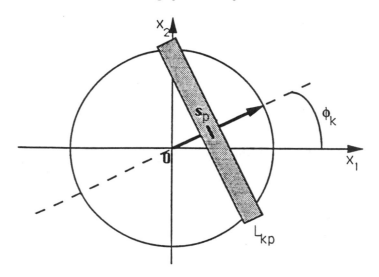

Figure 1: Measurements geometry: strip case

1.2 Algebraic approach

The modelisation we use for our tomography problem is the usual one: the measurements y are supposed to be integrals over strips of the unknown function f:

$$y = Rf \text{ where } y_{k,p} = \int_{L_{k,p}} f(x)dx \ k = 0,\dots,K-1; \ p = 1,\dots,P, \qquad (2)$$

where $L_{k,p}$ is the strip of width h centered on s_p orthogonal to the line generated with the unit vector $\theta_k = (\cos\phi_k, \sin\phi_k)$ (see figure 1).

$$x \in L_{k,p} \Leftrightarrow s_p - h/2 < \langle\theta_k, x\rangle \leq s_p + h/2$$

The usual starting point for estimating f from (2) is to compute $f^\dagger$ the minimal norm least squares solution in L_2.

$$f^\dagger = R^\dagger y = R^*(RR^*)^\dagger y, \qquad (3)$$

where $R^\dagger$ is the usual generalised inverse of R, R^* is the adjoint of R; namely $R^*y = \sum_{k,p} y_{k,p} l_{k,p}$, $RR^*_{k,p,k',p'} = \langle l_{k,p}, l_{k',p'}\rangle$ where the $l_{k,p}$ are defined by:

$$l_{k,p}(x) = \mathbb{1}_{L_{k,p}}(x) = \begin{cases} 1 & \text{if } x \in L_{k,p} \\ 0 & \text{else.} \end{cases}$$

The computation of (3) is generally very instable, so we generally have to introduce regularization. A common approach is to solve $\min_{f \in L_2} \|Rf - y\|^2 + \tau\|\Delta f\|^2$, where the operator Δ is chosen for its regularization feature and also for having a good condition number in solving the problem. $\tau > 0$, the regularization parameter, balances regularity and the least squares criterion. A wide work has been done around the automatic choice of this parameter (see Girard 1989, and references therein).

Regularization is just filtering when Δ and RR^* have the same eigenvectors. The usual low pass filter is also frequently used (and is our favourite algorithm):

$$f_\tau = R^* f_\tau \text{ with } f_\tau = (RR^*)^{\tau\dagger} y, \tag{4}$$

where

$$(RR^*)^{\tau\dagger} = U D^{\tau\dagger} U^t \text{ with } D^{\tau\dagger}{}_{ii} = \begin{cases} 1/D_{ii} & \text{if } D_{ii} \geq \tau \max_i D_{ii} \\ 0 & \text{otherwise} \end{cases}, \tau > 0. \tag{5}$$

(the D_{ii} are the eigenvalues of RR^*).

The measurements are done for different θ and s. One of the crucial question of tomography concerns the best choice of the parameters θ and s, i.e. the choice of the sampling scheme.

2 EFFICIENT SAMPLING SCHEMES

The interlaced scheme has been proposed for the first time by Cormack (1978) in the case of the algebraic approach with a very elegant geometrical argument, as a more efficient scheme than the standard one. Some recent studies using algebraic techniques have been done about the projections information content in tomography (Kazantsev 1991, Desbat 1991). Nevertheless, the analytic approach seems much more powerful for answering the question of efficient schemes.

2.1 The analytic approach

The choice of the "best" sampling scheme can be solved in the lack of a priori information by the application of the Petersen and Middleton theorem (see Petersen and Middleton 1962). Suppose that the support of $\hat{g}$, the Fourier transform of the function $g:\mathbb{R}^n \longrightarrow \mathbb{R}$,

$$\hat{g}(\xi) = \int_{\mathbb{R}^n} g(x) e^{-i(x,\xi)} dx$$

is a subset of $S \in \mathbb{R}^n$. The generalisation of the classical Nyquist condition to the case of sampling on lattices , i.e. sets of the form $\Lambda = \{Wl, l \in \mathbb{Z}^n\}$ where W is a non-singular real (n, n)-matrix, is the following one:

$$\text{the sets } S + 2\pi(W^{-1})^t l, \, l \in \mathbb{Z}^n \text{ have to be mutually disjoint.} \tag{6}$$

It has been shown (Rattey and Lindgren 1981, Natterer 1986) that the support of Fourier transform of the radon transform of an essentially b-bandlimited function (in a suitable sense, see Natterer 1986) is small outside the set:

$$S(\vartheta, b) = \{(\nu, \sigma) \in \mathbb{Z} \times \mathbb{R} : |\sigma| < b, |\nu| < \max(|\sigma|/\vartheta, (1/\vartheta - 1)b)\}, \tag{7}$$

where $0 < \vartheta < 1$, ϑ can be chosen arbitrary near to 1.

2.1.1 The standard scheme

The Petersen and Middleton condition can be applied to the standard sampling (see Natterer 1986): $(\theta_k, s_p) = (\pi k/K, ph), k = 0, ..., 2K - 1; p \in \mathbb{Z}$ such that $|ph| \leq 1$. This is the lattice $\{W_S l, l \in A_{W_S}\} \cap T \times [-1, 1]$ $(A_{W_S} = \{k \in \mathbb{Z}^2; W_S k \in [0, 2\pi) \times \mathbb{R}\}$, $T = \mathbb{R}/2\pi\mathbb{Z}$) with:

$$W_S = \begin{pmatrix} \pi/k & 0 \\ 0 & h \end{pmatrix}, k \in \mathbb{N}, h > 0.$$

The sampling conditions are thus $K \geq b/\vartheta$ and $h \leq \pi/b$ (the optimal values consist of choosing K the first integer bigger than $\pi/h = b$).

2.1.2   The interlaced scheme

In tomography, the Petersen and Middleton condition can be achieved with a much more efficient sampling scheme (Rattey and Lindgren 1981, Natterer 1986) with the matrix:

$$W_I = \begin{pmatrix} 2\pi/K & -\pi/K \\ 0 & h \end{pmatrix}$$

As can be seen in the figure 2, the matrix W_I is sufficient (according to the Petersen and Middleton condition) for sampling the Radon transform of a b-bandlimited function.

Note that the efficiency of a scheme for sampling a function can be characterised by the area of the elementary parallelogram of the lattice: $\det W$. The bigger it is, the less are the number of points necessary for covering the plane. The efficiency of the interlaced scheme is optimal and twice better than those of the standard scheme: $\det W_I = 2 \det W_S$.

2.1.3   Some new efficient schemes

Efficient sampling with the use of too coarse lattices is possible in tomography (Faridani 1990). The use of two grids generated by:

$$W_1 = \begin{pmatrix} 2\pi/K & 0 \\ 0 & 2h \end{pmatrix}, \ K \in \mathbb{N}, \ h > 0.$$

can yield as efficient sampling schemes as the interlaced scheme. Using the theory developped in Faridani (1990) and introducing $S_e \supset S$ (see Desbat 1992):

$$S_e(\vartheta, b) = \{(\nu, \sigma) \in \mathbb{Z} \times \mathbb{R}; \ -b \le \sigma < b, -\nu_{max}(\sigma, \vartheta, b) \le \nu < \nu_{max}(\sigma, \vartheta, b)\},$$

where $\nu_{max}(\sigma, \vartheta, b) = \min(\lfloor b/\vartheta \rfloor, \max(|\sigma|/\vartheta + (1/\vartheta - 1)b/2, (1/\vartheta - 1)b))$ (see figure 2), the use of $2NM$ translated grids generated by:

$$W_{N,M} = \begin{pmatrix} 2N\pi/K & 0 \\ 0 & 2Mh \end{pmatrix}, \tag{8}$$

can yield as efficient sampling geometries as the interlaced scheme.

2.2   The algebraic approach

2.2.1   The standard scheme

Let us denote:

$$\phi_k^o = \frac{k}{K}\pi, \quad \theta_k^o = (\cos\phi_k^o, \sin\phi_k^o) \quad k = 0, \ldots, K-1 \tag{9}$$

$$h = \frac{2}{P} \tag{10}$$

$$s_p^o = -1 + h/2 + (p-1)h = -1 + \frac{(2p-1)h}{2} \quad p = 1, \ldots, P \tag{11}$$

In order to have a regular structure, we reorganize the measurements functions $l_{k,p}^o$ and the corresponding data. Let us denote $\lfloor a \rfloor = n$ if $n \le a < n+1$, $\lceil a \rceil = n$ if $n-1 < a \le n$ with $a \in \mathbb{R}, n \in \mathbb{N}$:

$$l_{k,p} = \begin{cases} l_{k,p+\lfloor P/2 \rfloor}^o & p = 1, \ldots, \lceil P/2 \rceil, \ 0 \le k \le K-1 \\ l_{k-K,\lceil P/2 \rceil-p+1}^o & p = 1, \ldots, \lceil P/2 \rceil, \ K \le k \le 2K-1 \end{cases}$$

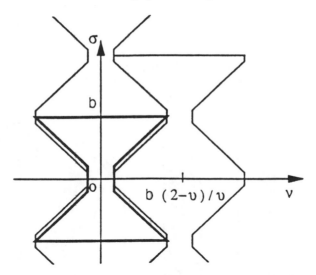

Figure 2: Support S (bold) and S_e: $S \subset S_e$. The sets $S_e + 2\pi(W_I^{-1})^t l$, $l \in \mathbb{Z}^2$ tile the Fourier plane.

In this case the matrix RR^* is block-circulant. This property can be used for computing (3) or (4) using Fourier transform, in order to block-diagonalize the matrix RR^*. Remark that if P is odd, the central strips $L_{k,1}, \forall k$ are used twice in order to obtain the rotational invariance and thus the corresponding $l_{k,1}, y_{k,1}$ should be divided by $\sqrt{2}$ for solving the same least squares problem (see Natterer 1980 and Girard 1987 for efficient algorithms).

2.2.2 The interlaced scheme

In algebraic approach, the link between standard and interlaced schemes was not clear until Klaverkamp's work (Klaverkamp 1991). In particular the original Cormark interlaced scheme does not lead to the same reconstruction as the one produced in the corresponding standard scheme. For Klaverkamp, the measurements functions of the interlaced sampling scheme in algebraic approach are just the half of those in the corresponding standard scheme chosen with k and p odd and k and p even (see figure 3), or equivalently k odd and p even, and k even and p odd. For example, the interlaced scheme we use corresponds to the set of measurements functions: For $k = 0, \ldots, 2K - 1$:

$$l_{k,p}^{+,o} = \begin{cases} l_{k,2p-1} & \text{if } k \text{ even, for } p = 1, \ldots, \left\lceil \frac{P}{4} \right\rceil \\ l_{k,2p} & \text{if } k \text{ odd, for } p = 1, \ldots, \left\lceil \frac{P}{2} \right\rceil - \left\lceil \frac{P}{4} \right\rceil \end{cases}$$

The second possible interlaced scheme is just the complementary scheme to the previous in the standard scheme:

$$l_{k,p}^{-,o} = \begin{cases} l_{k,2p-1} & \text{if } k \text{ odd, for } p = 1, \ldots, \left\lceil \frac{P}{4} \right\rceil \\ l_{k,2p} & \text{if } k \text{ even, for } p = 1, \ldots, \left\lceil \frac{P}{2} \right\rceil - \left\lceil \frac{P}{4} \right\rceil \end{cases}$$

Each interlaced measurements function set is just the half of the corresponding standard set:

$$\bigcup_{\epsilon\in\{+,-\}}\bigcup_{k=0}^{K-1}\bigcup_{p=1}^{\lceil\frac{P}{2}\rceil} l_{k,p}^{\epsilon} = \bigcup_{k=0}^{K-1}\bigcup_{p=1}^{\lceil\frac{P}{2}\rceil} l_{k,p}$$

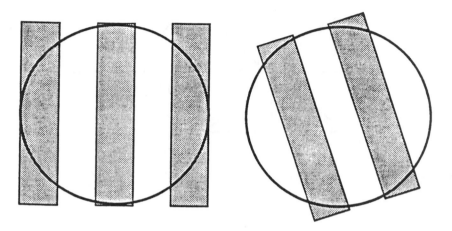

Figure 3: Measurements functions in the interlaced scheme ($l_{k,p}^{i,o}$): left: even direction (here θ_0), right: odd direction (here θ_1).

Remark: in order to have an interlaced scheme, if P is even then K has to be odd, if P is odd then K has to be even.

3   ALGORITHMS

Filtered backprojection algorithms for interlaced data yield good reconstructions (see Faridani 1990, and references therein). The way to deal with interlaced samplings in algebraic reconstruction is more recently due to Klaverkamp (see Klaverkamp 1991).

3.1   Klaverkamp's algorithm

Most of the idea for dealing with interlaced schemes in direct algebraic reconstruction are due to Klaverkamp. He proposed a very clever algorithm based on mathematical properties of the singular value decomposition of the Radon transform. Using the standard matrix, replacing the non-measured data by 0 and solving the problem with a truncated generalised inverse (5) yield essentially the same result as the standard scheme. τ must have the right value (see Klaverkamp 1991): τ has to be a bit less than the smallest eigenvalue of the first block corresponding to the zero frequence in the block-diagonalization).

3.2   A modified version

In the following we propose an alternative algorithm in which the choice of the cut-off parameter τ is not so critical. The natural idea is to use the standard scheme (with KP functions) as reconstruction geometry for the interlaced problem ($K\lceil P/2\rceil$ measurements). Remember that we have only half of the standard data, i.e. the dimension of the interlaced data y^+ is $KP/2$ (in the following $K\lceil P/2\rceil$ in order to produce an efficient algorithm). We want first to reorganize the measurements for efficiency.

For $k = 0,\ldots,K-1$:

$$l_{k,p}^+ = \begin{cases} l_{2k,p}^{+,o} & \text{for } p = 1,\ldots,\left\lceil\frac{P}{4}\right\rceil \\ l_{2k+1,p-\lceil\frac{P}{4}\rceil}^{+,o} & \text{for } p = \left\lceil\frac{P}{4}\right\rceil+1,\ldots,\left\lceil\frac{P}{2}\right\rceil \end{cases}$$

Thus we want to solve:

$$\min_{f\in\mathbb{R}^{KP}} \sum_{k=1}^{K}\sum_{p=1}^{\left\lceil\frac{P}{2}\right\rceil}\left(\left\langle l_{k,p}^+, \sum_{k'=0}^{2K-1}\sum_{p'=1}^{\left\lceil\frac{P}{2}\right\rceil} f_{k',p'}l_{k',p'}\right\rangle_{L_2} - y_{k,p}^+\right)^2$$

or equivalently:

$$\min_{f^+,f^-} \sum_{k=1}^{K}\sum_{p=1}^{\left\lceil\frac{P}{2}\right\rceil}\left(\left\langle l_{k,p}^+, \sum_{k'=0}^{K-1}\sum_{p'=1}^{\left\lceil\frac{P}{2}\right\rceil} f_{k',p'}^+l_{k',p'}^{i+} + \sum_{k'=0}^{K-1}\sum_{p'=1}^{\left\lceil\frac{P}{2}\right\rceil} f_{k',p'}^-l_{k',p'}^{i-}\right\rangle_{L_2} - y_{k,p}^+\right)^2$$

where the complementary scheme has also been reorganized: For $k = 0,\ldots,K-1$:

$$l_{k,p}^- = \begin{cases} l_{2k,p}^{-,o} & \text{for } p = 1,\ldots,\left\lceil\frac{P}{4}\right\rceil \\ l_{2k+1,p-\lceil\frac{P}{4}\rceil}^{-,o} & \text{for } p = \left\lceil\frac{P}{4}\right\rceil+1,\ldots,\left\lceil\frac{P}{2}\right\rceil \end{cases}$$

The $K\lceil P/2\rceil \times 2K\lceil P/2\rceil$ matrix of the last least squares problem has the following regular structure:

$$\begin{pmatrix} L^{+,0} & L^{+,K-1} & \cdots & L^{+,1} & L^{-,0} & L^{-,K-1} & \cdots & L^{-,1} \\ L^{+,1} & L^{+,0} & \ddots & \vdots & L^{-,1} & L^{-,0} & \ddots & \vdots \\ \vdots & \ddots & \ddots & L^{+,K-1} & \vdots & \ddots & \ddots & L^{-,K-1} \\ L^{+,K-1} & \cdots & L^{+,1} & L^{+,0} & L^{-,K-1} & \cdots & L^{-,1} & L^{-,0} \end{pmatrix}.$$

where $L^{\epsilon,k}$ are $\left\lceil\frac{P}{2}\right\rceil \times \left\lceil\frac{P}{2}\right\rceil$ matrix such that $L_{p,p'}^{\epsilon,k} = \left\langle l_{k,p}^+, l_{0,p'}^{i\epsilon}\right\rangle_{L_2}$. Both circulant parts can be block diagonalized by Discrete Fourier transforms of order K yielding the K independant least squares problems:

$$\min_{\hat{f}^{+,k},\hat{f}^{-,k}} \|\hat{L}^{+,k}\hat{f}^{+,k} + \hat{L}^{-,k}\hat{f}^{-,k} - \hat{y}^{+,k}\|^2, \quad \forall k = 0,\ldots,K-1$$

where $y_p^{+,k}$ is just $y_{k,p}^+$, $f_p^{\epsilon,k} = f_{k,p}^{\epsilon}$ and for x a vector and L a matrix:

$$\hat{x}_p^k \stackrel{\text{def}}{=} \sum_{j=0}^{K-1} e^{-2\pi ijk/K}x_p^j \quad \text{and} \quad \hat{L}_{p,q}^k \stackrel{\text{def}}{=} \sum_{j=0}^{K-1} e^{-2\pi ijk/K}L_{p,q}^j.$$

4 NUMERICAL EXPERIMENTS

4.1 Modelisation

In the following we give reconstructions of a simple model of the solid catalyst concentration in a cross section of a circulating fluid bed reactor for gas oil cracking with a perturbation (A in figure 4). When using the right parameter $\tau = .04$ (Klaverkamp proposes to choose τ a bit less than the smallest eigenvalue of the first block in the block-diagonalization) we have the almost the same results from interlaced data (i.e. with twice less data) as from standard. This result holds for both algorithms. The Klaverkamp algorithm is very interesting because we do not have to write any line of code (we use our favourite algebraic code for standard schemes). But the choice of the optimal τ is not so easy when dealing with so few data. In particular, the meaning of "a bit less than the smallest eigenvalue of the first block in the block-diagonalization" depends on the value of K and P. (note that K must be a bit bigger than $\pi P/2$). It was a sufficient reason to propose a modified version of this algorithm. Reconstructions with a smaller τ is stable only in the case of the algorithm proposed in this paper (see E and F in figure 4).

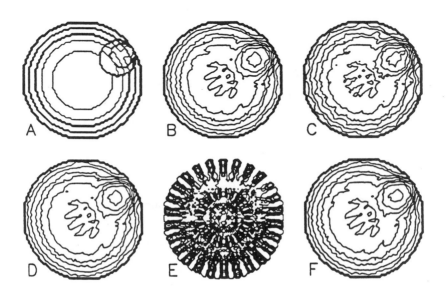

Figure 4: Comparison of standard and interlaced schemes. (A) Original model, (B) standard reconstruction with $K = 26, P = 15$ (i.e. from 390 data) using a standard algebraic algorithm $\tau = .04$, (C) reconstruction from interlaced data (i.e. from 195 data) using the Klaverkamp algorithm $\tau = .04$, (D) reconstruction from interlaced data using the modified algorithm with $\tau = .04$, (E) reconstruction from interlaced data using the Klaverkamp algorithm $\tau = .02$ (this bad result comes from a bad use of the Klaverkamp algorithm: τ values under .04 necessary yield big errors), (F) reconstruction from interlaced data using the modified algorithm with $\tau = .02$.

4.2   Reconstruction from true data

In figure 5 we present reconstructions from true data. These measurements were done on a real model of a reactor for gas oil craking (used for chemical research) in a standard geometry with $K = 24$, $P = 15$. The first reconstruction (A) is done with all the data with our usual algebraic algorithm for standard scheme with $\tau = .039$. Then reconstructions are provided with only the half of these data (in an interlaced scheme). We can see very small variations in the center of the image because of the noise in the data and because the region is very flat. When using $\tau = .036$ only the reconstructions D and F are usable.

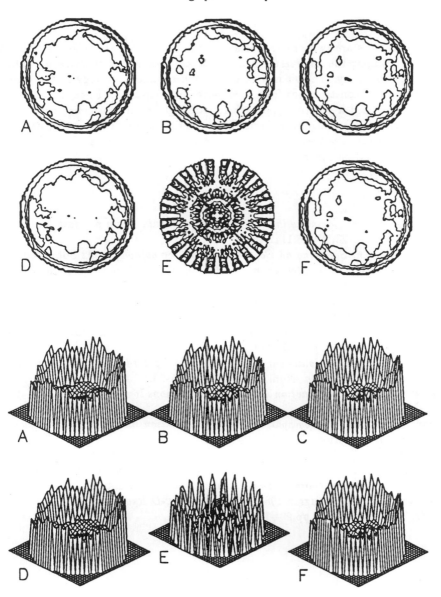

Figure 5: Comparison of standard and interlaced schemes on true data. (A) standard reconstruction with $K = 24, P = 15$ (i.e. from 360 data) using a standard algebraic algorithm $\tau = .039$, (B) reconstruction from interlaced data (i.e. from 180 data) using the Klaverkamp algorithm $\tau = .039$, (C) reconstruction from interlaced data using the modified algorithm with $\tau = .039$, (D) standard reconstruction with $K = 24, P = 15, \tau = .036$ (E) reconstruction from interlaced data using the Klaverkamp algorithm $\tau = .036$ (again this bad result comes from a bad use of the Klaverkamp algorithm: τ values under .039 necessary yield big errors), (F) reconstruction from interlaced data using the modified algorithm with $\tau = .036$.

5 CONCLUSION

Interlaced schemes are twice more efficient as the usual standard schemes. This means that you can achieve the same result as in a standard geometry with twice less data, when they are not too noisy. Thus it is a very good measurement strategy in the case of few data. Algebraic reconstructions from these schemes are possible since the Klaverkamp's work. We proposed a different approach for solving the direct algebraic problem from interlaced scheme. Our algorithm is useful in the case of small truncation parameter τ. Interlaced schemes have been shown to be powerful in the context of few data both on simulated data and on real data.

REFERENCES

A.M. Cormack 1978. *Sampling the Radon Transform with Beam of Finit Width.* Phys. Med. Biol., Vol. 23, No. 6,1141-48.

L. Desbat. *Efficient Sampling on Coarse Grids in Tomography.* 1992 Submited.

L. Desbat, P. Turlier 1991. *Measurements Optimisation in Tomography.* IMACS91, pp. 1523-1524, Dublin (1991).

A. Faridani 1990. *An application of a multidimensional sampling theorem to computed tomography.* Comtemporary Mathematics, vol. 113, pp. 65-80.

D. Girard 1987. *Optimal regularized reconstruction in computerized tomography* SIAM J. Sci. Stat. Comput., 8, pp. 934-950.

D. Girard 1989. *A fast 'Monte-Carlo cross-validation' procedure for large least squares problems with noisy data.* Num. Math., 56, pp. 1-23.

I.G. Kazantsev 1991. *Information Content of projections* Inverse Problems, 7, pp. 887-898.

W. Klaverkamp 1991. *Tomographische Bildrekonstruktion mit direkten algebraischen Verfahren* Dissertation.

F. Natterer 1986 *The Mathematics of Computerized Tomography* Wiley.

D.P. Petersen and D. Middleton 1962. *Sampling and reconstruction of wawenumber-limited functions in N-dimensional euclidean space* Inf. Control, 5, pp.279-323.

P.A. Rattey and A.G. Lindgren 1981. *Sampling the 2-D Radon transform,* IEEE Trans. ASSP-29, pp.994-1002.

Measurement of Mixing Phenomena in Gas and Liquid Flow

D. Mewes, A. Fellhölter, R. Renz

Institut für Verfahrenstechnik, Universität Hannover,
Callinstraße 36, D-3000 Hannover 1

ABSTRACT: This paper describes measurements of concentration fields in mixing processes by tomography. The concentration profiles are three-dimensional and instationary.
The measurements are taken by interferometric holography
and light absorption. Pictures from four directions are
used for tomographic reconstruction by the ART-Method.
Results are presented from experiments on liquid jet mixing
in vessels and gas mixing in a duct of rectangular cross-
section.

1. INTRODUCTION

The four-beam optical tomography by interferometric holography
as well as light absorption was developed for single phase
transparent liquid and gas flows. Mayinger and Lübbe (1984)
measured three-dimensional temperature fields by interferometry and examined the time and location-dependent mixing of a
liquid component in a stirred vessel. Ostendorf and Mewes
(1988, 1991) extended these kinds of measurements using
viscous liquids in order to visualize temperature fields
created by turbulent mixing and dissipative heating. Haarde
(1990) developed an experimental setup for the observation of
non-steadystate mass exchange processes occuring during jet
mixing. He observed the concentration profiles of a dye by the
intensity change of light beams. The experimental results
were recorded with diverging light in the form of transillumination projections from four angles of view.

In continuation of these experiments the interferometric holography was used to record concentration fields by parallel
coherent monochromatic light beams from four directions in
single phase gas flow. The concentration fields were reconstructed by tomography during the mixing process in ducts of
large cross-section. The results were used for the development
of mixing-divices with very low pressure-losses.

The mixing of liquids by jet flow of one component was
observed in order to develop an energency system for large
reactor vessels and tanks. In case of an exothermic chemical
reaction a small quantity of liquid reaction stopping agent
has to be distributed homogeneously through-out a large volume

of reacting liquid. A system of discontinous operating jets
was developed by consideration of the experimental results
from the tomographic reconstruction of the instationary
concentration fields. Colored jets were used spreading in
optical transparent liquids of different viscosity.

2. METHODS OF MEASUREMENT

The investigations related to gas phase mixing are carried out
in a transparent, open circuit wind tunnel with a square cross
sectional area according to **Figure 1**. The lateral length of
the channel is 85 mm. The channel is positioned vertically and
has a total length of 1190 mm. The carrier gas flow is sucked
through the channel by a roots compressor. Ambient air is
accelerated into the channel through a specially designed
nozzle. Carbon dioxide can be injected into six different
areas of the channel. Thus it is possible to measure the
concentration fields in different distances from the point of
injection by optical tomography.

The method of measurement is divided into two steps:

1. Recording of measured values by holographical
   interferometry.
2. Tomographical reconstruction of concentration fields.

With the holographical interferometry the phase shift of two
light waves due to the change of refractive index can be
measured. the refractive index depends on the concentration of
carbon dioxide in the carrrier gas flow.

The optical setup is shown in **Figure 2.** The light beam emitted
from the argon-ion laser reaches a beam splitter (BS), where
it is divided into an object beam and a reference beam. The
ratio between the intensity of the object beam and the intensity of the reference beam can be varied with this beam
splitter. The next beam splitter divides the object beam into
two portions, each of which is again divided into two object
waves of identical value via two large beam splitters, after
passing through the enlargement optics (BE). Thus, they

irradiate the wind tunnel at displacement angles of 45°. The
object waves are then bundled with lenses (L), which results
in an increase of the intensity of the light in the holographic plane (H). By this the exposure times for the holograms are reduced, which is of special importance for the
recording of non-steadystate processes. Two object waves can
be projected onto a holographic plate with mirror (M). The
reference beam is also enlarged. It bypasses the wind tunnel
and is divided into two reference beams for one holographic
plate each with. The holographic plates are installed in
clamped frames and fixed mountings with three-point bearings.
This makes an exact repositioning of the holograms after the
development possible. Pictures of the interferograms located
behind the holographic plates are taken from a motor-driven
camera with synchronized shutter release.

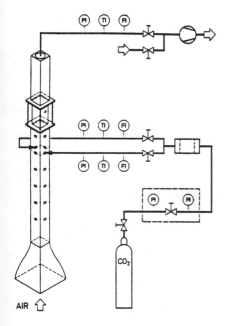

Carbon dioxide is injected into
the channel. The refractive
index, that depends on the
concentration of carbon dioxide,
changes. As a result the optical
pathlengths of the object beams
differ from those of the object
beams which are recorded on the
hologram plates without carbon
dioxide injection. Due to this
phase shift the fringe patterns
are deflected.

Fig. 1: Experimental facility for
gas mixing experiments

Fig. 2: Experimental facility for
four beam interferometric
holography

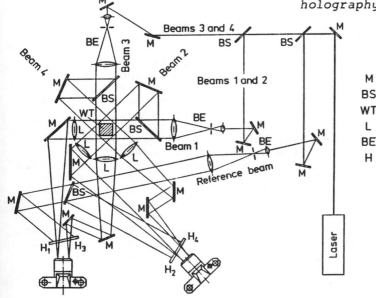

M - Mirror
BS - Beam splitter
WT - Wind tunnel
L - Lens
BE - Beam expander
H - Hologram

These are digitiled and used for the evaluation of the
concentration field of one cross sectional area. If there were
projection data only from one direction, only symmetrical
concentration fields can be reconstructed. Three-dimensional,
asymmetric concentration fields are reconstructed from optical
pathlength measurements using multidirectional holographic
interferometry. Projection datas of four different directions
over a 180° angle of view are necessary to reconstruct the
local concentrations by use of the algebraic reconstruction
technique.

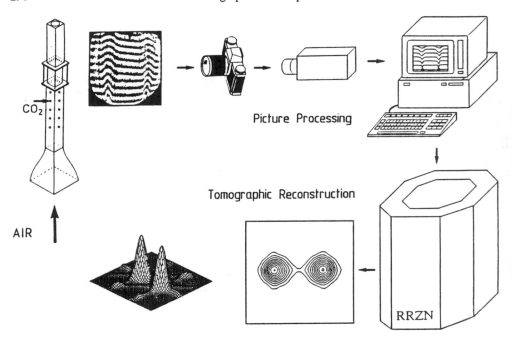

Fig. 3: Procedure of tomographic reconstruction of
        concentration fields

The experimental procedure is shown in **Figure 3.** The interferogram is recorded from each direction of illumination
during the injection of two coflowing jets of carbon dioxide.
Four interferograms which are taken simultaneously from four
different directions of view are recorded for picture processing using a video camera. The interferograms are digi-
tied, filtered and sceletted. The interferograms of the
reference beams and the phase shifted beams are superposi-
tioned and the phase shifts due to changes in refractive index
are measured. The interferograms of the four different directions are evaluated and the files containing the measurement
datas are transmitted to a Cyber 990-computer, where the
concentration fields are reconstructed tomographically in
discrete cross sectional areas of the channel. These data can
be used to draw isometric plots of the concentration fields.
The maximum concentration can be determined in order to
evaluate the quality of mixing.

The measurements of temperature fields are restricted to
optically transparent liquids of constant partial concentrations of the components on one hand side and to constant temperature if concentration fields are measured on the other
hand side as long as monochromatic light from one laser source
is used. To overcome this difficulty which restricts interferometry to small sized vessels, Haarde and Mewes (1990)
developed the experimental setup shown in **Figure 4** for the
observation of non-steadystate mass exchange processes
occurring during jet mixing. In this setup, the concentration

profiles of a dye can
be observed with the use of optical tomography. The dyes are
either injected or they develop during a color change reaction. They cause a decrease of the light intensity inside the
cylindrical mixing vessel. The experimental results are recorded with diverging light in the form of transillumination projections from four angles of view with divergent light. The
axes of the light bundles cross each other in the center of
the vessel at an angle of 45° each. Thus the light bundles
cover a range of 180°. The light is guided through the
measurement chamber from four directions via mirrors and two
beam splitters. With cylindrical lenses, the vessel can be
illuminated in sections of 50 mm (overall) height each. For
this purpose, the measurement chamber, which is about 200 mm
in high and has a diameter of 200 mm, must be divided up into
four sections that are located above each other. The cylindrical measurement chamber is located inside an octagonal
measurement chamber. The space between the octagonal exterior
chamber and the cylindrical interior chamber is filled with
water. By this total reflection is suppressed as much as
possible. After penetrating the chamber, the beams hit projection screens. Photographs of the four screens are taken with
synchronized, motor-driven microphotographic cameras. The
negatives are fed into a picture processing unit and the film
density is digitazed.

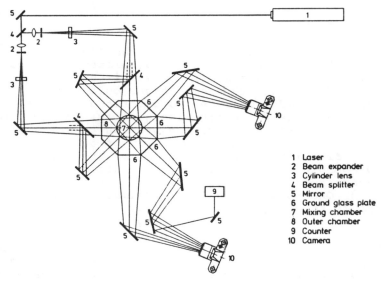

1   Laser
2   Beam expander
3   Cylinder lens
4   Beam splitter
5   Mirror
6   Ground glass plate
7   Mixing chamber
8   Outer chamber
9   Counter
10 Camera

Fig. 4: Experimental facility for the measurement of insta-
        tionary jet mixing processes inside large vessels by
        light intensity variations

The three-dimensional concentration field obtained with the
use of tomographic reconstruction is shown in **Figure 5** for
several planes. Renz (1991) used instationary operated jets,

which operated from different points of injection simultaneously during short intervals of time.

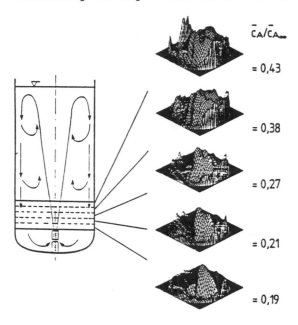

$\bar{c}_A / \bar{c}_{A\infty}$

= 0,43

= 0,38

= 0,27

= 0,21

= 0,19

Fig. 5: Concentration
profiles of a dye colored
instationary operated
liquid jet in different
horizontal planes at one
moment of time.

3. TOMOGRAPHIC RECONSTRUCTION

The tomographic reconstruction was done by the Algebraic
Reconstruction Technique (ART) which was developed by Gordon,
Bender and Herman (1970). Because of the small number of
directions of the different traversing beams only the combination with the so called Sample-Method described by Sweeney
(1972) gives considerable reconstruction quality. The computer
time limitation restricts the iteration process to areas of
200 x 200 mm which are broken down to a grid of 50 x 50 area
elements. Nearly five minutes of computer time are necessary
on a Cyber 990-computer to run through 6 iterations in order
to keep the reconstruction quality below an average systematic
deviation of 5 %. One possibility to preestimate the number of
iteration steps is to observe the quality of reconstruction by
the number of iteration processes selecting test functions.
Two-dimensional analytic functions are used for test purposes.
The values of these functions and the number of extreme values
in the investigated range correspond with the course of the
assumed field parameter. The applied functions should have no
symmetrical axes in the direction of the beam and are
integrated along defined paths. The obtained integral values
represent simulated experimental results, which reconstruct
the required analytic functions with the use of the mentioned
method. The quality of the obtained reconstructions depends on
the number of completed iteration processes. When the desired
quality of reconstruction is achieved, the determind number of
iteration steps can be used as a measure for the number of

*iterations required for the calculation of the field function
from experimental results. In **Figure 6** the average deveation
is given as the number of iteration processes varies for two
different test functions. The number of iterations has to
be determined individually for each application and the
required quality of reconstruction.*

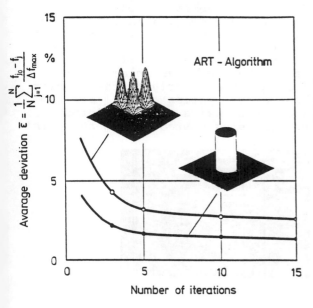

*Fig. 6: Two different
test functions: there
influence on the number
of necessary iterations*

4. DISCUSSION OF EXPERIMENTAL RESULTS

*The tomographic method was applied on mixing processes in
single phase gas and liquid flows. The results of the measurments are explained first in gas flow mixing. Mixing of gases
with different temperatures and concentrations is of great
significance in the chemical and the power plant industry. The
intention of research in this area is to realize homogeneous
concentrations and temperatures in ducts and channels of very
large as well as smaller sized cross sections after short
mixing lengths of gas flow. Technical applications are the
mixing of ammonia into large quantities of flue gas in order
to minimize nitrogen oxid emissions or the reheating of gas
flows entering into a catalytical conversion process by mixing
with small quantities of gas with higher temperatures.*

*The mixing of gases by coflowing jets requires long channel
lengths to ensure complete homogenization. The injection of*

*carbon dioxide perpendicular to the carrier gas will improve
the degree of mixing (**Figure 7**). At the outlet of the nozzle
the flow pattern is similar to the flow around a cylinder. An
eddy flow develops in the tail of the jet, which is axisymmetric in this initial section. Due to shearing forces at the
edge of the jet a circularity flow is induced in the jet
itself. As a result of pressure and shearing forces peripheral
fluid elements of the jet are more forcefully bent by the
deflecting flow, which leads to the development of a cross
sectional area that is shaped like a kidney. With increasing
distance from the point of injection the jet flows parallel to
the carrier gas flow. The different cross sectional areas of a
jet injected perpendicularly into a carrier gas flow are
depicted in the interferograms. The presented interferogram
results from two jets injected perpendicularly to the carrier
gas flow. In the kidney shaped cross section of the jets the
deflection of the fringes shows two maxima and one minimum.
The minimum disappears with increasing distance from the point
of injection.*

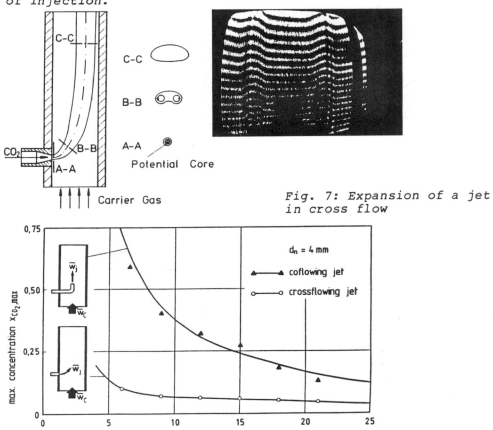

*Fig. 7: Expansion of a jet
in cross flow*

*Fig. 8: Maximum of concentration in cross-sections at differen
       distances from the nozzle outlet for coflowing and
       cross-flowing jets.*

The concentration fields of a single jet injected perpendicularly were reconstructed in several areas of the mixing
channel. A comparison of the maximum concentration between a
crossflowing and a coflowing jet is given in **Figure 8**. The
diameter of the nozzles is 4 mm, the velocity ratio is the
same in both experiments. While the maximum concentration of
the coflowing jet decreases slowly, the cross sectional area
of the jet, injected perpendicularly, is deformed extremely
due to the greater momentum exchange between jet and carrier
gas flow. As a result, the maximum concentration of the crossflowing jet is smaller than that of a coflowing jet at the
same mixing length.

In order to investigate the interaction betweeen multiple
jets, concentration fields are measured, which result from
four jets discharging into the carrier gas flow. The nozzles
are located peripherally. The distance between two nozzles is
42,5 mm. The tomographically reconstructed concentration
fields in two different cross sectional areas are presented in
Figure 9. The concentration fields in the left part of **Figure 9** are scaled to the maximum concentration of carbon dioxide
in the respective cross sectional area. The maximum concentration is 11 % of the initial value at the distance of 15 mm
downward of the injection point while at the distance of 50 mm
the maximum concentration is still 7 %.

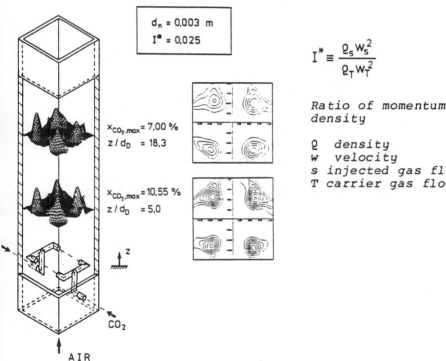

$d_n = 0,003 \ m$

$I^* = 0,025$

$$I^* \equiv \frac{\varrho_s w_s^2}{\varrho_T w_T^2}$$

Ratio of momentum flow·
density

ϱ density
w velocity
s injected gas flow
T carrier gas flow

$x_{CO_2.max} = 7,00 \ \%$
$z / d_D = 18,3$

$x_{CO_2.max} = 10,55 \ \%$
$z / d_D = 5,0$

CO_2

AIR

Fig. 9: Concentration fields of four crossflowing jets in
        different sections of the channel

304   Tomographic Techniques

In the area of jet deformation the maximum concentration of
carbon dioxide decreases rapidly. The concentration exchange
slows down, if jet and carrier gas are flowing parallel and
velocity differences are small.

The quality of mixing can be improved by increasing the ratio
of momentum flow between jet and carrier gas flow. This is
illustrated by **Figure 10** showing the intensity of segregation
upon the dimensionless distance from the nozzle for different
ratios of momentum flow. The intensity of segregation considers the deviation of the concentration from the mean concentration at every point of the cross sectional area of the
channel. The intensity of segregation becomes unity for complete separation and zero for homogeneous mixing of the two
components.

A higher quality of mixing can be achievedfor an increased
ratio of momentum. **Figure 10** also gives the intensity of
segregation for jets in counterflow. Due to the higher momentum exchange between jet and carrier gas flow the quality of
mixing can be improved even further.

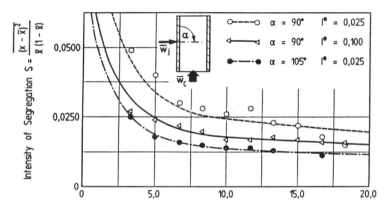

dimensionless distance from the nozzle z / d$_n$

Fig. 10: Intensity of segregation in dependence of the
         distance from the point of injection for different
         ratios of momentum flow and differnt angles of
         injection

The second application of tomographic measurements was done in
liquids with the aim of theproper sizing of a jet mixing
system for large storage vessels and tank farms responsible
for cooling or mixing. In case of an emergency it is normal
that the ordinary mixing and cooling systems are out of
operation. Then a possible exothermic chemical reaction might
have to be stopped. In this case small amounts of liquids have
to be injected by jets in order to stop the chemical reaction.
The injected small liquid volume has to be distributed among
the large vessel volume homogeneously without any additional
power input. Strong differences in viscosity might occur
because of polymerisation reactions.

The concentration fields are visualized by dyes which are
injected together with the liquid jet flows. **Figure 11** gives a
qualitative impression of the mixing process by one single
operating jet during a short period of time and different
ratios of viscosity. Quantitative measurements were done by
tomography using the light absorption technique. Results are -
given in **Figure 12.** The progress in mixing depends on the
viscosity ratio as well as on the angle of inclination of the
nozzle axis and the time period the jets are in operation.

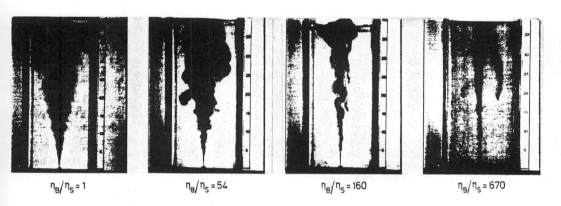

$\eta_B/\eta_S = 1$ $\eta_B/\eta_S = 54$ $\eta_B/\eta_S = 160$ $\eta_B/\eta_S = 670$

Fig. 11: Instationary operation of a jet during a short period
         of time at different ratios of viscosity of the two
         mixing liquids

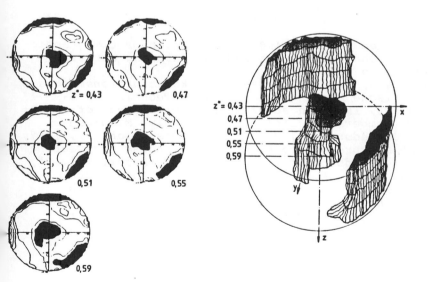

Fig. 12: Concentration fields in a storage tank due to
         instationary jet mixing taken from four directions by
         light absorption and tomographic reconstrucion

5. CONCLUSIONS

In this paper two methods of measurement are described in order to observe concentration profiles in optical transparent single phase gases and liquids. The concentration fields are three dimensional and non-stationary. The tomographic reconstruction of considerable accuracy is possible by projections of different bundles of parallel light beams traversing the whole volume from four different directions. The experimental results are presented for the jet-mixing process of liquids in large vessels and tanks as well as in the continous flow of gas-mixtures inside channels of large cross section.

ACKNOWLEDGMENT

The authors acknowledge the AIF and DECHEMA as well as the DFG, BMFT and Degussa AG for supporting this work by financial grants.

REFERENCES

1) Gordon, R., Bender, R., Herman, G. T., 1970, Algebraic reconstruction techniques (ART) for three-dimensional electron microscopy and X-ray photography; J.of Theor. Biol. 29, 474-481
2) Haarde, W., Mewes, D., 1990, Das Vermischen geringer Stoffmengen in großvolumigen Lagertanks und chemischen Reaktoren; Chem. Ing. Technik 62, 52-53
3) Mayinger, F., Lübbe, D., 1984, Ein tomographisches Meßverfahren und seine Anwendung auf Mischvorgänge und Stoffaustausch; Wärme- und Stoffübertragugn 18, 49-59
4) Mewes, D., 1991, Measurement of temperature fields by holographic tomography; Exp. Therm. and Fluid Sci 4, 171-181
5) Mewes, D., Ostendorf, W., 1986, Application of tomographic measurement techniques for process engineering studies; Int. Chem. Engng. 26, 11-21
6) Mewes, D., Renz, R., 1991, Meß- und Rekonstruktionsmethoden für tomografische Messungen; Chem. Ing. Technik 63, 699-715
7) Sweeney, D. W., 1972, Interferometric measurement of three-dimensional temperature fields; Diss., Univ. Michigan
8) Mewes, D., Ostendorf, W., Haarde, W., Friederich, M., 1989, Tomographic measurement techniques for process engineering studies; in: "Handbook of Heat and Mass Transfer, Vol. 3", p. 961/1021, Ed. N. P. Cheremisinoff, Gulf Publishers
9) Herman, C., Mewes, D., Mayinger, F., 1992, Optical in transport phenomena; in "Adavances in Transport Processes", Vol. 8, A.S. Mujumdar, R.A. Mashelkar (Ed.), Elsevier Science Publ., Amsterdam und New York, p. 1-58

STUDY OF BED VOIDAGE IN PACKED BED FLOWS USING PHOTON TRANSMISSION TOMOGRAPHY

M. E. Hosseini-Ashrafi[+], U. Tüzün[+] and N. MacCuaig[++]

+ Department of Chemical & Process Eng., Surrey University, Guildford, UK.
++ SMIS ltd., Allan Turing Rd., Surrey Research Park, Guildford, UK.

ABSTRACT: A specially constructed multiple source transmission
tomography scanner rig is used to produce consecutive tomograms of the
horizontal planes at different heights of the granular beds flowing in
both cylindrical and conical vessels. In a series of experiments
involving axial-symmetric flow of mono sized and binary fills of powder
materials, the transients in the cross sectional voidage profiles are for
the first time quantified to within a spatial accuracy of 1 mm.

Experimental results to date with near spherical particles indicate
highly reproducible correlations between particle size distribution and
bed porosity in both static and flowing beds. Spatial and time transients
of the porosity resulting from interstitial fluid drag are also studied.
The results show clear evidence of a cyclic propagation of a
counter-current voidage wave accompanying solids discharge from the
hopper.

1.   INTRODUCTION

The porosity of a packed bed of particles is determined largely by the
single particle properties such as particle size and shape distributions
(Cumberland et al [1987]) as well as particle surface properties such as
surface roughness and hardness. The effect of geometric constraints such as
a wall boundary is known to be confined very locally to within a distance
of a few particle diameters (Laohakul [1978]).

There is , however, little experimental literature investigating the
effects of single particle properties on the voids structure of flowing
granular beds. The need for such measurements is long established in
industrial applications such as extrusion, tabletting, agglomeration,
mixing and blending, dosing and metering of granular materials. Problems
range from the lack of control on solids flow rates, build up of adverse
pore pressures during solids discharge, to the prevention of particle
segregation and attrition during bed compaction and shearing and to
achieving desired bulk density specification of the products. The extent
and the frequency of these problems are believed to be closely linked to
the transients of the bulk voidage experienced by the particle assemblies
during handling in the respective process units.

The interstitial pore structure of static assemblies of mono size, binary
and ternary mixtures of spheres has been the subject of many theoretical
studies; see for example the reports by Dodds [1980], Yu and Standish

[1988] and Arteaga and Tüzün [1990]. There is yet to emerge a completely analytical method to predict the so-called "packing efficiency" of different size spheres as a function of particle size ratio and relative volume fraction (McGeary [1961]). There are also theoretical studies such as those by Stovall et al [1986] and Ouchiyama et al [1989], of the mean field values of the bulk density of materials corresponding to different continuous functional forms of the particle size distribution. In contrast, non spherical particle shape or indeed particle shape distributions have received very little attention.

Measurements of flowing bed voidage have not met with much success in the past largely due to the lack of technology which currently exists in remote imaging. Photography could only be used to visualize voidage patterns next to a transparent wall surface such as in a 2D or a semi-cylindrical vessel see for example Tüzün and Nedderman [1982]. The X-ray radiography technique used in the seventies by such investigators as Bransby and Blair-Fish [1975], relied on the use of lead markers for the identification of deformation patterns during flow. The hazards associated with high energy radiation and the practical difficulty of developing numerous radiographic plates to cover a few seconds of flow have seriously hindered progress.

The use of probe techniques such as laser, acoustic or fiber optics; (see Tüzün et al [1982] for a comprehensive review) can provide local information around the vicinity of the probe but often with rather poor spatial accuracy. The electrical capacitance measurements of the granular beds have also been used with some success by workers such as Hancock [1970] to monitor voidage changes during flow. Usually, the measurements of voidage are averaged across the bed cross section since the accuracy of the capacitance reading deteriorates as one moves from the vessel walls into the center of the bed. Moreover, to detect changes of voidage on a number of cross sectional planes, it is necessary to set up integrated wire circuits on the holding vessel. Thus, in general, the spatial accuracy afforded by the capacitance technique limits its use to the detection of large bubbles or cavities (of the order of centimeters) while monitoring the relative volume fractions of the solid and fluid phases passing through the circuits.

The transmission tomography technique employed in the present study has allowed us to quantify interstitial voidage profiles to within 1 - 2 mm of spatial accuracy while allowing consecutive scans of many cross sectional planes at various stages of discharge from an axially - symmetric holding vessel. Engaging a system of multiple parallel radiation sources for scanning has ensured that the scan times are reduced to within a few minutes. The high spatial accuracy of the voidage readings provided by the current technique is essential for detecting the effects of the single particle properties discussed above on the void structure of the packed beds. Our measurements to date have already revealed reproducible trends in both the horizontal and vertical variations of voidage in different flow regimes corresponding to different stages of batch discharge from a holding vessel.

2.   EXPERIMENTAL APPARATUS

Fig. 1 shows a schematic of the model hopper rig used together with a detailed layout of the scanner ring shown as an insert.

2.1 Mobile Multiple Source Scanner

The scanner employs six [153]Gd emitted, parallel geometry photon beams in conjunction with six collimated CsI scintillation detectors arranged on a circular gantry which is placed around the object to be scanned. The availability of two energies per emission provides the additional opportunity of dual energy transmission tomography and the high specific activity of the sources allows the utilization of high photon fluxes. Collimators with two different aperture widths i.e 1 mm and 2 mm were used in the present study to scan 3 mm thick cross sectional slices of the powder beds.

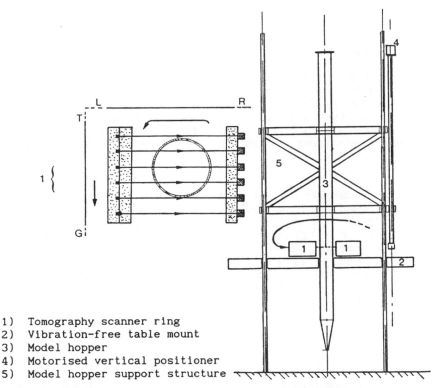

1) Tomography scanner ring
2) Vibration-free table mount
3) Model hopper
4) Motorised vertical positioner
5) Model hopper support structure

Fig.(1)   Schematic of the experimental apparatus and the rotating scanner ring comprising six parallel geometry photon beams; also showing the L-R and T-G axes.

2.2 Model Hopper Rig

A 2 m tall perspex cylinder of 96 mm inner diameter is mounted on a conical hopper section of 10^0 half angle and a 10 mm diameter orifice so chosen to achieve "mass flow" condition. The flow experiments to date were carried out under open top condition; future work will consider flows in closed top bins.

The scanner is fixed on a vibration free stone table and is therefore restricted to imaging on a fixed horizontal plane. To allow for scans at different heights , the model hopper is mounted on an aluminium frame which is driven by a computer controlled stepping motor.   The stone table has a hole drilled to match the central opening of the scanner rig , thus

allowing the hopper to travel up and down a vertical distance of about 850 mm.   The versatility of the hopper rig ensures that scanning experiments can be run in one of three modes :
i)   Sequential scanning at different heights in start-stop flow mode to maximise reconstructed image quality,
ii)   Sequential scanning at a fixed height during continuous discharge to produce different time averaged voidage profiles,
iii) Continuous discharge and simultaneous upwards hopper travel at a specified speed to match the flow velocity of the particles.   This brings the particles moving at the same speed as the hopper travel to relative stagnation and therefore into 'focus' during imaging.

Only results of experiments of type (i) are reported here.

3.   PROCEDURE FOR IMAGE EVALUATION

The best resolution currently achievable is given by 1 mm square pixel of 3 mm thickness. With granular materials of different particle sizes in the field of view, two possibilities exist : i) Individual particle sizes are larger than the pixel size in which case the boundaries of individual particles may be observed directly, and ii) the particle sizes are smaller than the resolving element when no particle boundaries will be observed and a volume averaging over each pixel between the particle and the surrounding medium occurs.

Figs.2(a) and (b) compare the reconstructed images of the same horizontal plane across a static granular bed with mono-sized (850- 1000 μm) acrylic beads set against a binary mixture of 8.3 ÷ 1 size ratio of 30 % by weight of fines (90 - 125 μm) .   Since the individual particle sizes are less than the spatial resolution of the scans, it is not possible to distinguish between these two images by visual inspection.   Fig.3(a) compares the line profiles of the scaled attenuation coefficients , G.S. across the centers of the two images seen in Figs.2 (a) and (b) respectively.   In this case, the difference between the two beds is more apparent with somewhat higher values of the attenuation coefficient for the binary mixture bed.

 a

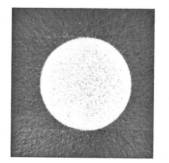 b

Fig.2   Reconstructed images of the same horizontal plane across two different static beds. (a) Mono-size static bed of spherical particles; (b) Binary mixture bed of spherical particles.

Given that no useful information could be obtained by visual inspection of the two images, an analytical procedure was developed to extract from the photon attenuation maps , the numerical values for the fractional solids content of each pixel within the field.   The linear attenuation coefficient at a given discrete photon energy is a strong function of the atomic number of the material's constituting elements as well as its solid density.   If particles of the same material are used, the attenuation coefficients will be linearly related to the density and the following equation may be used to calculate the fractional solids content, at position [x,y], η [x, y] of a single pixel;-

$$\eta[x,y] = \frac{\mu_{[x,y]} - \mu_{AIR}}{\mu_{SOLID} - \mu_{AIR}} = 1 - \varepsilon[x,y] \tag{1}$$

where $\mu_{[x,y]}$ represents the reconstructed linear attenuation   coefficient value of the pixel with the unknown solids content and μ_{air} and μ_{solid} are the reconstructed linear attenuation coefficient values of air and solid filled pixels respectively. In practice, μ_{air} and μ_{solid} are determined by averaging   the   reconstructed   attenuation   coefficient   values   of   a representative sample of pixels which are filled totally by air or solid respectively.   Both values have therefore associated standard deviations , which in turn may affect the calculated $\eta[x,y]$ values.

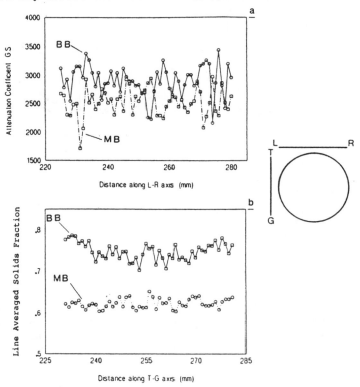

Fig. (3)   Line scans along the L-R and T-G axes at the same horizontal plane with two different static beds; BB: Binary Bed, MB: Mono-Bed.

Fig. 3(b) compares the profiles of solids fraction along the T-G axes of the reconstructed images seen in Figs. 2(a) and (b). These profiles were calculated by averaging the $\eta[x,y]$ values obtained from eqn. 1 for each successive line across the L-R axis. The difference in the solids contents of the mono and the binary beds is now quite apparent as seen in Fig. 3(b).

The computer software has been developed to extract from the calculated linear attenuation coefficient maps the line profiles of the interstitial voidage both on the cartesian and polar coordinates. The Cartesian coordinate system maintains consistency with the pixel geometry, Fig. 4(a), whilst the polar coordinate system ensures consistency with the hopper geometry, Fig. 4(b). In the Cartesian coordinate system the average void fraction is calculated on the L-R axis and is plotted in the T-G axis. In the polar coordinate system however, the average values are calculated for a pre-selected radius and plotted for various angles , β, in steps of 1° and from zero to 360°. Furthermore, the necessary software has been developed to calculate averaged void fraction values for equal area strips spanning radially away from the center of the hopper cross-section, Fig. 4(c). It is thought that the results together from the three complementary analysis routines provide a complete data set allowing features such as axial asymmetry and radial variations to be recognised and quantified.

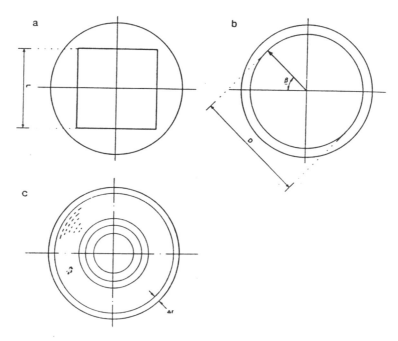

Fig. (4) The coordinate systems for the calculation of the mean voidage values at the hopper plane excluding the wall region; a): Cartesian coordinates; b): Polar coordinates; c): Annular segment coordinates.

The plane mean void fraction, E over n number of pixels per horizontal plane is calculated by ;-

$$E = \left(\sum_{i=1}^{n} \varepsilon [x_i, y_i] \right) / n = 1 - \left(\sum_{i=1}^{n} \eta [x_i, y_i] \right) / n \qquad (2)$$

where n is the number of pixels in a given planar section and η is the solids fraction of each pixel as defined in eqn. 1 above. It must be emphasized here, however, that each reconstructed image represents a cross sectional slice of the object with a finite thickness. The thickness of the slice is determined by the aperture height of the collimator which is kept at 3 mm at the present study. Therefore, the values of ε and η used in eqn. 2 are averaged over each volume element.

The plane mean void fractions presented here were calculated by considering a central circular region of interest as seen in Fig. 4(b) where the minimum distance between the region of interest and the bin perimeter, Δr is not allowed to be smaller than 8- 10 particle diameters thereby excluding the 'wall effect' on the values of the voidage obtained; see for example the report by Laohakul [1978]. Further work will address the voidage variations near the walls as a function of wall roughness and hopper half-angle.

4.   AXIALLY-SYMMETRIC FLOW EXPERIMENTS

4.1 Materials
The particles used throughout the study were polymethyl methacrylate spheres. They had an original size range of 90 to 1000 μm and were sieved into the required size classes. Quantimetric analyses were performed on representative samples from each particle batch, the results of which are shown in Table I.

Table I: Material Properties.

Particle size class	Mean particle diameter $\pm \sigma$ (μm)[*]	Mean sphericity $\pm \sigma$ (%)[**]
90 to 125 μm	110 $\pm$ 13	85.2 $\pm$ 12.6
125 to 212 μm	179 $\pm$ 25.8	84.3 $\pm$ 7.3
850 to 1000 μm	915 $\pm$ 80.6	88.8 $\pm$ 6.0

[+]   (4 x surface area/π)$^{1/2}$
[++] Sphericity(%) = $4\pi K$ x 100; K = surface area/ (perimeter)^2

4.2 Experiments
In a series of experiments involving batch discharge of granular materials from the model hopper unit, (see Fig. 1), the interstitial voidage transients occurring in cylindrical and conical hopper sections have been monitored as a function of the duration of discharge. Cross-sectional line profiles in the polar coordinate system of voidage were generated to within 1° spatial accuracy at various heights along the model silo using both mono-dispersed and binary mixture beds. In a series of start - stop flow experiments, the same horizontal planes were scanned consecutively, in time steps of 5 - 10

seconds over a period of 1- 2 minutes of discharge. Further work will aim
to compare these results with the time averaged voidage profiles obtained
during continuous flow experiments.

5.   ANALYSIS OF EXPERIMENTAL RESULTS

The experimental scans have been analysed :
i) to provide comparison between the static and flowing voidage profiles
across different horizontal planes in both the conical and cylindrical
hopper sections,
ii) to generate height profiles of planar void fraction at different stages
of discharge.

5.1 Comparison of Static Voidage Profiles
Fig.5 shows some typical data obtained on the variation of the plane mean
voidage with height in a static bed of mono-sized particles in comparison
with a binary mixture of 25 % by weight of fines of 5.1 ÷ 1 size ratio.
Both sets of results were obtained in the model silo rig shown in Fig.1.
Each data point in Fig.5 was calculated using the procedure described in
section 3 and given by eqn.(2) above. The data obtained over several runs
were found to be reproducible to within ± 2 % as indicated in Fig.5. It is
not possible to comment quite how much of this is due to the accuracy of
the scanner data analysis and how much is due to the intrinsic assembly
fluctuations within the packed beds characteristic of the batch filling
technique used.

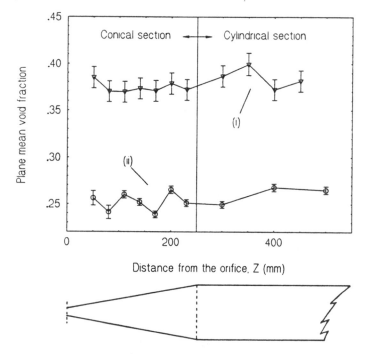

Fig.(5)   Comparison of the static voidage profiles of:
(i) mono-sized bed of 125-212 µm diameter spheres and (ii) binary
bed of 75% b.w. of 850-1000 µm and 25% b.w. of 125-212 µm diameter
spheres.

The static bed values of the solids fraction are found not to alter
significantly with height in both the cylindrical and conical sections of
the model hopper. Fig.5 demonstrates this point, and the mean value of the
plane mean solids fractions obtained at 13 different heights in static
condition is reported in Table II. However, there is a somewhat visible
increase in voidage in going from the conical to the cylindrical section of
the silo rig in line with the previously measured trends in bulk stress
fields set up during filling; see for example Tüzün and Nedderman [1985].
Similarly, voidage also appears to increase with approach to the orifice in
Fig.5; however, the present apparatus arrangement makes it impossible to
record data closer than about 50 mm ($\cong$ 5 D_o). Work is currently underway
to gather data at the vicinity of the orifice plane which is known to
affect significantly the mass discharge rates from hoppers; see for example
Nedderman et al [1982].

Table II: Solids Fractions of Binary Mixtures of Finite Particle
Size Ratios (i.e Φ_R < 10)

Φ_R	X_f	$(\eta_{mix})_{exp}$	X_{fl} *	$(\eta_{mix})_{max}$ *
5.1 : 1	0.25	0.75 $\pm$ 0.02	0.44	0.79
8.3 : 1	0.30	0.78 $\pm$ 0.02	0.33	0.83

*   Comparison   of   plane   mean   solid   fractions   obtained   with   gamma-ray
transmission   tomography   with   predictions   by   Arteaga   and   Tüzün   (1990)   of
maximum solid fractions of randomly packed binary mixtures.
X_{fl} = Predicted weight fraction of fines at maximum solids fraction.

5.2 Comparison of Flowing Voidage Profiles
Flow experiments were conducted in the experimental rig seen in Fig.1 both
with mono-sized and binary mixture samples.   A series of cross sectional
scans of the silo contents were obtained at various heights during batch
discharge. The static bed height was set at about 700 mm above the orifice
prior to each run and the material top surface was found to descend to a
height of about 400 mm during a 60 second discharge time.   As expected, no
significant coning of the top surface was observed during its descend in
the cylindrical section of the silo.

Figs.6(a) -(c) show some typical sample data on the flowing voids fraction
profiles obtained in different coordinate systems using the three analysis
routines discussed in section 3 above.As indicated in Fig.6, the data
showing line variation (Fig.6(a)) and angular variation (Fig.6(b)) of void
fraction across a given horizontal plane exhibit large ($\leq \pm$ 10 %) pixel
to pixel fluctuation.   More importantly, the present technique is able to
detect asymmetry about the center of the flow in both line and polar scan
data.

The noise in the voidage scan data is reduced considerably in the example
given in Fig.6(c) when the voidage values are calculated over annular
segments of equal cross-sectional area across the hopper.   The damping

effect of averaging voidage fluctuations in flow over distances of some
tens of particle diameters rather than a few at a time is self evident and
is demonstrated clearly in Fig. 6(c).

Fig. 7(a) – (c) compares the height profiles of plane mean values of voidage
obtained at various stages of batch discharge of a mono bed of fine
particles. Similar data are shown in Fig. 8(a) – (c) for a binary mixture
comprising the same fine particles in the presence of a 75% by weight of
large granules of 5.1 + 1 size ratio.

Considering firstly the mono bed of fines data in Fig. 7; two main features
emerge: i) There appears to be a well-defined voidage maximum within the
conical section whose position is shown to propagate up the silo with
continued discharge; ii) The interstitial voidage attains a minimum value
within the cylindrical section close to the cylinder/cone transition plane.

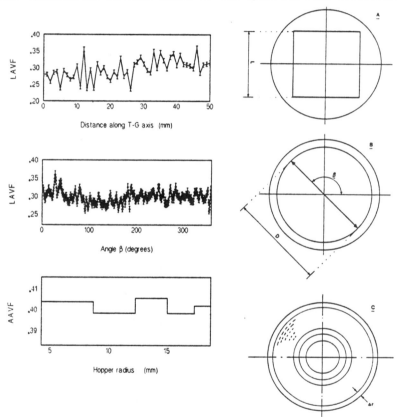

Fig. (6)   Cross sectional profiles of flowing voidage in Axially-symmetric
flow: (a) Line scan data for a binary bed of 75% b.w. of 850-1000 μm   and
25% b.w. of 125-212 μm diameter spheres after 5s of discharge at Z=230 mm,
(b) Polar scan data for the same binary mixture bed as in (a) but after
60s of discharge and at Z=400 mm and (c) Annular segment scan data for a
mono-sized bed of 125-212 μm diameter spheres after 7s of discharge and at
Z=140mm.   (L. A. V. F. = Line Averaged Void Fraction & A. A. V. F. = Annular
Averaged Void Fraction).

Similar observations are also applicable to the profiles seen in Fig.8(a) –
(c) with the binary mixture. However, this time, the positions of voidage
maxima and minima are much more sharply defined. An important feature of
Fig.8 is the dynamics of the voidage maximum in the conical section. It
has been assumed by many workers previously that the position of the
voidage maximum is a static feature of the fully developed flow fields in
conical hoppers where the position is altered only by altering the hopper
half- angle and the level of surcharge on the conical section; see for
example Spink and Nedderman [1978], Gu et al [1991]. In Fig.8, we observe
the position of the voids maximum to propagate up the cone with a decaying
magnitude while a second maximum is seen to emerge behind it with an
increasing amplitude. This clearly indicates a dynamic wave behaviour
strongly linked to the material properties of the flowing beds as well as
the percolation behaviour of the interstitial air through the bed.

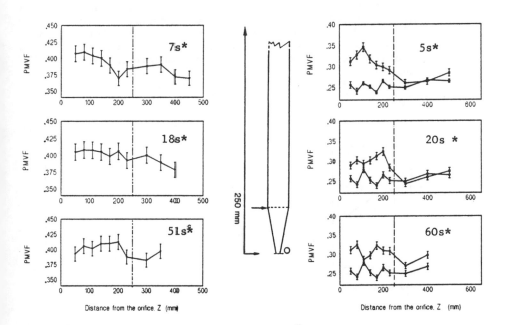

*   Discharge times in seconds

Fig.(7) Vertical profiles of the
plane mean voidage in the model
silo during batch discharge of a
mono-sized bed of 124–212 μm dia.
spheres.

Fig.(8): Vertical profiles of the
plane mean voidage in the model
silo during batch discharge of a
binary mixture of 75 % b.w. of
850–1000 μm and 25% b.w. of 125–
212 μm dia. spheres.

(P.M.V.F. = Plane Mean Void Fraction)

6.   COMPARISON WITH THEORY

6.1 Comparison of Experimental and Theoretical Values of Mean Voidage
Table II compares the statistical average of the plane mean values of the

static solids fraction obtained from the tomographic scans at 13 different heights with the theoretical maxima predicted by Arteaga and Tüzün [1990] for the corresponding particle size ratios. Details of their calculations are given elsewhere (Arteaga and Tüzün [1990] and Tüzün and Arteaga [1991]) and will therefore not be repeated here. The agreement between theory and experiment is encouraging especially in the case of Φ_R= 8.3 as is also revealed by Fig.3(b) above.

6.2 Calculation of Propagation Velocity of Voidage Maximum During Flow

Using the type of data presented in Fig.8, an empirical procedure was adapted to calculate the voidage maximum propagation velocity within the conical hopper. Fig.9(a) shows a second order polynomial fit to data used to calculate the position of the voidage maximum as a function of the discharge time.   The results are shown in Fig.9(b) where the position of the voidage maximum is plotted against the 60 second discharge time. Here the data point corresponding to the 60 second discharge time was generated by fitting a third order polynomial to the voidage profile in Fig.8(c) due to the pronounced second peak following the first one.   Furthermore, data presented in Fig.9(b) is fitted with another second order polynomial so as to allow the calculation of the velocity of void propagation as a function of discharge time.

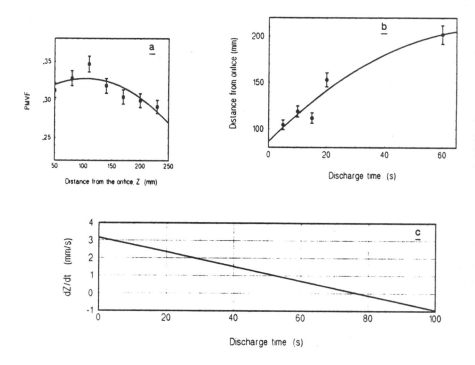

Fig.(9) Calculation of propagation velocity of the voidage maximum during batch discharge of a binary mixture bed of 75% b.w. of 850-1000 μm and 25% b.w. of 125-212 μm diameter spheres.   a) Variation of Plane Mean Void Fraction (P.M.V.F.) in the cone section   after 5s of discharge;   b) Point of maximum void vs discharge period; c) Velocity of maximum void vs discharge time.

Fig.9(c) shows a plot of void maximum propagation velocity versus the discharge time obtained by differentiating the curve in Fig.9(b). Extrapolation to zero time results in a maximum value of the propagation velocity of about 3.2 mm s^{-1}. Similarly, propagation velocity is reduced to zero after about 75 seconds of discharge. Clearly, flow times in excess of 75 seconds are required in this case to verify the time constants for these voidage transients. These will be the subject of a further study.

7. CONCLUSIONS

A novel computerised scanner featuring a multiple source and detector ring for gamma ray transmission tomography is developed specially to measure static and flowing voidage profiles of granular beds in axially-symmetric containers. The present equipment provides spatial resolutions of 1- 2 mm in imaging combined with scan times of the order of a few minutes. These features make it ideal for its use in continuous imaging of flowing particle beds in a number of modes as described above.

The paper describes a set of preliminary experiments with mono-sized and binary beds of particles of near spherical shape during gravity flow in a model hopper rig. In a series of scans taken at several consecutive time intervals during batch discharge of the material bed, the cross sectional profiles of solids fraction at different heights as well as the corresponding plane mean values of the voids fraction could be obtained in both cylindrical and conical hopper sections. These data are in turn used to generate the profiles of plane mean voidage prevailing at different times in the model silo.

The values of solids fractions obtained in static and flowing beds compare well with the theoretical values corresponding to the random packings of mono-sized and binary mixtures of spheres. The error analyses carried out on the accuracy and the reproducibility of the tomographic scan data have revealed less than ± 1.5 % error on the values of the plane mean voidage and less than ± 4 % on the values of the solids fraction calculated per pixel volume along the cross sectional line profiles taken over scan times of the order of a few minutes.

The voidage profile data generated in the model silo are used to identify the planes of maximum and minimum voidage as well as that of the propagation velocity of the voidage maximum as a function of the time of discharge. These results agree well with the expected initial flow transients and the subsequent flow regime transitions in the cylindrical and conical sections of the model silo. Further study of the voidage wave propagation described here should prove valuable in modelling the interstitial fluid and particle percolation patterns in packed bed flows.

ACKNOWLEDGEMENTS :

The authors would like to thank Surrey Medical Imaging Systems Ltd., Surrey University Research Park for the design and construction of the CAT Scanner Facility and the associated software. The SERC major equipment grant and the research funding provided under the Specially Promoted Programme in Particle Technology are also gratefully acknowledged.

Notation:

D_o	diameter of the outlet orifice
d	particle diameter
E	plane mean void fraction
^{153}Gd	Gadilinium isotope of atomic mass number 153
Δr	minimum distance between region of analysis & silo wall
β	Angle defining the polar coordinate system
ε	interstitial void fraction
Φ_R	particle size ratio
μ	linear photon attenuation coefficient
η	interstitial solid fraction

REFERENCES

Arteaga P. and Tüzün U. (1990) "Flow of Binary Mixtures of Equal-Density Granules in Hoppers - Size Segregation, Flowing Density and Discharge Rates" *Chem. Eng. Sci.* **vol.45** p.205.

Bransby P.L. and Blair-Fish P.M. (1975) "Initial Deformation During Mass Flow from a Bunker: Observation and Idealization" *Powder Technology* **vol.11** p.273.

Cumberland D.J. and Crawford R.J. (1987) "The Packing of Particles" *Handbook of Powder Technology* **vol.6** p.59. Elsevier Amsterdam.

Dodds J.A. (1980) "The Porosity and Contact Points in Multi-Component Random Sphere Packings Calculated by a Statistical Geometric Model" *J.Colloid and Interface Sci.* **vol.77** p.317.

Gu Z.H., Arnold P.C. and McLean A.G. (1991) "Prediction of Air Pressure Distribution in Mass Flow Bins" *Powder Technology*, in press.

Hancock A.W. (1970) "Stress on Bunker Walls" *Ph.D. Thesis,* University of Cambridge, UK.

Laohakul C. (1978) "Velocity Distribution of Flowing Granular Materials" *Ph.D. Thesis,* University of Cambridge, UK.

McGeary R.K. (1961) "Mechanical Packing of Spherical Particles *J. Am. Ceramic Soc.* **vol.44** p.513.

Nedderman R.M., Tüzün U., Savage S.B. and Houlsby G.T. (1982) "The Flow of Granular Materials-I: Discharge Rates from Hoppers" *Chem. Eng. Sci.* **vol.37** p.1597.

Ouchiyama N. and Tanaka T. (1989) "Predicting the Densest Packings of Ternary and Quaternary Mixtures of Solid Particles" *Ind. Eng. Chem. Res.* **vol.28** p.1530.

Spink C.D. and Nedderman R.M. (1978) "Gravity Discharge Rate Of Fine Particles from Hoppers" *Powder Technology,* **vol.21** p.245.

Stovall T., De Larrard F. and Buil M. (1986) "Linear Packing Density Model of Grain Mixtures" *Powder technology,* **vol.48** p.1.

Tüzün U. and Arteaga P. (1991) "Microstuctural Effects on Stress and Flow Fields of Equal Density Granules in Hoppers" *Proc. of the I. Mech. E (G.B.),* **vol.12** p.265.

Tüzün U., Houlsby G.T., Nedderman R.M. and Savage S.B. (1982) "The Flow of Granular Materials-II: Velocity Distribution in Slow Flow" *Chem. Eng. Sci.* **vol.37** p.1691.

Tüzün U. and Nedderman R.M. (1982) "An Investigation of the Flow Boundary During Steady-State Discharge from a Funnel-Flow Bunker" *Powder Technology* **vol.31** p.27.

Tüzün U. and Nedderman R.M. (1985) "Gravity Flow of Granular Materials Round Obstacles-II: Investigation of the Stress Profiles at the Wall of a Silo with Inserts" *Chem. Eng. Sci.* **vol.40** p.337.

Yu A.B. and Standish N. (1988) An Analytical-Parametric Theory of the Random Packing Of Particles" *Powder Technology* **vol.55** p.171.

Chapter 4

Process Monitoring and Control

DEVELOPMENT OF AN EIT SYSTEM
FOR
THERMAL MAPPING AND PROCESS CONTROL

Pär H Henriksson, BRR Persson, B Bladh, K Tranberg, P Möller

Request for reprints: Professor Bertil RR Persson, Radiation Physics Department, Lund University Hospital, S-221 85 Lund, Sweden.

ABSTRACT: In our previous and ongoing projects Electrical Impedance Tomography (EIT) has been evaluated as a tool for temperature monitoring during hyperthermia treatments. The image reconstruction used is based on a recently developed algorithm SPREAD. The amount of floating point arithmetic has been greatly reduced, the aim is to design a system working in "real time". Although further development is needed, we belive that the EIT method used in conjunction with conventional temperature measurements will form an important tool for deep penetration hyperthermia. The aim of the recently started work is to investigate the possibility to use the EIT method for monitoring thermal distribution and mixing properties during biological processes.

1. Introduction

Electrical Impedance Tomography, EIT, is a promising imaging method that can be used to study the dynamic behavior within a conductive body. The method is well suited for the reconstruction of relative maps describing the changes of resistivity. A possibility to reconstruct absolute images is also exists, the spatial resolution and accuracy presently however cannot compete with other imaging system available. The low complexity and moderate cost of an EIT system talks for absolute imaging system for portable use and as an complementary method.

The collection of each individual measurements takes only a short time, typically 1 mS or less depending on the frequency and data collection technique. It is possible to secure data from all individual electrodes in the system at the same time using a parallel front-end system. If 16 electrodes are used and all potentials are measured in parallel, the complete set of data can be collected in less than 16 mS.

The main advantage, besides low cost and simplicity, is the high measurement speed. To fully utilize the possibilities given, a fast image reconstruction method is vital. Instead of a straight beam that penetrates the object, as in most imaging systems, EIT uses a current which is injected through the matter. The resulting potentials are measured at pre-defined points on the surface. Each individual measurement will depend on the complete intersection. The commonly used and relatively fast back-projection algorithm and the further developed successors are not very well suited to solve this problem.

Previous work (Amasha H.M, Griffiths H 1987, Conway J. 1987, Blad B 1991) show that the EIT method can be used to calculate the temperature distribution within the treatment area. During these projects the method was evaluated in-vitro on test phantoms as well as in-vivo on patients.

2. ALGORITHMS AND SOFTWARE

We need to develop a method that can works on the whole intersection of the object at each projection keeping in mind that the object not necessary is circular nor homogeneous.

To be able to meet the needs for high speed performance making real time imaging possible, as many calculations as possible has to be made prior to the image reconstruction. The remaining arithmetic should if possible be restricted to integers only. The algorithm should be designed for future parallel processing.   .

Back projection and its further developed succesors are commonly used for image reconstruction. For system that uses some kind of beam to investigate the internal property of an object, these methods give a suitable quality and definition. The main problem with EIT is the fact that the current is spread throughout the object. This can studied and simulated in a tissue equivalent resistor mesh using a computer based electronic simulation tool (P Henriksson et al 1992).

In our case we will calculate and present the image as a 32 * 32 positions integer array. The selected spatial resolution of 64 * 64 pixels requires a total data size of 4096 elements or 16384 bytes. As the system is intended to present relative images, a reference frame with the same memory requirement is needed for normalization.

In each individual measurement, all elements in the cross-section will give their contribution to the measured potential. The influence from each element is calculated prior to the actual measurement using a simulation program. These data are stored in a multidimensional "distribution array" and will be used during the image reconstruction process. In a non homogeneous body the potential lines will be shifted compared to those in a homogeneous body. It is possible to describe this phenomena in the distribution array.

The image reconstruction process is simple and can be described using a Pascal "look alike" notation, figure 1.

Procedure Spread;

```
1   long integer image[0..63,0..63];
2   integer distr[0..15,0..15,0..63,0..63];
3   integer chan_out;
4   integer chan_in;
5   integer Xpos,Ypos;
6   integer data;

7   for(chan_out := 0 to 15)
8   begin
9     inject(chan_out);
10    for(chan_in := 0 to 15)
11    begin
12      data := readpotential(chan_in);
13      for(Xpos := 0 to 63)
14        for(Ypos := 0 to 63)
15          image[Xpos,Ypos] := image[Xpos,Ypos] +
16              data * dist[chan_out,chan_in,Xpos,Ypos];
17    end;
18  end;
```

Figure 1. The SPREAD algorithm

The image is stored in an array named "image" (line 1). The distribution array, calculated prior to the measurements, is stored in the multidimensional array "distr", (line 2). The procedure uses several loops, in the outermost loop (line 7), the signal is injected to all electrodes (line 9) in the system. I the next loop (line 10) the potential is measured on each electrode (line 12) the data is then distributed to the image array using two loops for X and Y dimension. The output from spread is a raw image which comprises the sum of the contribution of all projections. The relative image that will presented is normalized by subtraction of a background image.

One drawback is the amount of static data required for the distribution array. We intend to solve this problem temporarily by reducing the spatial and dynamical resolution. The resolution in the distribution array will be reduced to 32 * 32 elements. The data in the distribution array will be represented as a 4 bit integer giving a resolution of 0..15. The required amount of static data in the distribution array is thus reduced from 1 Mb to 64 Kb.

The distribution array data is stored on disk files using the original accuracy, when the data read into in memory the resolution is reduced to fit in memory.

3 Hardware

Two different systems have been used during the experiments, a third system is under development.

The first system is the well known serial system from Sheffield (Brown B.H. 1987). This system has been used by several groups in our studies and is used as a reference. The

Sheffield system works on 50 kHz and uses a non buffered
multiplexed technology.

The second system is a PC based parallel system (B Blad 1990)
developed in Lund. The system has 16 parallel channels with
buffers at the front end and a possibility to use 4 different
frequencies. Most experiments has been carried out using 50
kHz for comparative reasons.

The third system is serial and designed as a stand alone unit,
a built-in microprocessor is used for sequence control and
preprocessing of data. The microprocessor controlled 12 bit
signal generator can work on two frequencies, these
frequencies can be changed by replacing a crystal. The system
can communicate with a PC computer over two serial channels
for data and/or command interchange. Data processing and
presentation is made on the remote PC.

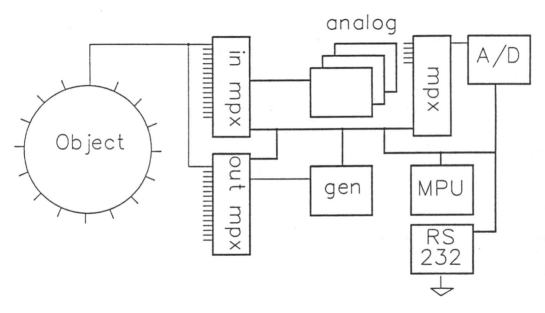

Figure 2 Block diagram

4 Results

Several different experiment has been carried out at Lund
university. We have decided to present two experiments, in
both the temperature changes in a phantom has been observed
using EIT.

4.1 Hot water interstitial heating

Electrodes are placed around a tissue equivalent phantom.
Water is circulated trough the phantom using small tubes, the
temperature of the water is controlled at 7 and 42 degrees
centigrade. The water flow is switched on and off using
valves.

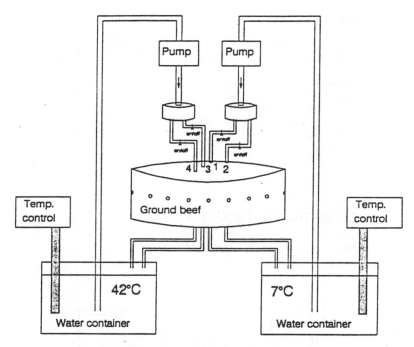

Figure 3 experimental setup

The experiment lasted for 20 minutes, during the first 10 minutes hot and cold water was flowing in the tubes. The following 4 minutes only the hot water was on, during the last part of the experiment both hot and cold water was left on. The resistivity change due to the temperature gradient was recorded. The results can be studied in figure 4.

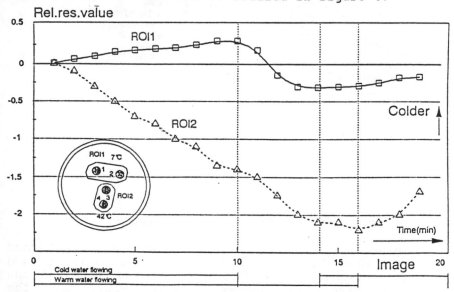

Figure 4. Recorded resistivity change in phantom.

3.2 Laserthermia

A surgical laser has been modified for external power on/off control from a PC computer equipped with a thermometry system.

During the experiment a phantom, pigs liver, is used. A thermistor i placed close to the laser tip. The laser is controlled from the computer, the aim is to keep the temperature in the surrounding tissue as close to 42.5 degrees centigrade as possible.

LASER THERMO THERAPY SYSTEM

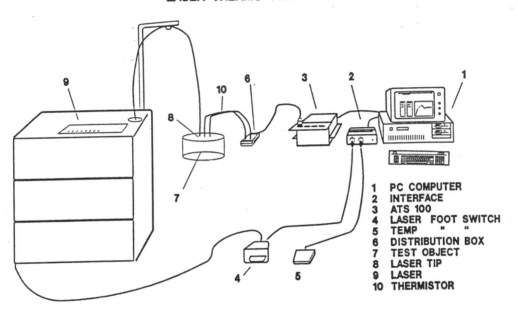

1	PC COMPUTER
2	INTERFACE
3	ATS 100
4	LASER FOOT SWITCH
5	TEMP " "
6	DISTRIBUTION BOX
7	TEST OBJECT
8	LASER TIP
9	LASER
10	THERMISTOR

Figure 5. Laser Thermo Therapy System

During the experiment the 16 EIT electrodes were attached symmetrically around the phantom. The heat distribution around the laser tip can observed in figure 6. At the start of the experiment, no effect can be seen (upper left). When the temperature increases a dark area becomes visible, (lower left, upper right and lower right).

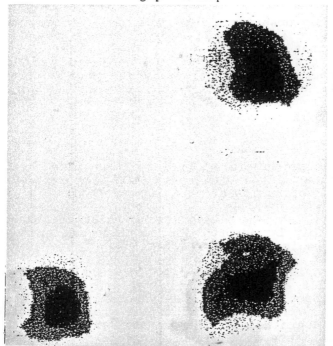

figure 6. Images of laserthermia phantom

The post analysis, figure 7, show that the impedance curve and temperature curve for specific points are similar. At the left the temperature recorded with thermistors at different distance from the laser tip is shown. At the right the resistivity change for the same positions is shown. It can be observed that curves are similar.

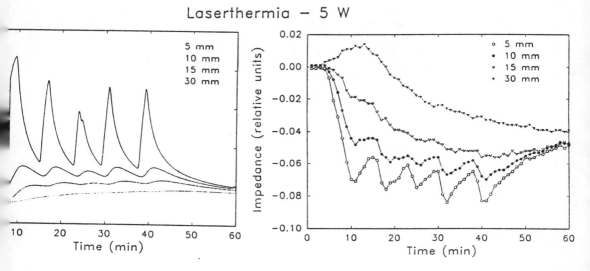

Figure 7. Impedance and temperature curve.

One intresting observation we have made is the fact that the
impedance curve is "tilted" compared to the temperature curve.
We belive that the this can have two major reasons, the
temperature gradient due to deposited energy or more likely
the permanent tissue change within the phantom. If the latter
is the case then the EIT system can be used not only for
temperature monitoring but also for monitoring the effect of
the treatment.

Conclusion

We have proposed a procedure for image reconstruction which
works on directly on the image array using pre calculated
arrays for distribution of data into the image.

The procedure has been designed for relative measurements but
can be probably be adapted for absolute measurements using a
simulated zero image for normalization.

The procedure is very well suited for parallel processing, the
image is built as a sum of several projections which can be
made independently. A parallel system with 16 identical input
sections and one main controller can be designed. The
summation of data can be done by hardware using the fact that
the image is the sum of the projections made at the 16 nodes.
Using relatively slow micro controllers for the task, (1
microsecond / instruction) the image reconstruction can be
completed i phase with the data collection. It is thus
possible to design a "real time" system capable of presenting
images at a frequency higher than 50 Hz.

Already in this first version effort has been made to make a
user friendly system environment. The program is written in
TURBO C which offers a large amount of pre written utility
procedures.

The different functions are blocked into pull-down menus as an
aid for the user to navigate within the system. Data can be
stored on files in "raw" form or in an image form for export
to other image processing systems. Directories are maintained
by the system to avoid the user from using non unique names or
accidently overwriting existing data.

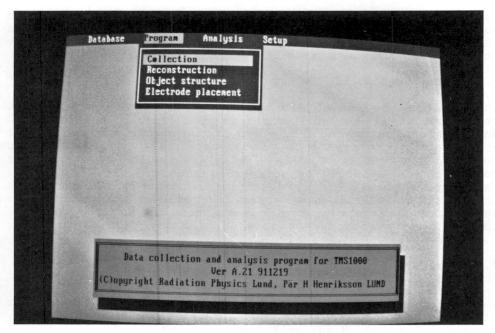

Figure 7. Main screen.

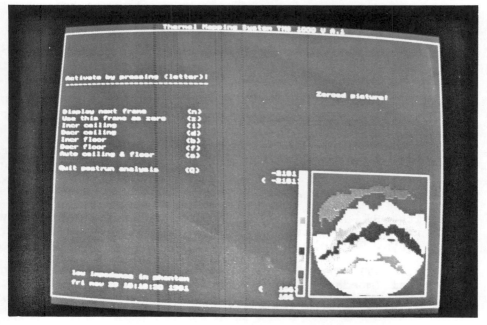

Figure 8. Graphical presentation

Image reconstruction can be made on-line or as a post analysis. Data is presented as a 64 times 64 matrix with 16 colors. The scale used when presenting data can selected automatic or manually by the user. Data is also presented as a histogram over a cross-section of the object using the same scale as for the color image.

6. Future development

The work on the serial EIT system developed in Lund has not been completed. We will continue the development on both software and hardware if the required funding can be raised. Analog data processing is made on small printed circuit boards, five boards can be installed simultaneously. These boards can be selected by software, adaption to other objects is therfore possible. The multiplexor strategy together with the built-in intelligence, makes it possible to program the system for different measuring sequences. It is also possible to use fewer electrodes to speed up the process when a lower image resolution is needed.

7. References

Amasha H.M., Anderson A.P.,Conway J., Barber D.C., 1988. Quantiative assessment of impedance tomography for temperature measurments in microwave hyperthermia. Clin. Phys. Physiol. Meas.,vol9,Suppl A;49-53.

Barber   D.C.,Brown   B.H.,   1984,   Applied   potential tomography. J. Phys. E Sci. Instrum. Vol.17, 723-733.

Blad B., Bertenstam L., Persson B., Holmer, N.-G., 1991, Eletrical impedance tomography, a non-invasive imaging system, for temperature monitoring. Acta Radiol. 32, Fasc. 1.

Brown B.H.,Seagar A.D.,1987, The Sheffield data collection system. Clin. Phys. Physiol. Meas. Vol. 8, Suppl. A, 91-97.

Conway   J.,   1987,   Eletrical   impedance   tomography   for thermal   monitoring   of   hyperthermia   treatment: an assessment using in vitro and in vivo measurments. Clin. Phys. Physiol. Meas., Vol. 8, Suppl. A, 141-146.

Griffiths H., Ahmed A.,1987, Applied potential tomography for non-invasive temperature mapping in hyperthermia. Clin. Phys. Physiol. Meas., Vol.8, Suppl.A, 147-153.

Blad B., 1991, Temperature Measuring in Hyperthermia using Eletrical Impedance Tomography. Internal report 7/91, Dep. of Eletrical Measurments. Lund Institute of Technology, LUTEDX/(TEEM-1045)/1-10/(1991).

Henriksson P H, Brockstedt S, Persson BRR (1992)

Transputer-based Electrical Capacitance Tomography for Real-Time Imaging of Oilfield Flow Pipelines

C. G. Xie*, S. M. Huang+, B. S. Hoyle†, C. P. Lenn+ and M. S. Beck*

*Department of Electrical Engineering & Electronics, Process Tomography Unit, UMIST, P.O. Box 88, Manchester M60 1QD.
+Schlumberger Cambridge Research, P.O. Box 153, Cambridge CB3 0HG.
†Department of Electrical & Electronics Engineering, University of Leeds, Leeds LS2 9JT.

ABSTRACT: This paper describes a transputer-based 12-electrode capacitance tomography system for imaging gas/oil flow pipelines. It is capable of reconstructing and displaying the distribution of each component of a flow over the pipe cross-section at 40 frames/s. The flow component fraction can be calculated and displayed, at the same speed, to an accuracy of 5% of full scale for most flow regimes (worst case about 10% for core flows). The image reconstruction algorithm is based on the filtered linear backprojection method and is implemented on a load-balancing transputer pipeline. The capacitance transducer incorporating an interface circuit with the remote transputer network can provide a data acquisition speed of 100 frames/s and a measurement resolution of 0.3 fF (it represents a 2% oil area-fraction change at the centre of an empty pipe).

1. INTRODUCTION

Oil wells often produce mixtures of oil, gas and water. Measurement of volume fraction of each component is required for well head control, production logging and, therefore, the optimal use of oil resources. The current technique is to separate the flow mixture first, and then measure each component using conventional single-component flowmeters. With the space on a production platform becoming increasingly costly, the use of conventional offshore separators, which are often very bulky, is becoming less desirable. There is, therefore, a strong incentive to develop a compact multi-component flowmeter for oilfield applications.

A 12-electrode electrical capacitance tomography system has been developed to meet the industrial demands [1-2]. This system can produce images of cross-sectional distribution of gas/oil flow components in the pipe, from which each component fraction can be obtained and the flow regime identified. Since flows in the pipe often travel at a few meters per second, this requires a flow imaging system to have high data acquisition and image reconstruction speeds. Fast capacitance measurement circuit and parallel processing technique using multiple transputers were chosen to accomplish these requirements.

The flow imaging system consists of three parts - the primary sensor, the sensor electronics and the transputer network for data acquisition, image reconstruction and display (Fig. 1).

The primary sensor is made by mounting 12 metal plates on the outer surface of a pipe section with an insulating pipe-liner (Fig. 4). The sensor can be designed to give an optimal image fidelity by using a finite element (FE) model implemented on transputers [2] or on a Sun workstation [3]. The FE model also accommodated the development of a linear backprojection algorithm for image reconstruction [2] (Section 3). The sensor electronics has incorporated an interface circuitry with a remote transputer network. It measures, in parallel, the capacitances between any two of the 12 electrodes in all possible combinations (there are 66 independent measurements, calculated from $N(N-1)/2$ where N is the total number of electrodes). The measured 66 capacitance values, whose amplitudes depend on the permittivity distribution of a gas/oil flow in the pipe, are sent to the transputer network via an electrical/optical link for image reconstruction. The design of the capacitance transducer electronics is described in Section 2. The transputer network is configured as a load-balancing pipeline. An imaging speed of 40 frame/s has been achieved and this has met the industrial requirement of real-time performance (Section 4). The on-line test of the imaging system on a 6-inch flow rig at SCR has been performed, and some typical experimental results will be presented in Section 5.

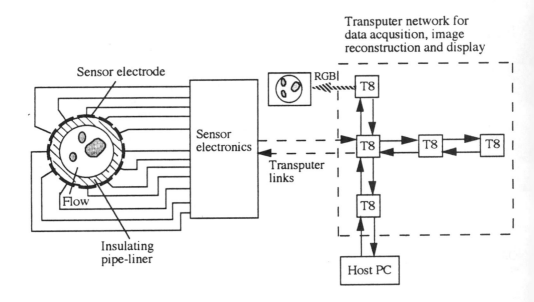

Fig. 1 *Transputer-based electrical capacitance tomography system for flow imaging*

2. THE CAPACITANCE MEASUREMENT CIRCUIT

For a 12-electrode system, the minimum standing capacitance (between two diagonally separated electrodes when the pipe is empty) is as small as 0.015 pF, and the measurement resolution required when imaging oil/gas flows is often 2% of this standing value (0.3 fF). To resolve such a small capacitance change, the sensor electronics must be designed to provide high sensitivity, high SNR, low baseline drift and large dynamic range. Additional requirements by industrial real-time applications include fast dynamic response (100 frame/s), support for high speed communication with the transputer system placed at a remote distance (up to 250 metres) from the sensor, fully software controlled circuit adjustment and compliance with the industrial safety standards. The design of the sensor electronics circuit which satisfies all the above requirements is described below.

2.1. Circuit Principle
The basic capacitance measuring circuit is based on the charge transfer principle [4]. The principle of the circuit's operation can be explained with reference to Fig. 2. One electrode of the unknown capacitance (source electrode) is connected with a pair of CMOS switches, S1 and S2, and another (detecting electrode) is connected with switches S3 and S4. In a typical operating cycle, the switches S1 and S3 are first closed (S2 and S4 open) to charge the unknown capacitance, C_x, to voltage, V_c, and the charging current flows into the input (at virtual earth potential) of the detector CD1 where it is converted into a negative voltage output. In the second half of the cycle, switches S2 and S4 close (S1 and S3 open) to discharge C_x to earth potential. The discharging current flows out of the current detector CD2, producing a

positive voltage output. This typical charge-discharge cycle repeats at a frequency f (1.25 MHz or 625 kHz), and the successive charging and discharging current pulses are averaged in the two current detectors, producing two dc output voltages:

$$V_1 = -fV_cR_fC_x + e_1 \qquad (1)$$
$$V_2 = fV_cR_fC_x + e_2 \qquad (2)$$

where R_f is the feedback resistance value of the current detectors, and e_1 and e_2 are output offset voltages of CD1 and CD2 caused mainly by the charge injection effect of the CMOS switches (Section 2.2). The capacitors C_{in} (0.1 µF) ensure that the virtual earth potentials at the inputs of CD1 and CD2 remaining stable during the high speed charge and discharge operation. Since during the operation, the source electrode is always connected with low impedance supplies (V_c and earth), and the detecting electrode always at virtual earth potential, stray capacitances have no significant effect on the measurement.

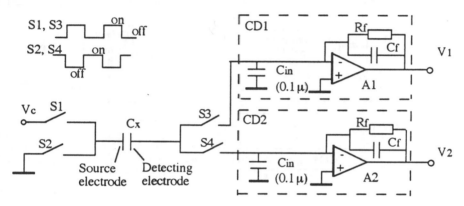

Fig. 2 *The basic capacitance measurement circuit*

The differential output voltage, $V_1 - V_2$ is taken as the output signal of the basic circuit. From eqn. 1 and 2,

$$V_2 - V_1 = 2fV_cR_fC_x + e_2 - e_1 \qquad (3)$$

The complete sensor electronics circuit for a 12-electrode imaging system is given in Fig. 3. Each measurement channel, which consists of the two current detectors shown in Fig. 2, is connected to a sensor electrode via a 4066 quad CMOS switch IC (providing S1 to S4 in Fig. 2), except electrode 1, which is connected only with two switches (S1 and S2). Electrodes 2 to 11 can be selected as either the source electrode by setting S1 and S2 active, or as the detecting electrode by activating S3 and S4; electrode 1 can be selected as either the source or idle (earthed), while electrode 12 always works as a detecting electrode. By using this arrangement, capacitances between any two of the 12 electrodes can be measured and a total number of 66 independent measurements can be obtained. The 11 channel outputs are selected one by one by a multiplexer followed by intermediate amplification and A to D conversion.

A problem associated with the sensor structure shown in Fig.1 is that the standing capacitances and sensitivity of different electrode pairs can be very different. The standing capacitance (when the pipe is empty) between two adjacent electrodes is about 50 to 100 times larger than that between two diagonally separated electrodes. This causes difficulties for the capacitance measuring circuit which has a relatively limited dynamic range. To avoid circuit saturation, the gain of the circuit must be kept at a level that is too low for measurement of two diagonally separated electrodes. To compensate for the differences in the standing value and sensitivity, an offset control unit and a gain control unit are incorporated into the design. Both units are controllable by the remote transputer. When measuring the capacitance of a pair of the electrodes, the transputer programs the units to provide offset (standing value) balance and gain (sensitivity) balance appropriate to this particular configuration. This approach provides the sensor electronics with a dynamic range of 76 dB (from 0.3 fF to 2 pF).

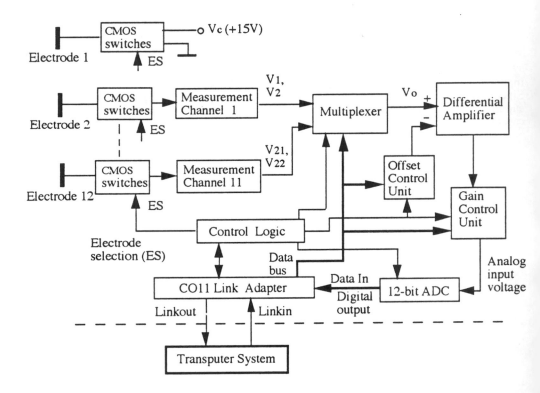

Fig. 3 *The principle block diagram of the sensor electronics circuit*

The sensor electronics interfaces with the transputer system via an INMOS CO11 link adapter. The link adapter is built into the sensor electronics, and is connected with the transputer system via a pair of (bi-directional) high-speed serial communication links (10/20 Mbits/s). The control signals from and the measured data to the transputer system are transmitted via the links, which are usually optical fibres for distances larger than 15 metres. The maximum distance supported is 250 metres, and this enables the transputer system to be placed in a less hostile environment far from where the primary sensor and sensor electronics are installed.

2.2. Circuit Performance
The performance of the sensor electronics, characterised by its baseline stability, measurement resolution and dynamic response, is limited mainly by the level of noise voltage generated in the circuit and the baseline drift of the circuit. Noise voltages in the circuit are generated mainly from: (i) the noise of the operational amplifiers, in particular, the first stage current detectors, (ii) ground interference due to ground current returns from the switching part of the circuit, and (iii) 50/100 Hz mains frequency interference. In this design, low noise amplifiers ($e_n < 4$ nV/$\sqrt{Hz}$ at 1kHz) are chosen as the first stage amplifiers. Separate ground returns are used for the analogue and digital parts respectively, and large area ground planes are used. To limit the noise bandwidth, the response time of the circuit is limited to no more than what is required to

achieve 1 frame measurement data in 10 ms. These measures enable a RMS noise level of 0.07 fF to be achieved. The baseline drift of the circuit is mainly attributed to the temperature dependency of the charge injection effect of the CMOS switches (caused by the feed-through of gate control signals of semiconductor switches via the gate-channel capacitance). In Fig. 2, the gate control signals for switches S3 and S4 inject unwanted charge into the current detectors, resulting in offset voltages at their outputs. The offsets were equivalent to a measured capacitance of about 0.1 pF when a MC14066 CMOS switch IC was used to provide the switches S3 and S4. The magnitude of the charge injection is temperature dependent. Over a temperature change of 10°C, the drift measured on the differential output was equivalent to an input capacitance change of 5 fF (» 0.3 fF). To solve this problem, a self-baseline correction mode is incorporated into the circuit operation. In this mode the source electrode is earthed while the switches S3 and S4 remain operational, and the output offset due to the charge injection is measured. The circuit is then restarted and the offset value obtained in the checking are subtracted from each measurement value obtained after the check. The time needed for the checking is 1 ms. Laboratory test of the industrial version of the electronics shows that the RMS value of the noise is equivalent to an input capacitance of 0.07 fF and peak value of the noise (Gaussian) is estimated as 0.21 fF (with 99.7% confidence) which is better than the required resolution. No drift with time is observed over a 5-hour period. The acquisition time for the 66 measurement data is 9.8 ms which satisfies the requirement of 100 frame/s.

3. SYSTEM MODEL AND IMAGE RECONSTRUCTION ALGORITHM

3.1. System model: the forward problem

A two-dimensional (2D) model of the imaging system has been established based on the finite element method (FEM). It is characterised by Possion's equation (assuming no free charge):

$$\nabla \cdot \left[\varepsilon_0 \varepsilon(x, y) \nabla \phi(x, y) \right] = 0 \tag{4}$$

and the associated boundary conditions (the Dirichlet boundary conditions), when electrode i is the source electrode ($i = 1, 2, ..., 11$), are

$$\psi^{(i)} = \begin{cases} V_c & (x,y) \subseteq \Gamma_i \\ 0 & (x, y) \subseteq \text{all } \Gamma_k \ (k \neq i) \text{ and } (x,y) \subseteq \left(\Gamma_s + \Gamma_{pg} \right) \end{cases} \tag{5}$$

where $\phi(x, y)$ and $\varepsilon(x, y)$ are, respectively, the 2D potential and dielectric constant distributions, and ε_0 the free-space permittivity. $\Gamma_1, \Gamma_2, ...,$ and Γ_{12} represent the spatial locations of the 12 electrodes, Γ_s that of the sensor screen, and Γ_{pg} that of the 12 projected guards (Fig. 4).

The forward problem is to determine the 66 capacitance measurements for a known profile of dielectric constant $\varepsilon(x, y)$ of a flow (for gas $\varepsilon = \varepsilon_{gas} = 1$ and for oil $\varepsilon = \varepsilon_{oil} = 3$). To achieve this, eqn. 4 must first be solved to obtain the potential distribution $\phi(x,y)$. Since flow distribution $\varepsilon(x,y)$ is, in general, very irregular, there is no analytical solution to eqn. 4. Therefore, a numerical method based on the FEM is used. To obtain a FE solution, the region shown in Fig. 4 is divided into P four-noded quadrilateral elements corresponding to Q nodes. The unknown gas/oil distribution can be expressed by a vector ε^*, which is the subset of the vector $\varepsilon = (\varepsilon_1, \varepsilon_2, ..., \varepsilon_P)$ representing the dielectric constant of the P elements. When electrode i is the source electrode ($i = 1, 2, ..., 11$), the resulting nodal potentials are expressed by a $Q \times 1$ vector $v^{(i)}$, and it can be shown that [5]

$$A v^{(i)} = b^{(i)} \tag{6}$$

where $b^{(i)}$ is a $Q \times 1$ vector incorporating the boundary conditions expressed by eqn. 5, and A a sparse $Q \times Q$ matrix whose entries depend on the element dielectric constants ε (therefore ε^*), as well as on the element topology. Since matrix A is symmetric and positive-definite, there exists a non-singular upper triangular matrix U, with unit diagonal matrix D, such that

$$A = U^T D U \tag{7a}$$

After performing the matrix factorisation indicated by eqn. 7a (this is only done once for all of the 11 source electrodes as indicated by eqn.5), the solution to eqn.6 is carried out by

(i)   forward reduction: $U^T z = b^{(i)}$ (7b)

(ii) diagonal scaling: $Dy = z$ (7c)

(iii) back substitution: $Uv^{(i)} = y$ (7d)

After solving node potentials from eqn. 6 and 7, the capacitance of the electrode pair $i - j$ can be calculated by performing the following line-integration numerically:

$$C_{i,j} = \frac{Q(\Gamma_j)}{V_c} = -\frac{\varepsilon_o}{V_c}\int_{(x,y)\subseteq\Gamma_j} \varepsilon(x,y)\nabla\phi^{(i)}(x,y)\bullet d\vec{\Gamma}_j \tag{8}$$

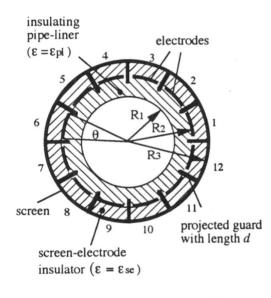

insulating pipe-liner ($\varepsilon = \varepsilon_{pl}$)

electrodes

screen

screen-electrode insulator ($\varepsilon = \varepsilon_{se}$)

projected guard with length d

Fig. 4 *Schematic diagram of a 12-electrode capacitive primary sensor*

where $Q(\Gamma_j)$ is the charge sensed by detecting electrode j ($j = i + 1, ..., 12$), and $\phi^{(i)}(x, y)$, represented by $v^{(i)}$ in a discrete form, is the potential distribution when electrode i is the source electrode and when a flow $\varepsilon(x, y)$, represented by vector ε (and therefore ε^*) in a discrete form, is present.

The finite element model of the 12-electrode system is implemented in OCCAM-2 running on T800 transputers. For a 2000-node system model, for example, one transputer (25 MHz) completes the 66 capacitance calculations ($C_{i,j}$, $i = 1, 2, ..., 11, j = i + 1, ..., 12$) within 60 seconds. Obviously, this calculation time can be reduced by distributing the finite element calculation processes over several transputers running in parallel.

3.1.1. Calculation of capacitance field sensitivity distribution
The field sensitivity distribution of electrode pair $i - j$, $S_{i,j}(k)$, is defined as

$$S_{i,j}(k) = \left[C_{i,j}(k) - C_{i,j(gas)}\right] / \left[\Delta C_{i,j} \Delta\varepsilon \beta(k)\right] \tag{9a}$$

where

$$\Delta C_{i,j} = C_{i,j(oil)} - C_{i,j(gas)} \quad \text{and} \quad \Delta\varepsilon = \varepsilon_{oil} - \varepsilon_{gas} \tag{9b}$$

and where $C_{i,j}(k)$ is the capacitance when k th in-pipe element (the element inside the circle with radius R_1) has dielectric constant ε_{oil} and the rest of the in-pipe elements all have that of ε_{gas} (in our model, there are 900 in-pipe elements, i.e. the vector ε^* has 900 entries; $k = 1, 2, ..., 900$). $C_{i,j(gas)}$ and $C_{i,j(oil)}$ are, respectively, the capacitances when the pipe is filled with gas and with oil; $\Delta C_{i,j}$ is, therefore, the full-scale capacitance change. Note that $C_{i,j(gas)}$ are called the system standing capacitances. $\beta(k)$ is the fractional area of the k th in-pipe element (with respect to the pipe cross-sectional area).

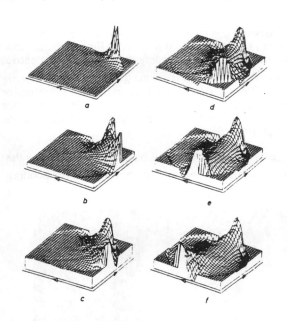

Owing to the property of symmetry, only 6 out of 66 distributions of the field sensitivity need calculating; they are $S_{1,2}$, $S_{1,3}$, $S_{1,4}$, $S_{1,5}$, $S_{1,6}$ and $S_{1,7}$ (type 1 to type 6). This can significantly reduce computation time since the rest of the 60 sensitivity distributions can be obtained by simple rotation transformation (see below). To make these six sensitivity distributions accessible by the image reconstruction process, a procedure is used to transform them from the FE domain (which has 900 in-pipe elements of different areas distributed irregularly) to the image domain (for 32 x 32 image-display format, there are 812 in-pipe square picture-elements or pixels having the same area), i.e.

$$\Omega_{i,j}(p) = T\left\{S_{i,j}(k)\right\} \tag{9c}$$

Fig. 5 *Capacitance sensitivity distributions of six typical electrode pairs calculated for the model sensor (see text).*

(a) adjacent electrode pair, $\Omega 1,2$

(b) electrode pair separated by one electrode, $\Omega 1,3$

(c) electrode pair separated by two electrodes, $\Omega 1,4$

(d) electrode pair separated by three electrodes, $\Omega 1,5$

(e) electrode pair separated by four electrodes, $\Omega 1,6$

(f) diagonally separated electrode pair, $\Omega 1,7$

where $\Omega_{i,j}(p)$ are the transformed sensitivity distributions in the image domain and p the pixel number ($p = 1, ..., 812$).

$T\{\cdot\}$ denotes the transformation operator. The linear transformations involved are scaling (the sensor geometry has different units in two domains), and interpolation or extrapolation of sensitivity values for each pixel p.

Fig. 5 shows the typical six transformed sensitivity distributions $\Omega_{1,2}$ to $\Omega_{1,7}$ (type 1 to type 6), for a sensor with $R_1 = 76.2$ mm, $R_2 - R_1 = 15$ mm, $R_3 - R_2 = 7$ mm, $d = 9$ mm, $\theta = 26°$, $\varepsilon_{se} = 4$ and $\varepsilon_{pl} = 5.8$ (this sensor is called the *model sensor* below). It shows that the field sensitivity is higher near the pipe wall than in the middle of the pipe, and in some areas the sensitivity exhibits positive response, otherwise it is negative (the sunken areas) or zero. The area of positive response interrogates different parts of the pipe cross-section for different electrode pairs.

To obtain the other 60 sensitivity distributions, rotation transformations are further employed in the image domain (the centre of the pipe is the centre of rotation), i.e.

$$\Omega_{m,n} = R\left\{\Omega_{i,j} ; \gamma\right\} \tag{9d}$$

where $R\left\{\cdot\right\}$ is an operator representing the rotation transformation. Eqn. 9d is interpreted as that $\Omega_{m,n}$ is obtained by rotating $\Omega_{i,j}$ anti-clockwise by γ degree. Note that $\Omega_{m,n}$ and $\Omega_{i,j}$ must be of the same type [2].

3.1.2. Calculation of capacitance measurements due to various gas/oil flow distributions

Realistic flow models of different 'regimes', such as stratified flow, core flow, annular flow, gas-bubble flow and oil-droplet flow, can be produced by assigning the corresponding entries of the vector $\boldsymbol{\varepsilon}^{*}$ with either ε_{gas} or ε_{oil}. Flows of different oil fractions (β), various orientations of gas/oil interfaces in the case of stratified flows, different numbers and sizes of bubbles or droplets can be generated. The corresponding responses of a sensor, i.e. the 66 capacitance data, are then calculated (eqn.8), serving as the flow measurement data for evaluating the performance of the image reconstruction algorithm (Section 3.2).

Fig. 6a shows an example of a stratified gas/oil flow, where the oil phase is represented by the high grey level ($\beta=0.603$) and the gas phase by the low one. Fig. 6b shows the corresponding

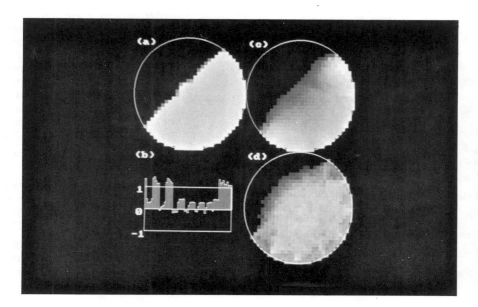

Fig. 6 *Comparison of images reconstructed using different algorithms.*
(a) a stratified gas/oil flow model, where the high grey level represents the oil phase and the low the gas; *(b)* the corresponding 66 normalised capacitances $\lambda_{i,j}$ of the flow model *(a)* calculated for the model sensor (see text); *(c)* image reconstructed using $\lambda_{i,j}$ and the improved backprojection algorithm using full sensitivity data as shown in Fig. 5; *(d)* image reconstructed using the '0/1 algorithm'.

66 normalised capacitances $\lambda_{i,j}$ of the model sensor, $\lambda_{i,j}$ is defined as

$$\lambda_{i,j} = \left(C_{i,j(m)} - C_{i,j(gas)}\right)/\Delta C_{i,j} \tag{10}$$

where $C_{i,j(m)}$ is the capacitance measurement due to a gas/oil distribution model. For a linear system, $0 \le \lambda_{i,j} \le 1$. Fig. 6b indicates that, there may be $\lambda_{i,j} < 0$ (called 'undershooting') or $\lambda_{i,j} > 1$ (called 'overshooting'). The magnitude of overshooting is, in general, larger than that of the undershooting. This non-linearity in the capacitance data is caused by the effects of the guard electrodes and the discontinuity in the distribution of dielectric constants ε^*. With respect to the situations when there is only gas or oil in the pipe, the presence of a gas/oil mixture will redistribute the electric flux lines in the system. This redistribution may cause some detecting electrodes to absorb more (or less) electric flux lines than when the pipe is filled with oil (or gas), resulting in overshooting (or undershooting) effects.

3.2. Image reconstruction algorithm: the inverse problem

For a capacitance tomography system, the inverse problem is to determine the distribution of dielectric constants of gas/oil components (the vector ε^*) from the measured 66 capacitances $C_{i,j}$, i.e. to find the inverse of eqn. 8. It should be pointed out that there is no analytical solution to such an inverse problem. Important features associated with the capacitance sensing field are that, the electric flux lines, expressed by field vector $-\varepsilon(x, y)\nabla\phi(x, y)$, tend to spread, and worst of all, are related to the object $\varepsilon(x, y)$ to be imaged (eqn. 4 and 8). Therefore, the capacitance field is called a 'soft field', and this field is inherently non-linear. To solve the inverse problem for capacitance tomography, some approximation methods are needed. Note that, in general, the number of unknowns in the system (e.g. the 812 image pixels) is more than that of the knowns (e.g. the 66 capacitance measurements), so that the system is under-determined. Some *prior* knowledge of the system, such as the field sensitivity distributions, may be used to alleviate the problem. In principle, to correct the field distortion, an iterative method should be used to obtain an accurate solution, however, its implementation often demands intensive computations and, in some cases, convergence cannot be guaranteed. Therefore, a non-iterative method, although less accurate, is used.

An image reconstruction algorithm based on a simple backprojection method has been developed in the past for capacitance tomography [6]. When the backprojection process was carried out, only the binary information of the capacitance sensitivity distributions (as shown in Fig. 5) was used, i.e. $\Omega_{i,j} = 1$ if $\Omega_{i,j} > 0$, otherwise $\Omega_{i,j} = 0$ (this is called the '0/1 algorithm' below for brevity). A direct consequence of this method is that the reconstructed image is seriously distorted (see, for example, Fig. 6d). To alleviate this problem, the backprojection algorithm is modified, in which the precalculated full sensitivity information $\Omega_{i,j}$ is used. Let a reconstructed image be represented by pixel grey-level $G(p)$ approximating the vector ε^*; $G(p)$ is calculated from the following equation:

$$G(p) = \sum_{i=1}^{11}\sum_{j=i+1}^{12}\lambda_{i,j}\Omega_{i,j}(p) \bigg/ \sum_{i=1}^{11}\sum_{j=i+1}^{12}\Omega_{i,j}(p) \qquad (p = 1, 2, ..., 812) \tag{11}$$

For a linear system, the normalised capacitance data $\lambda_{i,j}$ should fall within the interval $[0, 1]$, so should the resulting image grey-level $G(p)$. Since a capacitance tomography system exhibits non-linearity, $\lambda_{i,j}$ may have overshooting or undershooting values, so may $G(p)$. Therefore, some processing on $G(p)$ is needed before the grey-level image is displayed. Overshooting in $G(p)$ is eliminated by using a truncation operation, i.e. in eqn. 11, $\lambda_{i,j} = 1$ if $\lambda_{i,j} > 1$. Under-shooting is dealt with by using a threshold operation described below.

The use of a threshold operation can reduce the low grey-level artefacts present in an image. It has been observed that the level of thresholding is dependent upon the flow distribution and the flow component fraction, so an adaptive threshold operation is required. Numerical experiments have suggested that the following threshold operation is suitable (in our imaging system, 256 integer grey-levels, 0 - 255, are used).

$$G_t(p) = \begin{cases} 0 & \text{if } G(p) < \eta \\ 255 G(p) & \text{otherwise} \end{cases} \tag{12a}$$

where the threshold level η $(0 \le \eta \le 1)$ is,

$$\eta = (1 - 0.5\,\alpha)\,\zeta \tag{12b}$$

and where

$$\alpha = AVG\left(\lambda_{i,j} \ \{\lambda_{i,j} = 1 \quad \text{if } \lambda_{i,j} > 1\}\right) \tag{12c}$$

$$\zeta = AVG\left(G(p) \ \{\text{for } G(p) > 0\}\right) \tag{12d}$$

where $AVG(\cdot)$ denotes an average operator and $\{\cdot\}$ a conditional statement.

To illustrate the effectiveness of this algorithm, Fig. 6c shows the reconstructed image using the capacitance data shown in Fig. 6b, which closely resembles the flow model (Fig. 6a). The image reconstructed using the '0/1 algorithm' and a similar threshold operation is shown in Fig. 6d; it has poorer fidelity in comparison with Fig. 6c.

4. PARALLEL IMPLEMENTATION OF IMAGE RECONSTRUCTION ALGORITHM

The image reconstruction algorithm described in Section 3 is implemented using a transputer-based system. It takes about 100 ms for one T801 transputer (25 MHz) to complete one image reconstruction; this is equivalent to an imaging rate of about 10 frame/s. To increase the speed further, multiple transputer-based processors are used in parallel to implement the back-projection algorithm (Fig. 7).

The transputer network consists of a host processor on a PC card (INMOS B004 compatible, T800-20 MHz, used also as the Transputer Development System - TDS), a master processor (T801-25 MHz), a graphics processor (T800-25 MHz), and three slave processors (T801-25 MHz). The host handles the external I/O for the transputer network. It distributes the codes (developed under TDS) to the appropriate processors in the network, presents data on PC's VDU, selects program options via keyboard input, loads data (e.g. sensitivity distributions) from the PC hard-disk into the slave processors, and saves data (e.g. the captured streams of 66 capacitance data sent by the master) to the PC hard-disk for future use. The master processor in the network controls the remote sensor electronic circuit (e.g. gain and offset adjustments) and performs acquisition of capacitance measurements (see Fig. 3); it also distributes the tasks (a stream of captured 66 capacitance measurements) to the slave processors, collects and passes on the results (the calculated flow component fractions and/or the reconstructed images) to the graphics and the host processors. Each slave processor in the task farm executes the same serial program - the backprojection algorithm - on its own data set. In this load-balancing pipeline [2], several buffer processes (the 'throughput' and the 'feedback') carrying tasks to workers and results to the display are also run on each slave, ensuring that whenever a slave completes one task another task is immediately available. The graphics processor displays grey-level images of flows on a graphics monitor via RGB outputs.

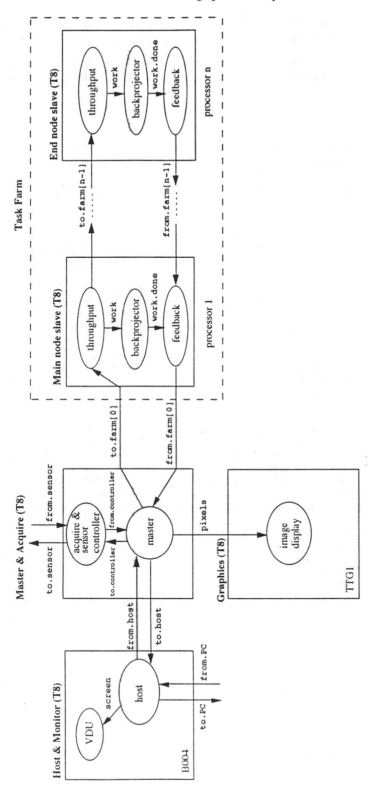

Fig. 7 *Transputer-based multi-processor system with task farm configuration for parallel implementation of the backprojection image reconstruction algorithm*

It also displays the 66 normalised capacitance measurements (a useful diagnostic aid of the imaging system) and the trend diagram of oil fraction change with time (see Fig.10b).

The imaging frame rate when different numbers of slave processors are used is shown in Fig. 8. Fig. 8a indicates that, when the image is reconstructed and displayed using 20 x 20 pixels,

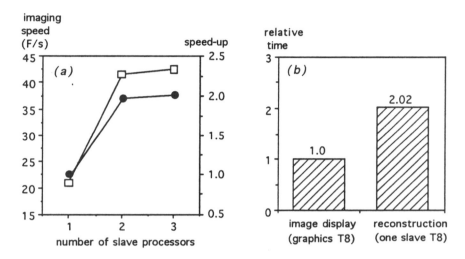

Fig. 8 *Performance of transputer network for parallel image reconstruction.*
(a) Imaging speed (—□—) and speed-up (—●—) vs number of slave processors.
(b) Comparison of time for image display and reconstruction.

over 40 frame/s speed is achieved when 2 slaves are in use. From one slave to two, the speed-up is quite linear (speed-up $= N_n /N_1$, where N_n and N_1 are the frame-rate achieved by one slave and n slaves, respectively). This is because the time taken for one slave to reconstruct an image is about 2 times that for the graphics transputer to display it (Fig. 8b), so when the third slave is added to the task farm the imaging rate is only increased slightly (Fig. 8a). This indicates that the bottleneck of the whole transputer network comes from the graphics transputer. To achieve a higher imaging speed, a faster graphics transputer should be used.

5. TYPICAL TEST RESULTS

The performance of the imaging system has been extensively tested, including tests under static conditions using physical phantoms, and under dynamic conditions - various gas/oil flow rates and pipe inclinations - on a 6" flow loop at SCR. The details of the static test are reported in a separate paper [7], so only one typical result is given in Fig. 9. It shows the calculated oil fraction β_1 versus the true oil fraction β for core, annular and stratified flows. The error term, $\beta_1-\beta$, is also plotted. Here the oil fraction β_1 is obtained by processing the 66 normalised capacitance measurements $\lambda_{i,j}$:

$$\beta_1 = AVG\left(\lambda_{i,j} \ \{\lambda_{i,j}\text{'s excluding those from the 12 adjacent electrode pairs}\}\right) \qquad (13)$$

Fig. 9 indicates that, for stratified and annular flows, the maximum value of $\beta_1-\beta$, i.e. the full-scale error, is 5%, whereas for core flow this value becomes larger (10%). In most cases, the oil fraction for core flow is underestimated ($\beta_1-\beta < 0$), whereas for annular flow, it is over-estimated ($\beta_1-\beta > 0$), due to the inherent non-uniformity of the capacitance sensitivity distribution over the pipe cross-section. To increase the accuracy of volume fraction measurement further, better data processing methods may be used.

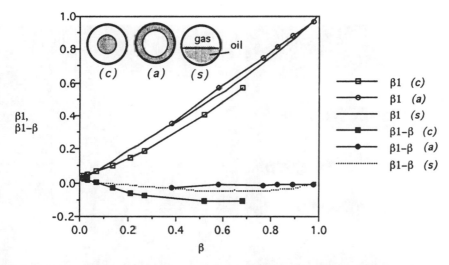

Fig. 9 *Static test results of the 12-electrode capacitance imaging system for measuring oil volume fraction.* 'c', 'a' and 's' in the legends are for core, annular and stratified flow models, respectively. β is the oil fraction of the flow model, and β_1 that calculated from the mean of the 54 normalised capacitances (eqn.13). $\beta_1-\beta$ is the error term.

Fig. 10 shows one typical dynamic test results at SCR. The test conditions were: the 6" I.D. flow pipe was 6° from horizontal; the flow rate of oil (kerosene) was 2.7 m³/hr and that of gas (compressed nitrogen) was 28 meter-reading (exact flow rate unknown). Images in Fig. 10a show the evolution of gas slugs on the top part of the pipe. The variation of oil fraction β_1 with time is given in the right half of Fig. 10b, where 2500 instantaneous readings are displayed. From this the pseudo-periodic nature of gas slugs is clearly visualised, and the frequency of occurrence of gas slugs and the mean oil fraction can be readily derived. The instantaneous 66 capacitance measurements λ_{ij} are also displayed at the bottom left, and the corresponding reconstructed flow image is displayed at the top left. This integrated display has provided a powerful means of visualising the dynamics of gas/oil flows.

6. CONCLUDING REMARKS

This paper has demonstrated the capability of a transputer-based 12-electrode capacitance tomography system for imaging gas/oil flows. The capacitance transducer is able to resolve a capacitance change as small as 0.3 fF. This represents a 2% oil volume fraction at the centre of an empty pipe [7]. A data acquisition speed of 100 frame/s has been achieved. The sensor electronics has an interface circuit with the remote transputer network so that all the circuit adjustments (e.g. offset and gain) are software controllable.

The linear backprojection algorithm has been improved. Methods for determining component fraction from capacitance data have been investigated. The errors are 5% of full scale for stratified and annular flows and 10% for core flows. Further research is needed to improve the image reconstruction algorithm and to reduce errors in component fraction measurement.

The transputer network can reconstruct and display flow images at 40 frame/s. The bottleneck of the network lies in the graphics transputer. To achieve a higher imaging speed, a faster graphics transputer should be used. By using INMOS's new generation transputers - T9000, which is ten times faster than T800 series, a 100 frame/s imaging speed can be readily achieved. The system model based on the FEM will also benefit, running ten times faster.

(a)   *(b)*

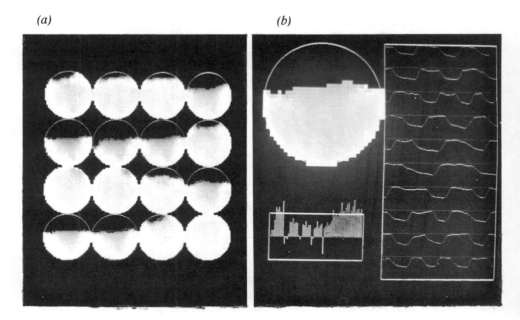

Fig. 10 *Typical dynamic test results. (a)* The evolution of the gas slugs (displayed in dark grey levels). Time interval between successive images: 80 ms. Order of images: left to right, top to bottom. *(b)* Right half: the variation of oil fraction $\beta1$ with time (2500 instantaneous reading: time interval between successive readings: 10 ms). Bottom left: the instantaneous 66 capacitan measurements $\lambda_{i,j}$ (the 2500*th* set of data in this particular case). Top left: the corresponding reconstructed flow image.

ACKNOWLEDGEMENT

The research work described in this paper was supported by the Science and Engineering Research Council and the Department of Trade and Industry under the LINK scheme.

REFERENCES

[1] Huang S M, Xie C G, Thorn R, Snowden D and Beck M S 1992 *IEE Proc.G* **139** (1) 83-88
[2] Xie C G, Huang S M, Hoyle B S, Thorn R, Lenn C, Snowden D and Beck M S 1992 *IEE Proc.G* **139** (1) 89-98
[3] Khan S and Abdullah F 1992 *Proc. ECAPT'92*
[4] Huang S M, Green R G, Plaskowski A B and Beck M S 1988 *IEEE Trans. Instrum. Meas.* **IM-37** (3) 368-373
[5] Silvester P P and Ferrari R L 1990 *Finite element for electrical engineers* (New York: Cambridge University Press) 2nd Edition
[6] Xie C G, Plaskowski A and Beck M S 1989 *IEE Proc.A* **136** (4) 173-191
[7] Huang S M, Xie C G, Vasina J, Lenn C, Zhang B F and Beck M S 1992 *Proc. ECAPT'92*

Experimental evaluation of capacitance tomographic flow imaging systems using physical models

S M Huang*, C G Xie*, J Vasina*, C Lenn+, B F Zhang† and M S Beck*

* Department of Electrical Engineering & Electronics, Process Tomography Unit, UMIST, P.O. Box 88, Manchester, M60 1QD
+ Schlumberger Cambridge Research Ltd., P.O. Box 153, Cambridge, CB3 0HG
† Department of Automation, Tsinghua University, Beijing 100084, China

ABSTRACT: This paper describes an experimental method for evaluating the performance of capacitance tomographic flow imaging systems. Criteria such as spatial and permittivity resolution, accuracy (system errors) and signal to noise ratio are defined to characterise the performance of the systems. Static physical models simulating typical flow distribution patterns are used as standard phantoms and the criteria are quantified by comparing the reconstructed images with the standards. Systems with 8 and 12 electrodes have been tested and the results compared to show the improvement obtained with the increased number of electrodes.

1. INTRODUCTION

Capacitance-based tomography systems (Fig. 1) are useful for imaging two-component processes, where two components have significantly different dielectric constants, such as oil/gas and solids/gas flows. Since the development of the first working model based on an 8-electrode capacitance sensor [1], a 12-electrode industrial pre-prototype system with improved sensor electronics and image reconstruction algorithm has been developed for oil-field applications [2-3]. Contemporary work by the US Department of Energy has resulted in a capacitance tomography system for fluidized bed imaging [4]. The oil-field flow imaging system has been successfully tested on a 6" oil/gas pipe at Schlumberger Cambridge Research. It produced images (at 40 frame/s) which appeared to be similar to the actual flow pattern. However, we are unable to say quantitatively how well the reconstructed images can represent the real distributions under different flow conditions. More generally, an analysis or test procedure for quantitative evaluation of capacitance tomographic imaging systems is needed in order to quantify the errors of the systems under different flow conditions and to compare the effects of different sensor structures, number of electrodes and reconstruction algorithms.

The objective of this work is to develop an experimental test method for quantitative assessment of capacitance tomographic flow imaging systems. Since standards for dynamic calibration are not available, static physical models which simulate typical flow distribution patterns are used for the evaluation. Criteria characterising system performance are quantified by comparing the reconstructed images with the physical models. With this approach, the effects of different primary sensors, sensor electronics, reconstruction algorithms as well as complete systems can be compared. In the following sections, the definitions to the criteria are first given, then the experimental system and physical models for the tests are described, test results for different distribution patterns presented, and finally conclusions on the performance limitations of capacitance tomographic flow imaging systems are drawn.

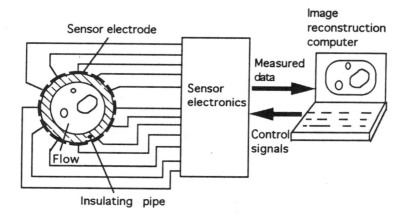

Fig. 1 *Capacitance-based tomographic flow imaging system*

2. DEFINITIONS

The quality of a tomographic flow imaging system can be judged by comparing the reconstructed cross-sectional image (two-dimensional) of a physical model with the actual model. To perform the comparison on the image reconstruction computer, a standard image of the model can be generated on the computer, which closely matches the cross-section of the model (dependent upon the fineness of the image display pixels). The image plane, representing the cross-section of the flow conveying pipe, can be divided into M square image pixels, and an image of two-component distribution is fully defined by assigning the grey level (or colour code) of each pixel, $G(i)$, with an appropriate value for $i = 1, 2, ..., M$. For the standard image,

$$G_s(i) = \begin{cases} G_m & \text{at pixels occupied by the cross-section of the physical model} \\ 0 & \text{elsewhere} \end{cases} \qquad (1)$$

where G_m is a grey level value proportional to the permittivity of the model material. For a two-component flow imaging system, G_m is often chosen to be the maximum grey level of the display (e.g. 255), representing the permittivity of the component with higher dielectric constant.

For the reconstructed image, $G_r(i)$, the grey level values of the M pixels are determined by all the independent capacitance measurements through the image reconstruction algorithm. In our systems, the algorithms used are based on the filtered backprojection method in which a threshold filter is always used to remove the artifacts produced by the backprojection. The function of the threshold filter is shown by the following expression [3]

$$G_r(i) = \begin{cases} 0 & \text{if } G_n(i) < \eta \\ G_m G_n(i) & \text{otherwise} \end{cases} \qquad \text{for } i = 1, 2, ..., M \qquad (2)$$

where $G_n(i)$ is the normalised grey level of the ith pixel on the "raw" image obtained from the backprojection operation, which satisfies $0 \le G_n(i) \le 1$ (or $0 \le G_m G_n(i) \le G_m$) and η is the filter threshold defined by

$$\eta = (1 - k\alpha)\alpha \qquad (3)$$

where α is the average value of all the independent measurements (28 and 66 for 8- and 12-electrode sensors, respectively) for reconstructing an image and k is a coefficient ranging from 0 to 1 which can be determined experimentally. The threshold filtering results in a reconstructed image consisting of pixels with grey-level values either above the threshold or equal to zero, i.e. $\eta G_m \leq G_r(i) \leq G_m$ or $G_r(i) = 0$.

For an ideal tomographic imaging system, the reconstructed image should be identical to the standard image. In practice, this rarely happens and the reconstructed image always differs from the standard. Obviously the departure from the ideal situation can be characterised by the difference image

$$D(i) = G_s(i) - G_r(i) \qquad (i = 1, 2, ..., M) \qquad (4)$$

While the difference image is a two-dimensional graphical presentation, it is practically more convenient to use some simple values to describe the quality of an imaging system. In this work, the following criteria are defined.

2.1. Spatial and permittivity errors

When imaging a physical model in the pipe, the reconstructed cross-section of the model may differ from the standard in area, average grey level, shape and position (e.g. weight centre). The differences in area, shape and position can be classified as spatial errors, whereas that in grey level is regarded as permittivity error. Here we define the *spatial image error* (*SIE*) of the system using the following expression :

$$SIE = \sum_{i=1}^{M} |G_s^*(i) - G_r^*(i)| \bigg/ \sum_{i=1}^{M} G_s^*(i) \qquad (5)$$

where

$$G_s^*(i) = \begin{cases} 1 & \text{where the model is} \\ 0 & \text{elsewhere} \end{cases} \quad \text{and} \quad G_r^*(i) = \begin{cases} 1 & \text{if } G_r(i)/G_m > \eta \\ 0 & \text{otherwise} \end{cases}$$

SIE represents the spatial error information as one would see on the difference image. It contains all the spatial errors such as those in shape, cross-sectional area and position of the reconstructed object. In practice, the error in the cross-sectional area of the reconstructed object is often a good representation of the spatial image error, and it is easier to be estimated than the *SIE*. This area error is defined by the following formula:

$$AE = \left(\sum_{i=1}^{M} G_r^*(i) - \sum_{i=1}^{M} G_s^*(i) \right) \bigg/ \sum_{i=1}^{M} G_s^*(i) \qquad (6)$$

To reduce the effect of random noise (see Section 2.3), when calculating the *SIE* or *AE* the reconstructed image, $G_r(i)$, is obtained from a time-average of 100 consecutive frames of real time images.

The *permittivity error* (*PE*) of the system is defined as the difference between the average grey level, G_r, of the reconstructed object and that of the standard, G_s, divided by G_s, i.e.

$$PE = (G_r - G_s)/G_s \qquad (7)$$

In this system, G_s is usually chosen to be G_m and G_r can be calculated from

$$G_r = \sum_{i=1}^{M} G_r(i) \Big/ N_r \tag{8}$$

where N_r is the number of the pixels with non-zero grey level values on the reconstructed image. (Note that only N_r non-zero values of $G_r(i)$ are actually summed here). G_r is also time-averaged to reduce its random fluctuation.

2.2. Component fraction measurement error

Component fraction (e.g. oil volume fraction in an oil/gas flow) is an important parameter of two-component flow. One objective of flow imaging is to provide a method of measuring this from the cross-sectional image of the two-component flow. In our system, the component fraction, β_r, is calculated by averaging the normalised grey level values of all image pixels over the pipe cross section [3]:

$$\beta_r = \sum_{i=1}^{M} \left(\frac{G_r(i)}{G_m} \right) \Big/ M \tag{9}$$

From eqn. 8, this can be rewritten as

$$\beta_r = N_r G_r / (M G_m) \tag{10}$$

The *component fraction measurement error* (*CFME*) of the system is defined as

$$CFME = \beta_r - \beta_s \tag{11}$$

where β_s is the real concentration defined by

$$\beta_s = N_s G_s / (M G_m) \qquad (G_s = G_m) \tag{12}$$

where N_s is the number of pixels with non-zero grey level values on the standard image. To reduce random errors, the time average value of β_r is used in eqn. 11.

CFME shows the combined effect of *SIE* and *PE*. However, a small *CFME* does not necessarily mean that the *SIE* and *PE* are small because their contributions may tend to cancel each other.

2.3. Signal to noise ratio

Due to noise generated by the sensor electronics of capacitance tomography systems [2], the area and grey level of the reconstructed image and the calculated value of β_r always fluctuate randomly with time, even when the component distribution in the pipe is stationary. In capacitance tomography, the signal that causes the sensor to respond is the component fraction change. Here we choose the time average value of the component fraction (eqn. 9), β_r, as the signal and define the *signal to noise ratio* (*SNR*) of the system as:

$$SNR = \beta_r / RMS\left(\beta_r(t)\right) \tag{13}$$

where $RMS\left(\beta_r\left(t\right)\right)$ is the root-mean-square value of the time variable $\beta_r(t)$, representing the amplitude of the random fluctuation.

2.4. Input signal resolution

Resolution is a term frequently used for describing the performance of an imaging system. For an image display, it means the spatial resolution determined by the size of image pixels. For a measurement system, on the other hand, it means the smallest input signal that will cause an identifiable output change [5]. With the presence of noise, an output change is identifiable only if it is clearly above the noise level. Therefore the resolution of a measurement system is related to the noise level of that system. For a capacitance tomographic flow imaging system, which can be regarded as a measurement system with the component fraction β_s as its input and reconstructed image as output, we define its *input signal resolution* (ISR) as **the smallest component fraction change that can be identified on the reconstructed image**. This criterion represents the capability of the system to detect the presence of small changes in component fraction, and it should not be confused with the spatial accuracy of the system which has been defined in Section 2.1 by eqn. 5.

In this work, the reconstructed image of a dielectric object (in an empty pipe) is regarded as definite (identifiable) if its SNR (see eqn. 13) is no less than 3. In determining the ISR, only the simple situation where an object with higher permittivity appears in a homogeneous lower permittivity background (e.g. a plastic test rod in an empty pipe), is considered. In this case, if the reconstructed image has an SNR of 3, then the ISR of the system at that point on the cross section equals to the area-permittivity product of the test rod (the area of the rod is normalised against that of the full pipe).

It should be noted that all the criteria defined above are position dependent. For instance, the ISR at the pipe centre is different from that near the pipe wall. Therefore, it is meaningless to quote a criterion value without mentioning where on the pipe cross-section it applies. The position dependence of the criteria is experimentally investigated in Section 4.

3. EXPERIMENT SYSTEM AND PHYSICAL TEST MODELS

The industrial pre-prototype capacitance flow imaging system developed at UMIST [6] was used for the tests. Basically the system consists of three parts - the primary sensor, sensor electronics and image reconstruction computer (Fig. 1). Two different primary sensors were used for the tests. One had 8 electrodes on a 3" insulation pipe of 280 mm long (Fig. 2a) and the other had 12 electrodes on a 6" insulation pipe of 380 mm long (Fig. 2b). The length of the electrodes along the pipe axis is 100 mm. This length is considered necessary to provide the measuring electrode pairs with adequate sensitivities which are proportional to the electrode area. Projected guards are used in both sensors to reduce the standing capacitance between the adjacent electrodes [3]. For the 12-electrode sensor, these guards extend 2 mm into the insulating pipe liner, whereas in the 8-electrode sensor, the guards are flush with the liner surface. The guards at both ends of the electrode section are used to protect the electrodes from the interferences of external electrical fields. Their length is no less than the outer diameter of the insulation pipe, R_2 (Fig. 2).

The sensor electronics has a typical RMS noise level of 0.08 fF, which equals to the smallest sensor capacitance change caused by an approximately 0.5% component (permittivity = 3) fraction change (area change) at the pipe centre. The sensor electronics provides a data capture rate of 100 frames (6600 measurements) per second for the 12-electrode system and about 160 frames per second for the 8-electrode system. The image reconstruction algorithm used is based on the filtered backprojection principle. In this the normalised measurement values (normalised between empty-pipe and full-pipe capacitances), weighted by their corresponding sensitivity distribution functions calculated using the finite element method, are backprojected onto the pipe cross-section and the resultant image is filtered by a threshold operation (eqn. 2). For the tests described in the following section, the coefficient k in eqn. 2 is chosen as 0.5. The reconstructed image is displayed on an image plane consisting of 3228 pixels ($M=3228$). (The image is actually displayed using 64 x 64 pixels, with 868 pixels outside the pipe).

The physical models simulating different flow patterns can be divided into three types. The first of these are cylindrical rods of plastic (permittivity = 3). When placed at the pipe centre, they simulate the core flow pattern of different component fractions. The second are plastic tubes with different wall thickness simulating annular flow of different volume fraction. The stratified flow pattern with different volume fraction is simulated with the level of oil (kerosene, permittivity = 3) in a horizontally laid sensor pipe section. These models and their dimensions are shown in Fig. 3 and 4.

4. RESULTS AND DISCUSSION

4.1. Signal to noise ratio and input signal resolution

4.1.1. Signal to noise ratio

The *SNR* of the imaging system was tested for both the 8 and the 12-electrode configurations. The tests were performed by placing plastic rods of different sizes at 4 different positions in the pipe (*a, b, c* and *d* in Fig. 2b) and calculating the *SNR* for each set-up using

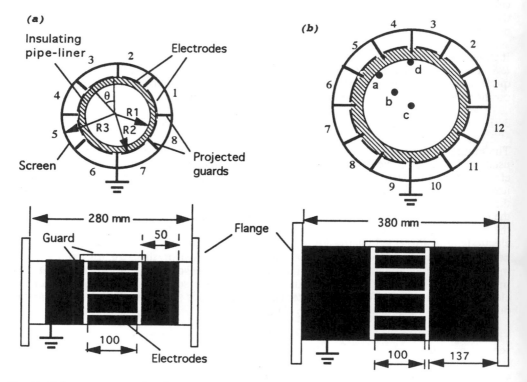

Fig. 2 *Primary sensors for the tests.* (a) 8-electrode sensor; R1=42.5 mm, R2–R1=5 mm R3–R2=5 mm, θ=39 deg.; Pipe-liner: perspex; Length of projected guard: 5 mm (b) 12-electrode sensor; R1=77 mm, R2–R1=15 mm, R3–R2=7 mm, θ=25.6 deg Pipe-liner: potting resin and Perspex; Length of projected guard: 9 mm.

(a)

Rod	#1	#2	#3	#4	#5	#6	#7	#8	#9	#10
D (mm)	9	15	20	27	40	57	70.5	80	111	127
A in the 6" pipe	0.34%	0.95%	1.69%	3.07%	6.75%	13.7%	21%	27%	51.95%	68%
A in the 3" pipe	1.12%	3.1%	5.5%	10.1%	22.1%	45%	68.8%			

(b)

Tube	#1	#2	#3	#4	#5	#6
Inner D (mm)	24.5	51	64.5	74	100	121
A of annular flow in the 6" pipe ('oil' fraction)	97.5%	89%	82.5%	76.9%	57.8%	38.3%

Fig. 3 *Physical models for the tests.* (a) Plastic rods. Material: Perspex. (b) Plastic tubes. Material: Perspex (when simulating annular flow, the gap between the outer surface of the tube and the pipe is filled with oil). *A* and *D* in the table stand for area and diameter, respectively.

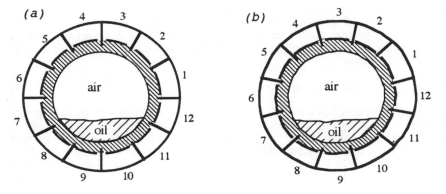

Fig. 4 *Stratified flow pattern.* (a) with electrode gap as central position; (b) pipe rotated 15 degrees from position shown in (a).

eqn. 13. The results are plotted versus the cross-sectional area fraction of the test rod in Fig. 5. Several observations can be obtained from Fig. 5:

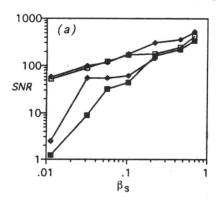
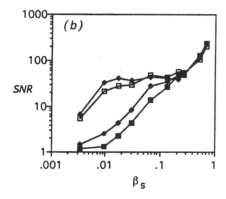

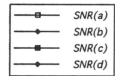

Fig. 5 *The SNR of the imaging systems tested with plastic rods at 4 different positions (a, b, c, and d in Fig. 2b) in the pipe versus the rod area fraction β_s.* (a) For 8-electrode configuration. (b) For 12-electrode configuration. (Note in the legend on the right, SNR(a) is for the SNR at position a, and so on).

(1) The *SNR* increases almost monotonically as the component fraction (rod size) β_r increases.

(2) The *SNR* improves as the rod moves from the pipe centre towards the pipe wall. For small rods, this improvement is more significant, indicating significant measurement sensitivity difference between the centre and the near wall area.

(3) The *SNR* of the 12-electrode configuration is about half that of the 8-electrode configuration. This is because for the sensor structure shown in Fig. 2, the area of each electrode reduces as the total number of electrodes increases, resulting in a reduction in capacitance signal level.

4.1.2. The input signal resolution

The *ISR* is closely related to the *SNR*. These tests were performed with small rods to find out the smallest size which satisfies the condition $SNR > 3$ (see section 2.4). *ISR* values (in terms of the percentage areas occupied by the rod) were obtained at the 4 positions mentioned above for both the 8 and 12-electrode configurations, and these are shown in Table 1. Note that, some of the figures, say less than 0.2%, in the table are obtained by extrapolating from Fig. 5, since rods of very small sizes were not available for the experimental tests (Fig. 3a).

Table 1. *Resolution of the imaging systems*
(plastic rod in empty pipe - area fraction)

Rod position	a	b	c	d
8-electrode sensor system	better than 0.1%	1.2%	2.0%	better than 0.1%
12-electrode sensor system	0.2%	1.5%	2.0%	0.15%

It can be seen from Table 1 that, the *ISR* of the 8-electrode sensor is better than that of the 12-electrode sensor. This is attributed to the larger *SNR* of the 8-electrode sensor (Section 4.1.1). The *ISR* of a capacitance imaging system is notably position dependent. Near the pipe wall (positions *a* and *d*), it is at least an order of magnitude higher than it is at the pipe centre (position *c*), due to the higher capacitance sensitivity near the pipe-wall area (Section 4.1.1). The *ISR* near the electrode-gap (position *d*) is slightly higher than that near the electrode centre (position *a*).

4.2. Imaging system errors

The imaging system errors include the *SIE* or the *AE* and the *PE* and these were calculated from the test results according to eqn. 5, 6 and 7.

4.2.1. Tests with plastic rods

Each time a rod was placed at positions *a*, *c* or *d* as shown by Fig. 2b, the errors *SIE*, *AE* and *PE* for this distribution were calculated. Results were obtained for different rod sizes shown in Fig. 3a, and for sensors with 8 and 12 electrodes. These results are plotted in Fig. 6, 7, 8 and 9 versus the area fraction of the rod β_s (with respect to the pipe cross-sectional area).

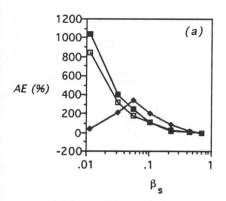 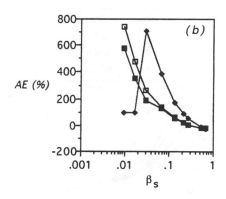

Fig. 6 *The cross-sectional area error (AE) of the test rods (Fig. 3a) at three positions in the pipe (a, c and d, see Fig. 2b) versus the rod area fraction β_s. (a)* For 8-electrode configuration. *(b)* For 12-electrode configuration. (Note in the legend on the right, *AE(a)* is for the *AE* at position *a*, and so on).

─□─	AE(a)
─◆─	AE(c)
─■─	AE(d)

Fig. 6 shows the *AE* values for both the 8 and the 12-electrode configurations. It is noted that *AE* is dependent on both the size and the position of the test rod. In general, the image error reduces as the rod size increases, and the error is significantly larger at the pipe centre than it is near the pipe wall, except for rods smaller than a few percent of pipe cross section, where the situation may reverse. It is unclear why the error at the pipe centre reduces as the rod size reduces towards its resolution limit.

The *AE* values for positions *a* and *d* are not very different for rod sizes larger than about 10%. For small rod sizes, there are some differences. For the 8-electrode configuration, there is *AE(a) < AE(d)*, whereas for the 12 electrode configuration, the situation is just opposite, possibly due to different sensor structures (Section 3).

Fig. 7 shows a comparison between the *AE* and the *SIE* for the 12-electrode configuration. Obviously the two criteria have a similar trend, although the values of *SIE* are larger than those of *AE* because *SIE* contains the errors in shape, position as well as cross-sectional area (Section 2.1). In calculating *SIE*, the precise position of the test rod in the pipe must be known in order to guarantee the accuracy of the calculation. However, with our simple experiment model, it was difficult to control precisely the position of the physical models. Therefore in the fóllowing sections, *AE*, instead of *SIE*, is mainly used to represent the spatial error of the reconstructed image.

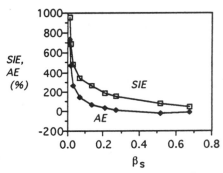

Fig. 7 *A comparison of the spatial image error (SIE) with the cross-sectional area error (AE), versus the area fraction β_s of the test rods, for the 12-electrode configuration (with test rods at position a).*

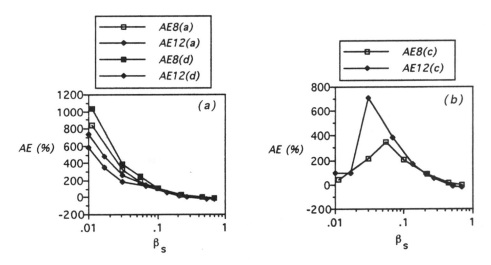

Fig. 8 *A comparison of the 12-electrode configuration with the 8-electrode configuration.* (a) Comparison of image error (*AE*) curves near the pipe wall. (b) Comparison of *AE* curves at the pipe centre. β_s is the area fraction of the test rods.

Fig. 8 compares the spatial image error of the 12-electrode configuration with that of the 8-electrode system. It is noted that, near the pipe wall (Fig. 8a), the 12-electrode system produces a smaller spatial image error than the 8-electrode system. This is more obvious when the size of the test rod is small. For instance at $\beta_s=0.03$ the average of *AE12(a)* and *AE12(d)* is about 65% that of *AE8(a)* and *AE8(d)*. At the pipe centre (Fig. 8b) and for $\beta_s >$ 0.1, the results of the two configurations are not very different. However the error of the 12-electrode system becomes larger as the rod size reduces because of increased random noise contribution to the spatial error.

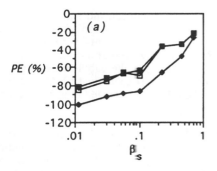

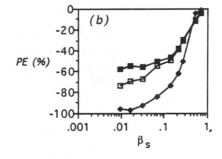

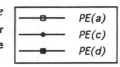

Fig. 9 *Permittivity error (PE) of the test rods at 3 positions in the pipe (a, c and d, see Fig. 2b) versus the rod area fraction β_s. (a) For 8-electrode configuration. (b) For 12-electrode configuration. The legend for the figures is on the right.*

Fig. 9 shows the *PE* for both the 8- and the 12-electrode configurations. The values of *PE* are all negative, indicating that the grey level of the reconstructed object is always lower than that of the standard. At the pipe centre, the error is at its largest, and it increases almost monotonically as the rod size reduces. By comparing Fig. 9a with Fig. 9b, it is noted that the 12-electrode system has a smaller *PE* (about 10% on average).

4.2.2. Tests with tubes

These tests were performed with the 12-electrode system only. A plastic tube (permittivity = 3) is placed at a given position (*a* or *c*) in the pipe, with the gap between its outer surface and the inner surface of the pipe wall filled with oil (permittivity = 3), simulating a cylindrical gas bubble in oil. The volume fraction of oil (and the bubble size) was changed by selecting tubes with different inner diameters. The maximum bubble size used was 62% as larger tubes were not available.

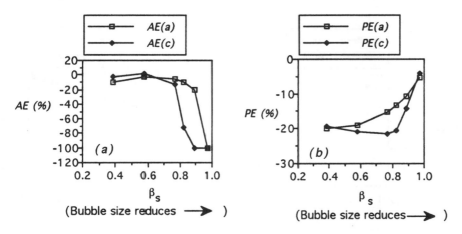

Fig. 10 *Cross-sectional area error (AE) and permittivity error (PE) of the 12-electrode system, tested with tubes (see Fig. 3b) at 2 positions in the pipe (a and c, see Fig. 2b), versus oil area fraction β_s. (a) AE. (b) PE.*

The *AE* of the bubble was calculated from the difference between the standard and the reconstruction bubble cross-section (divided by the standard cross-section). The results are plotted versus oil volume fraction in Fig. 10a. In Fig. 10a, the points with $AE=-100\%$ represent the situation when the reconstructed bubble size is zero (can not be seen on the reconstructed image). According to the figure, this happens when the bubble size reduces to about 3% near the pipe wall, and much worse at the pipe centre to about 12% (Actually, at the centre, bubbles smaller than 25% becomes blurred on the reconstructed image). For large bubbles (> 25%), *AE* is no more than 15% of the reading.

Compared with the results obtained with test rods (Section 4.2.1), where the minimum detectable rod size was about 2% (at pipe centre), the resolution of the system for gas bubble in oil is much poorer. In this work, the phenomenon that a low permittivity object is obscured by its surrounding high permittivity material is called the "dielectric screen effect". It was noticed that when the bubble was unrecognisable on the image, the changes in the 66 capacitance measurements were clearly observable. This means that the bubble presence was detected by the measurements, but our image reconstruction algorithm failed to reconstruct it. The situation was improved when the filter threshold was reduced by choosing $k=0.25$ in eqn. 2, but this resulted in greater image errors for other type of models (e.g. rod). Therefore $k=0.5$ was finally chosen as a compromise.

Fig. 10b shows the *PE* of the reconstructed bubble. Compared with Fig. 9, the values of *PE* in Fig. 10b are much smaller, and the error is smaller at the pipe centre than it is near the pipe wall. It is noted that the bubble-in-oil tests were performed in a region where β_s is relatively large, and there is more oil (high permittivity) in the more sensitive region of the sensor (near wall) when the bubble is at the centre. Therefore it is clear that the permittivity error depends on the input (capacitance) signal amplitude.

4.2.3. Tests with stationary oil

The tests were performed using the 12-electrode sensor. Oil was put into the horizontally laid sensor pipe to simulate the stratified flow patterns (see Fig. 4) and the amount of oil in the pipe was increased step by step to produce different oil fractions. Image errors *AE* and *PE* were obtained for the two different electrode orientations shown in Fig. 4a and 4b and these were plotted versus the oil fraction in Fig. 11.

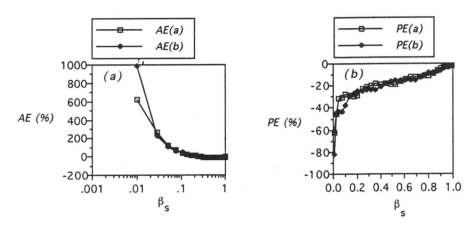

Fig. 11 *Cross-sectional area error (AE) and permittivity error (PE) of the 12-electrode system versus oil fraction β_s for stratified flow patterns with 2 different orientations (see Fig. 4). (a) AE. (b) PE. (AE(a)* for the orientation shown in Fig. 4a, and *AE(b)* for Fig. 4b, and so on).

Fig. 11a shows that, for stratified oil flow, AE is large at very low oil levels, and it reduces as the oil fraction increases. At oil fractions higher than 30%, AE becomes negative. The trend is similar to that shown by Fig. 8a. The trend of PE shown by Fig. 11b is also similar to that shown by Fig. 9b. The AE and PE values for the two different orientations are not very different except at low oil levels where the orientation shown in Fig. 4a produce less error because its higher sensitivity near the bottom of the pipe (near electrode gap [3]).

4.3. Component fraction measurement errors

$CFME$ errors for core, annular and stratified flow patterns were obtained from the reconstructed images according to eqn. 9 and 11. The core flow and annular flow of different component fractions were simulated by plastic rods and tubes of different sizes placed at the pipe centre. The stratified distributions were obtained in the same way as that in Section 4.2.3 with the electrode orientation as that shown by Fig. 4a. The errors are plotted versus oil area fraction in Fig. 12 and the maximum errors are about 17% (absolute) for all three flow patterns (core pattern with $\beta_s > 70\%$, annular pattern with $\beta_s < 35\%$ were not tested.). This shows that the accuracy of calculating component fraction from the reconstructed image is limited by the linear backprojection algorithm. Adjusting the threshold filter (eqn. 2) may improve the accuracy, but the threshold value is difficult to optimize for all the flow patterns. In order to improve the accuracy for component fraction measurement, better methods of image reconstruction and/or measurement data processing should be investigated. For example, Fig. 12b shows the $CFME$ calculated by using the average value of the 54 normalised capacitance measurements to replace the β_r in eqn. 11 (those from the 12 adjacent electrode pairs are excluded, since they are found prone to generate large overshoots or undershoots [3], leading to overestimated or underestimated measurements). Fig. 12b indicates that, using this method, the $CFME$ has significantly reduced to 5% (maximum) for annular and stratified flows, and to 12% (maximum) for core flow.

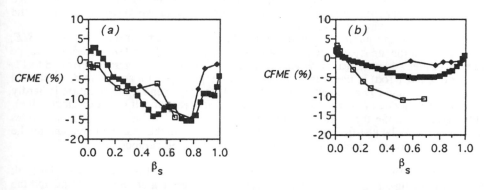

Fig. 12 *Component fraction measurement error (CFME) of the 12-electrode sensor versus the real component fraction β_s.*
(a) *CFME calculated from the reconstructed images (eqn. 9 and 10).*
(b) *CFME calculated from the average of the 54 normalised mea-surements (except those from the 12 adjacent electrode pairs)*

	core flow
	annular flow
	stratified flow

5. CONCLUSIONS

It is realized that it is very difficult to fully describe the performance of a capacitance imaging system. In this paper, a system is evaluated with only a number of simple distribution patterns. Although it is difficult to predict precisely the system errors for more complex distribution patterns, the criteria defined for the simple patterns do provide a quantitative way of describing some aspects of the system performance, as well as standards for comparing different systems and reconstruction algorithms. Referring to the definitions given in Section 2 and the results in Section 4, following conclusions can be drawn for the present UMIST 12-electrode system:

(1) For an object with a permittivity of about 3 in an empty pipe, its minimum size that the imaging system can resolve is 0.2% (of pipe cross-section) near the pipe wall and 2.0% at the pipe centre. These are the best *ISR* values that can be achieved with the current signal to noise ratio. For more complex distributions, the resolution might not be as good.

(2) The system errors such as the *SIE* and the *PE* are strongly position dependent and flow pattern dependent. From the results of the test with a 3% rod, near the pipe wall the *SNR*, *AE* and *PE* improve 6, 3 and 1.33 times respectively compared with their corresponding values at the pipe centre.

(3) Discrete objects formed by the low permittivity component tend to be obscured by the high permittivity component surrounding them. Similarly objects near the pipe centre tend to be masked by high permittivity component presented near the pipe wall. This is called, in this paper as the "dielectric screen effect". Due to this effect, objects of lower permittivity in the higher permittivity component are more difficult to detect than vice versa. The system errors are particularly large when gas bubbles at the pipe centre are imaged (Maximum reconstructable bubble size is around 20%.). The fact that the bubbles can be detected by the measurement circuit suggests that this effect may be reduced by using other image reconstruction algorithms which are more accurate than the linear backprojection method.

(4) When component fraction is estimated from the reconstructed image, the *CFME* errors can be large for all the simulated flow regimes (all at about 17% maximum). When component fraction is estimated from the average of the 54 normalised capacitance measurements (excluding those from the neighbouring electrode pairs), the *CFME* is significantly reduced (for stratified and annular flows to 5% maximum, for core flow to 12% maximum). In order to improve the accuracy further, either more accurate image reconstruction algorithms or an appropriate (adaptive and weighted) average of the capacitance measurements have to be used.

(5) The increase in the number of electrodes reduces the system errors such as the *SIE*, particularly in the areas near the pipe wall. However, the *SNR* and *ISR* deteriorate as the number of electrodes increases. When the number of electrodes is increased from 8 to 12, the *AE* (for a 3% rod) in the near wall area (the average of point *a* and point *d*) is reduced by about 30%, and *PE* by about 15%. However at the pipe centre, the situation is hardly improved or may be even worse due to the reduced *SNR* (about half of the original value). This agrees with the theoretical prediction by Seagar *et al* [7]. The use of 12 electrodes instead of 8 may be justified by the reduction of the errors in the near wall area and by the feasibility of further reducing the noise level of the sensor electronics [8].

ACKNOWLEDGMENT   This work is funded by the SERC and the DTI under the Link Scheme. S M Huang and B F Zhang wish to thank the Chinese Nature Science Fund and the British Council for their support which enables them to join the UMIST team for this research. Mr. R John of Tealgate Ltd is thanked for his assistance in designing and constructing the primary sensors for this test.

REFERENCES
[1] Huang S M, Plaskowski A B, Xie C G and Beck M S *Electronics Letters*, 1988 **24**, (7), pp. 418-419
[2] Huang S M, Xie C G, Thorn R, Snowden D and Beck MS *IEE Proc.G*, 1992, **139**, (1), pp. 83-88
[3] Xie C G, Huang S M, Hoyle B S, Thorn R, Lenn C, Snowden D and Beck M S *IEE Proc.G*, 1992, **139**, (1), pp. 89-98
[4] Fasching G E and Smith N S *Rev. Sci. Instrum.* 1991, **62** (9), pp. 2243-2251.
[5] Doebelin E O *Measurement Systems: Application and Design* (London: McGraw-Hill, 1983) 3rd Edition.
[6] Xie C G, Huang S M, Hoyle B S, Lenn C and Beck M S *Proc. ECAPT'92*.
[7] Seagar A D, Barber D C and Brown B H *Clin. Phys. Physiol. Meas.*, 1987, **8**, Suppl.A, pp. 13-31
[8] Yang W Q and Stott A L *Proc. ECAPT'92*.

APPLICATION OF CAPACITANCE TOMOGRAPHY
TO PNEUMATIC CONVEYING PROCESSES

K. Brodowicz, L. Maryniak, T. Dyakowski[*]

Institute of Heat Engineering Warsaw Technical University
00-065 Nowowiejska 25
Poland

[*] Department of Chemical Engineering,UMIST, P.O.Box 88, Manchester M60 1QD
United Kingdom

Abstract

Experimental results of monitoring a pneumatic process are presented. Capacitance sensors were used to provide 2-dimensional images and the results obtained have been applied in modelling the pneumatic conveying process. These results are presented in the form of a two phase flow map.

Nomenclature

A - cross sectional area of pipe
A_u - area above a stationary or moving bed of solid (from tomographic image)
A_{lm} - area of immovable part of slug (from tomographic image)
L - length of particles transported by the solid slug
T - time between appearance of slugs
V - average cross sectional air velocity
V_u average air velocity above a stationary or moving bed of solid
Q_s - flow rate of solid
ε - component fraction (from tomographic image)
ρ - density of solid
μ - loading factor (solid/air mass flow ratio)

Introduction

Process tomography is a new non-intrusive technique for investigating physical processes. This kind of monitoring is particularly useful for examining processes and flow patterns where density gradients take place. This is a feature of a two phase flows (Chang et al.,1989). Process tomography provides information about such processes in virtually real time. In the case of two-phase flows such rapid information is needed to determine the correct flow pattern. Significant advantages include the possibility of getting flow images in the form of slides for further study. These advantages and the dielectric properties of the two components used in this experiment indicate that capacitance tomography could be used for examining pneumatic transport.

Experiments were focussed on monitoring flow patterns. The experimental results gave significant information about the cross sectional packing of solid inside a conveying line. To give a full description of a flow, measurements of cross sectional average velocity of gas, mass flow rate of solid and pressure drop along the conveying line were made. These parameters were needed to draw a map of two phase flow.

Experimental stand

Figure 1 shows the experimental arrangement. The horizontal tubular test section was built of glass segments enabling the flow patterns to be observed. The external diameter tube diameter was D_0 = 96 mm and the internal D_i = 84 mm.

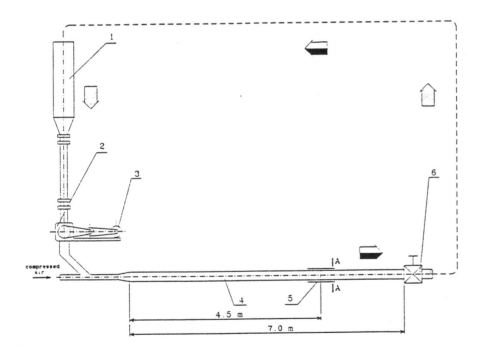

Figure 1 The experimental stand: 1) storage container,2) rotary feeder, 3) D.C.motor, 4) test section,5) capacitance sensor, 6) speed control valve.

The system was arranged so that the solids could be recycled; see Figure 1. In this experiment compressed air was used for transporting rape seeds (rape seeds are characterized by their nearly spherical shape of 1 mm radius and density about 1210 kg m^{-3}). To continuouslly regulate the seed mass flow rate a rotary feeder D.C. motor driven was used. In this way, the different flow patterns were obtained as a function of seeds mass flow rate. The pressure drops (along 3 m distance of the pipe) were measured by pressure gauges. The main items of the flow imaging system were as follows:

– an eight electrode capacitance sensor;

– a data collection and reconstruction system.

The capacitance sensor shown in Figure 2 was built of eight brass plates (length l=190 mm) mounted on the external surface of the glass pipe and screened.

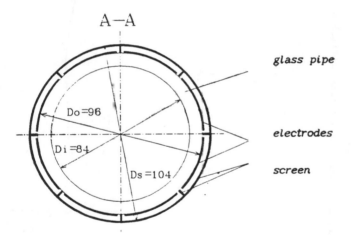

Figure 2 Section through the sensor.

The data collection system measured the capacitances between any two of the eight electrodes in all possible combinations. The measured values were converted into digital signals and a cross sectional of image of the flow pattern was reconstructed by using a linear back-projection algorithm (Huang et al., 1989 and Xie et al., 1989).

Experimental results

The application of capacitance tomography provided important tomographic images of the flow patterns. Both stratifed and slug flow patterns were investigated successfully using the technique but it failed to visualize a dilute dispersed flow. The reason for this was because the permittivity of the dispersed flow was nearly equal to the air permittivity and capacitance tomography could not detect it (Brodowicz et al., 1989, Dyakowski 1988). To compare the accuracy of the reconstructed tomographic images with the actual flow structures (as seen through the glass section) photographs were taken. The different flow structures are shown on the flow map shown in Figure 3.

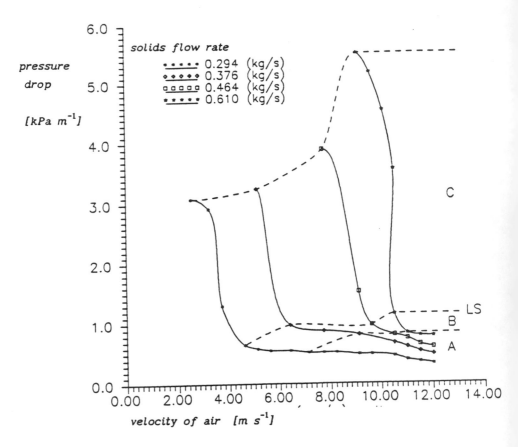

Figure 3 The map of gas solids flow pattern for horizontal test section: A) stratifed flow, B) dune flow, C) plug flow, LS) loosing stability line.

Stratified flow

Stratified flow with a sliding bed is shown in Figure 4. The high permittivity of this bed made detection possible.

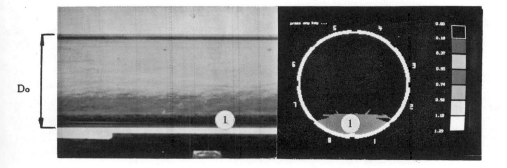

Figure 4 Stratified flow with sliding bed (A): 1)sliding bed (ε = 0.39).

When the air velocity (V) was reduced it caused greater settlement of the seeds which then formed a stationary bed. This process continued until a balance was achieved i.e. until V_u was sufficiently high to transport the seeds in the form of dunes above the stationary bed. Figure 5 shows the change in void fraction between dune flow (ε = 0.48) and the stationary bed (ε = 0.36).

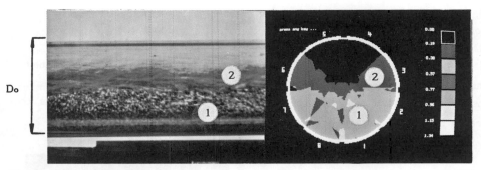

Figure 5 Stratified flow with moving dunes (B): 1) stationary bed (ε = 0.36), 2) moving dunes (ε = 0.48).

The above flow patterns are characterized by high energy consumption, significant damage to the seeds and erosion of the pipe wall (Govier and Aziz 1972, Konrad 1986, Kubuj and Talacha 1992). but will always occur in the transition period before a satisfactory flow pattern (slug flow) is achieved. Because of this it is worth calculating the conveying mass flow rate over a stationary bed.

According to Figure 6, from the simplified continuity equation the velocity of air and seeds mass flow rate are expressed as follows:

the velocity of air:

$$V_u = V \, (A/A_u) \tag{1}$$

seeds mass flow rate

$$Q_s = 2V_u \, R^2 \int_{\theta_b}^{\pi/2} \varepsilon \, \cos^2\theta \, d\theta \tag{2}$$

where ε is unknown function of θ.

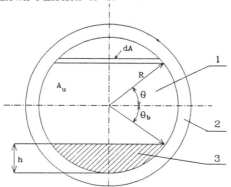

Figure 6 Stratified flow - cross section view: 1) dispersed phase, 2) glass pipe, 3) settled particles; infinitesimal area $dA = 2R^2 \cos^2\theta \, d\theta$.

Loss of stability

A further decrease of air velocity V plugged a section of pipe directly below the feeder. Transport of material ceased for a short time. Figure 7 shows the instant just before the stationary bed lost stability. Lack of air flow is the reason for a uniform void fraction ($\varepsilon = 0.36$).

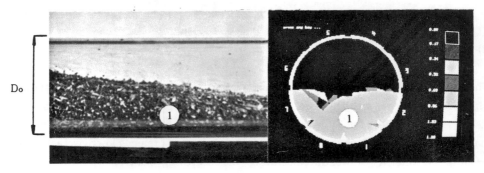

Figure 7 Loosing stability: 1) Stationary bed ($\varepsilon = 0.36$).

Slug flow

After the pipe blocked the air pressure increased. This causes the first appearance of slugs, Figure 8. Because of the high value of the loading factor μ (Wirth and Molerius 1985, Konrad 1986, Kubuj and Talacha 1992) this flow pattern is the most desirable. The tomographic images were reconstructed from data averaged over collecting time and the length of capacitance sensor. To a first approximation the seeds mass flow rate can be obtained from the formula:

$$Q_s = (A - A_{lm})\ (1-\varepsilon)\ \rho\ L\ /T. \tag{3}$$

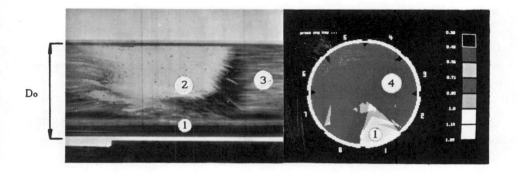

Figure 8 Slug flow: 1) immovable part of seeds ($\varepsilon = 0.30$), 2) gas slug, 3) solid slug, 4) averaged slug and slug image.

Conclusion

Application of capacitance tomography gives valuable information on the distribution of the conveyed material. For example, analysis of 2-dimensional images can give significant information about which part of a flow pattern structure is in motion and which is stationary. Combining measurements of cross sectional velocity and tomographic images enables the seeds mass flow rate to be calculated.

REFERENCES

Huang S.M., Plaskowski A.B., Xie C.G., and Beck M.S. 1989 Tomographic imaging of two-component flow using capacitance sensors *J Phys.E.Sci Instrum.* **22** 173-177

Xie C.G., Plaskowski A.B. Beck M.S., 1989 8-electrode capacitance system for two-component flow identification Part 1: Tomographic flow imaging Part 2: Flow regime identification *IEE Proc. A* **136** 173-191

Brodowicz K., Dyakowski T., Wierzbicki D.1989, Two-phase gas particle flow through venturi *Multiphase flow and heat and mass transfer Second International Symposium* Beijing, China 1159-1166

Dyakowski T. 1988   Optical method for measuring void fraction and particles velocity in dispersed particles-air flow *Second International Symposium on Two-phase Annular and dispersed flows* Oxford 129-132.

Chang J.S., Tofiluk W., Myint T.A., Hayashi N., and Brodowicz K., 1989 Time averaged particle fraction and flow patterns in gas-powder two-phase horizontal flow The Fourth Miami International Symposium on Multi-Phase Transport, USA

Wirth K.E.and Molerius O.1985 Critical solids transport velocity with horizontal pneumatic conveying *Powder Technology & Bulk Solids Technology* 9 17-24

Govier G.W. and Aziz K.,1972 The flow of complex mixtures in pipes *Litton Educational Publishing*

Konrad K. 1986 Dense-phase pnueumatic conveying *Powder Technology* 49 1-35

Kubuj G. and Talacha M.1992, Research on flow patterns in horizontal and inclined pneumatic transport using capacitance tomography M.Sc.Thesis, *Warsaw Technical University (in Polish)*

VELOCITY PROFILE MEASUREMENT IN TWO-PHASE FLOWS

D G HAYES, I A GREGORY, M S BECK

Process Tomography Group, UMIST, Manchester, M60 1QD, UK.

ABSTRACT: This paper describes real-time correlation techniques for determining the velocity profile in two-phase oil / gas flows. The computational requirements of this task are investigated and suitable algorithms presented. It is shown that a combination of efficient image buffering and a recursive correlation technique can reduce both the computational and memory requirements of this task. A general purpose transputer / DSP system can then provide a viable hardware implementation of a real-time velocity profile measurement system.

1. Introduction

Single-phase fluid flow measurement is now well developed and there are many possible methods to choose from. Examples are the Venturi meter, orifice plate, pitot tube, and various forms of mechanical, magnetic, ultra-sonic and correlation techniques. By a suitable choice of flowmeter, it is now usually possible to obtain accuracies of around 1% with 'simple' flows. However, although methods of measuring single-phase fluids are well developed, the problem of two-phase flow measurement is still a major problem. The methods traditionally used for single-phase flow measurement are not readily extended to more complex two-phase flows.

The basic problem with two-phase flow measurement is that both the concentration and velocity profiles vary considerably with time. This is because the different components can arrange themselves in many different ways. Recent developments in tomographic imaging can overcome the problems associated with concentration distributions. Here, the problems associated with velocity distributions are addressed. Because most of the current two-phase flowmeters are highly dependent on flow regime, this leads to significant errors. In favourable situations accuracies approaching 5-10% can be obtained, but 50% is not unknown. In the worst cases, results can not only be useless; they can be misleading.

In this paper there will be a particular bias towards oil / gas flows as encountered in the oil industry (much of it however, particularly the details concerning correlation and processing requirements is applicable to the wider case of two-phase flows in general). To give some idea of what is commercially available, some recently developed instruments can claim an accuracy of around 1-2% in measuring oil / gas void fraction (e.g. Endress & Hauser 'Aquasyst'), but unfortunately, they normally need a homogeneous flow to achieve this. The most reliable method of achieving around 1% accuracy is to separate the different components and then measure each component separately. This has the advantage that different types of flowmeter can be used for each component, each one being designed for specific flow conditions. Unfortunately, for off-shore oil platforms, the separation equipment is normally very large, occupying several cubic metres, and also very expensive. Another problem that arises with separation techniques is that they can be slow to respond to changes in flow conditions. This is particularly so when periodic, rather than continuous measurements are taken. It is hoped that the collected sample is representative of the long-time-averaged flow conditions, but this is not necessarily so and significant errors can still occur.

Yet another problem is the fact that most meters are intrusive. This not only affects the flow conditions that the meter is being used to measure; it also subjects the meter to general wear and tear. This is a greater problem when the substances to be measured are corrosive or abrasive. One other obvious advantage of the non-intrusive meter is the zero pressure drop caused by the meter. In addition, a non-intrusive imaging system allows for pigging of pipelines for cleaning and inspection purposes. The ideal instrument would be accurate, non-invasive, insensitive to the concentration profile, physically small and inexpensive.

Most previous work (e.g. Hammer (1983), Geraets & Borst (1987)) has been directed at averaging bulk effects over the cross-section of the pipe. This allows relatively simple systems to be used but the results tend to be dependent on flow regime. To overcome this, some recently developed instruments can obtain a 'tomographic image' of the flow; this potentially allows measurements to be independent of the flow regime. This paper examines how a capacitance imaging system developed by Xie et al (1991) can be used to obtain velocity profile measurements in real-time using efficient correlation techniques. This is seen to be a key step in the development of a two-phase oil / gas (and ultimately, 3-phase oil / gas / water) measurement system. The current capacitance transducer electronics system can collect a complete set of data at a rate of 100 frames per second (f/s). For two sensors the reconstruction rate must then be 200 f/s. A transputer/DSP based system has been designed to satisfy this requirement.

2. Principle of Velocity Profile Measurement

The principle of velocity profile measurement can be explained with reference to figure 1. Two imaging systems are placed a short distance apart along the pipe to be monitored. A computer system then reconstructs the images at the two planes (I1, I2). The concentration function at each plane $\beta_c(x,y)$ can thus be determined, where $\beta_c(x,y)$ is the concentration of component c at position (x,y) in the vessel. For a pipe of circular cross-section, the total concentration of component c can be obtained by integrating this function over the area of the pipe A.

i.e.
$$\beta_{tot,c} = \frac{1}{A} \int_{-r}^{r} \int_{-r}^{r} \beta_c(x,y)\, dx\, dy \tag{1}$$

By measuring the time taken for features at one plane to reach the second plane, the velocity v of the features can be obtained since:

$$v = \frac{L}{T}$$

where L is the distance between the image planes and T is the measured transit time. If the velocity profile $U_c(x,y)$ is known then the total volumetric flow rate of component c (Q_C) can be found.

i.e.
$$Q_C = \frac{1}{A} \int_{-r}^{r} \int_{-r}^{r} \beta_c(x,y)\, U_c(x,y)\, dx\, dy \tag{2}$$

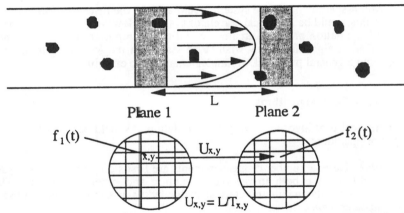

Features passing through
pixel (x,y) in plane 1
produce a signal $f_1(t)$

$f_2(t)$ will be similar to $f_1(t)$
but delayed by the transit
time $T_{x,y}$ and with added
noise.

Fig. 1 Image Cross Correlation

The velocity profile is found by cross correlating pixels in plane I1 with their corresponding
pixels in plane I2. This can be done in a variety of ways, but the most common technique,
described in detail by Beck and Plaskowski (1987), is to use the cross correlation function:

$$R_{12}(\tau) = \frac{1}{T-\tau} \int_{0}^{T-\tau} f_1(t)f_2(t-\tau)\, dt \qquad (3)$$

where $f_1(t)$ and $f_2(t)$ are the time signals (pixel values) produced by pixels in planes I1 and I2
respectively and T is the observation time. The transit time is given by the value of τ that
maximises the cross correlation function.

In discrete form, equation (3) is often written as

$$y(n) = \sum_{m=0}^{N-1-n} x_1(n+m)\, x_2(m) \qquad n = 0, 1, 2, ...N-1 \qquad (4)$$

where the factor outside the integral has been removed for simplicity.

In principle, for images consisting of P pixels, P correlation functions need to be calculated.
In practice however, the turbulent nature of many flows means that this is not necessarily the
case. Firstly, in some cases, e.g. inclined flows, it may be necessary to correlate pixel (x,y) in
plane 1 with pixels other than pixel (x,y) in plane 2. This would substantially increase the
number of correlation functions to be calculated. However, as the number of pixels in the
images are increased, there comes a point when correlating more pixels produces negligible
additional velocity information. This is because signals from adjacent pixels will in
themselves be highly correlated. Hence this would reduce the number to be correlated.
However, whichever pixels are to be correlated in a given system, it is clear that there is a
substantial processing requirement involved.

A dedicated, application-specific hardware system would achieve the fastest implementation (the extreme case of this would be an optical correlator system). However, a general purpose microprocessor implementation provides greater flexibility, an important feature of a new system in which different algorithms may wish to be tested. In the following text, some techniques for allowing a general purpose DSP implementation are examined.

3. Comparison of Real-Time Algorithms

This section examines real-time algorithms for pixel correlation. It should be noted that there are two basic types of operation:

i)   *Pseudo real-time* : Here, a number of measurements are first stored and then analysed later. This would involve both image reconstruction and pixel correlation. This procedure is repeated at the maximum rate sustainable by the processor system in use to give periodic updates, hence the term 'pseudo real-time'.

ii)   *True real-time* : This is exactly as the name suggests; the flow measurements are updated in true real-time fashion after each new set of measurements.

It is the latter that will be considered here, the reason being as follows. It may initially be thought that pseudo real-time operation would require less processing power than true real-time operation. This is not necessarily the case however. Consider case (i) and assume that a display of the velocity profile is to be updated a given number times per second. For each update, a set of data is stored and then analysed. This requires a complete set of correlation functions to be calculated. With reference to equation (4), it can be seen that each calculation requires a computation time approximately proportional to NM, where N and M are the number of delays and the number of samples used respectively. A true real-time system can make use of the redundancy in consecutive calculations of equation (4). Hence it is possible apply the following recurrence relation:

$$\text{new value = old value + new product - old product} \qquad (5)$$

Or, in algebraic terms

$$y_i(n) \;=\; y_{i-1}(n) + x_1(n+N-1+i).x_2(N-1+i) \;-\; x_1(n+i).x_2(i) \qquad (6a)$$

$$y_0(n) \;=\; \sum_{m=0}^{N-1} x_1(n+m)\,x_2(m) \qquad n = 0, 1, 2, ...N-1 \qquad (6b)$$

where $y_i(n)$ is the value of the ith correlation function at delay n.

This shows that once the first correlation function has been calculated ($y_0(n)$) using 6b, successive functions can be computed using the recurrence equation of 6a. In the following text, these two methods will be referred to as "complete" and "recurrent" correlations respectively. Now, in terms of processing requirements, addition is similar in complexity to subtraction. Hence, for computational comparisons, addition will be assumed to encompass subtraction. For N delays each recurrent correlation calculation then requires 2N multiplications and 2N additions. This is a considerable saving compared with a full computation and even compares very favourably to polarity correlation when both are implemented on a general purpose microprocessor. The actual processing time is now only proportional to N rather than NM (N=no. of delays, M=no. of samples)

One drawback with this technique is that more memory is required to store the values of the correlation functions at each value of delay n. For N delays and P correlation functions (pixels), an additional NP memory locations are required. It is possible to reduce the number of multiplications from 2N to N by storing all the products that have been calculated. However, there will be an even larger number of these (MNP for M delays, N samples and P pixels), and this will significantly increase the memory requirements, particularly for an image correlation using many pixels.

Using this technique, although the update rate for a set of correlation functions may be 100/s (the current sensor acquisition rate), instead of say, 10/s for pseudo real-time, the calculations can be done much faster. Thus, a true real-time system is preferred from this point of view.

4. Limits to the Number of Correlation Functions Used

In order to make real-time operation possible, there is a limit to the number of correlation functions (pixels (P)) that can be calculated. This is determined primarily by the image réconstruction rate (T_F), and the time taken to calculate a single correlation function when the recurrence formula is being used (T_R). Hence, the limiting condition is

$$T_R . P < T_F \tag{7}$$

or
$$P_{MAX} = \frac{T_F}{T_R} \tag{8}$$

Figure 2 shows the maximum number of pixels that can be correlated as a function of T_R. The three lines are shown for three different values of the frame rate T_F. The graph is plotted over the most useful range of values with respect to the performance obtainable by modern processors. Thus, to give an example, with the current frame rate of 10ms, a value of $T_R = 100us$ allows a maximum of 100 correlation functions to be calculated. This value of T_R is not unrealistic with high performance digital signal processing (DSP) chips. A device running at 10 million instructions per second (10 MIPS) can execute 1000 instructions in 100us. If there are 128 delays/correlation function then this allows a maximum of 7 instruction cycles to be used to calculate each *point*. of the correlation function. If the recursive algorithm is used this figure is obtainable with the use of DSPs due to their optimised architecture and complex instruction set. No account here has been taken of other overheads such as communication of data and results, or any other code that must be executed. However, the correlation calculations are the major processing burden. Also, the rating of 10 MIPS is now a minimum, conservative figure and the use of multiple processors can add further processing power.

5. Comparison of Image Buffering Techniques

The following section will investigate the time required to achieve real-time operation using the recursive algorithm. This situation will not normally be obtainable immediately on switching on the system. The reason for this is that the first set of correlation functions have to be calculated without the use of the recurrence relation. This process is relatively slow and unless the processor is exceptionally fast, or very few pixels are correlated, the complete set of correlations can not be completed in the time taken for the next set of data to arrive. Thus, any new sets of data are stored, or buffered, until the first set of correlations is complete. The faster, recursive calculations can then begin and gradually use up the stored data. If these faster correlations proceed at a rate greater than that with which new images arrive (currently 100/s from each sensor) then eventually all stored data will be used up. This is the point of real-time operation. The time taken to reach this point is very important for two main reasons:

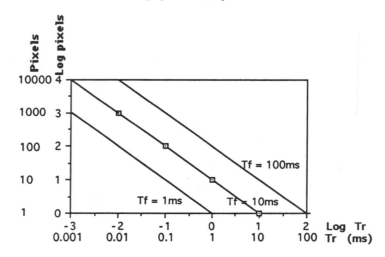

Fig 2 Maximum No. of Pixels that can be correlated
as a function of correlation parameters

i)   It determines how long the system, and therefore the operator, has to wait before real-time operation is obtained.

ii) It determines how many images need to be stored in a buffer, and therefore the memory requirements.

Of these, the second is of far greater importance than the first due to the high rate at which images are acquired.

Two possible image buffering algorithms will now be examined.

ALGORITHM A - BUFFERING WHOLE IMAGES

This algorithm is conceptually the simplest and entails collecting a sequence of complete images from two imaging planes, I1 and I2. The cross-correlation functions of the pixels in plane 1 with the corresponding pixels in plane 2 are then calculated. This is computationally intensive and is difficult to complete in the time taken to capture another image (typically 10ms). To overcome this, the incoming images are stored to be used later. Once the first set of complete correlation functions have been calculated the stored images are then used to calculate subsequent sets of correlation functions. These however, can be calculated using the recurrence relation described in section 3; this is very much faster. At the same time, any new images that arrive are stored. Now, if the rate of correlating a set of pixels in an image using the recurrence relation is greater than the rate at which new images are captured, then the number of stored images will decrease and eventually reach zero. At this point continuous real-time operation will have been reached.

Using some simple algebra, it can be shown that if

T_c = Time taken to calculate a single complete correlation function
T_R = Time taken to calculate a single correlation function using the recurrence relation
T_F = Time between image frames
P_c = No of pixels to be correlated

then the time (T_A) taken for algorithm A to reach real-time operation is:

$$T_A = T_c P_c \left[1 + \frac{P_c}{T_{FR} - P_c}\right] \tag{9}$$

where $T_{FR} = T_F/T_R$

There are a couple of points to note about this equation. Firstly, T_A is proportional to the time taken to calculate a complete correlation function without using the recurrence relation (T_c). Also of great importance is the dependence on T_{FR} and P_c. Because of the form of the last term in brackets, the total time rises very rapidly when T_{FR} is close to P_c. This will normally be the case if the maximum possible number of pixels are to be correlated. When T_{FR} and P_c are equal, T_A becomes infinite and real time operation can never be obtained.

Equation 9 is plotted in figure 3 for different values of T_R. This gives a visual indication of how many pixels can be correlated before the computation time rises rapidly. Values of $T_C=1ms$ and $T_F = 10ms$ have been assumed, but the readings can be scaled appropriately.

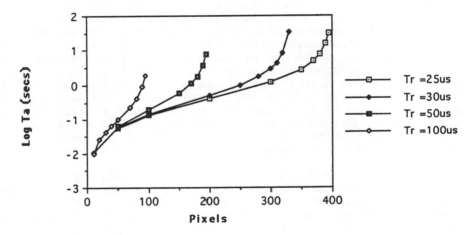

Fig. 3 Time taken for Algorithm A to reach real-time operation

The memory requirements of this simple algorithm can also be easily calculated. The number of images to be buffered is given approximately by the ratio $2T_A/T_F$ (the factor of 2 arises because there are two image planes). Substituting from (9), and assuming 1 byte / pixel, the buffer size for algorithm A (B_A) is given by:

$$B_A = \frac{2P_c^2 T_C}{T_F} \left[1 + \frac{P_c}{T_{FR} - P_c}\right] \quad \text{(bytes)} \tag{10}$$

This is a very substantial memory requirement for two main reasons. Firstly, there is the factor of P_c^2 in the numerator, and secondly, the second term in the brackets tends to infinity as P_c tends to the ratio T_F/T_R. The function is thus very sensitive to small changes in T_{FR} and

P_c. For correlating the maximum possible number of pixels, T_{FR} will be very close to P_c and hence the memory requirement will be substantial. With this in mind the benefits of a more efficient algorithm will be examined.

ALGORITHM B - BUFFERING PARTIAL IMAGES

This is a variation of algorithm A, but is intended to reduce both the time taken to achieve real-time operation and the memory requirements.

For this version, whole images are not buffered during the initial phase of obtaining the first set of correlation functions. Instead, only values of a few pixels are stored, the number increasing as more complete correlations are completed. Eventually there will come a point when all pixels have been included in the complete correlation calculation and all the pixels are stored when a new image is provided by the reconstruction software.

Figure 4 illustrates this technique for the simplified case of just four pixels per image. It is assumed here that two new images arrive in the time taken to perform a complete correlation using four pixels, or data points. First, four images (0-3) are collected but, only pixel 0 is stored from the first two and pixels 0 and 1 from the second two. This is because no other pixels from these images will be needed. The first correlation is done using pixel 0 in images 0-3. During this time, two more images (4 & 5) arrive and pixels 0-2 are stored. The next complete correlation is done using pixel 1 in images 2-5. Note that image 5 is the latest image to be collected and so the most up-to-date four point correlation function does not need pixel 1 from the first two images. In parallel with this, pixel 0 has its new correlation function calculated twice using the recurrence relation. The first time is done with pixels 1-4 and then with 2-5. These calculations are very much quicker however. Again, two more images (6-7) arrive but, this time all the pixels are stored since they will all be needed in later calculations. Since image 7 is now the latest, the third complete correlation function is calculated using pixel 2 from images 4-7. Again, pixel 2 data prior to image 4 is not needed and was not therefore stored. This process is repeated until four complete correlations have been calculated, each using the most recent four images. At this point, real-time operation is obtained. Subsequent correlations are then done using the recurrence formula.

It is evident that this method is both faster and uses less memory than algorithm A. It is faster because fewer complete correlation calculations are required. This is because only the latest images are used in calculating the first correlation function for a given pixel. The reason for less memory is obvious - fewer pixels are stored. For this algorithm, it can be shown that the time (T_B) taken to reach real-time operation for P_c pixels is given by:

$$T_B = \sum_{K=1}^{P_c} T_C \left[1 + \frac{K}{T_{FR} - K} \right] \qquad (11)$$

The corresponding buffer size for this algorithm (B_B) is significantly smaller than that for algorithm A; for this case, it is only necessary to buffer a sequence of pixels from a single pixel. It is readily shown that the maximum length of this sequence (and hence buffer size) is given by:

$$B_B = \frac{2(T_C + PT_R)}{T_F} \qquad \text{(bytes)} \qquad (12)$$

This is a substantial reduction when compared to the simplistic approach of buffering every image. However, it still allows identical performance once 'up to speed'. Figure 5 shows how

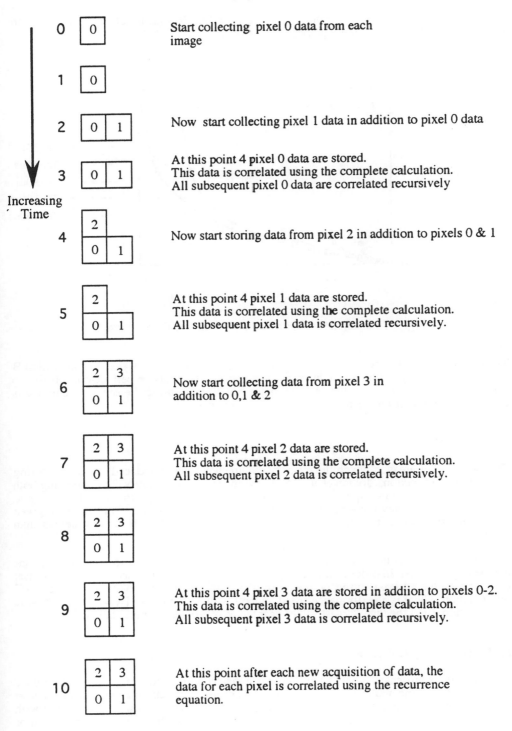

Fig. 4 Algorithm B - Buffering Partial Images

T_B varies as a function of T_{FR} for the case where T_C = 1ms. Results for other values of T_C are obtained by simply scaling these graphs appropriately.

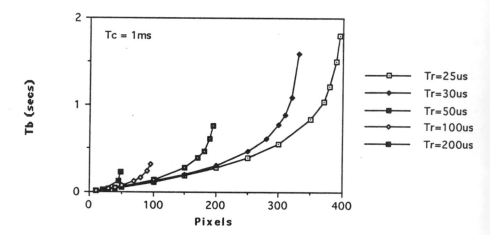

Fig. 5 Time taken for Algorithm B to reach real-time operation

The important factor to bear in mind when comparing T_A and T_B is not just that algorithm B reaches real-time operation much quicker than algorithm A. It may be perfectly acceptable to wait a few seconds for algorithm A. The major benefit from using the second technique is that a reduced time results is reduced memory requirements.

4. Other tricks

One of the other areas in which the memory requirements can be reduced is that for storing the correlation functions. Jordan et al (1989) describe several techniques for minimising both memory and processing requirements. One of the most promising for this application is to increase the time delay increments at the longer time-delay positions. This allows a given worst-case resolution in time delay estimation to be achieved with far few delays than otherwise required.

In order to provide better resolution, some form of interpolation of the correlation functions can be implemented. In order of increasing complexity, three possible techniques are to use: (a) a triangular approximation of the peak, (b) a parabolic interpolation, and (c) FFT interpolation. There is a performance/speed tradeoff with each method. However, a parabolic interpolation using the three largest values near the peak provides a useful balance.

5. Hardware Implementation

The techniques presented in this paper, provide a means of implementing a general-purpose system without using application specific devices. The use of a recurrence relationship can be fully exploited with general purpose processors, redundancy which is difficult to exploit with dedicated FFT devices and convolvers etc. As a result it is possible to use a combination of transputers and digital signal processors for the entire image reconstruction / correlation system.

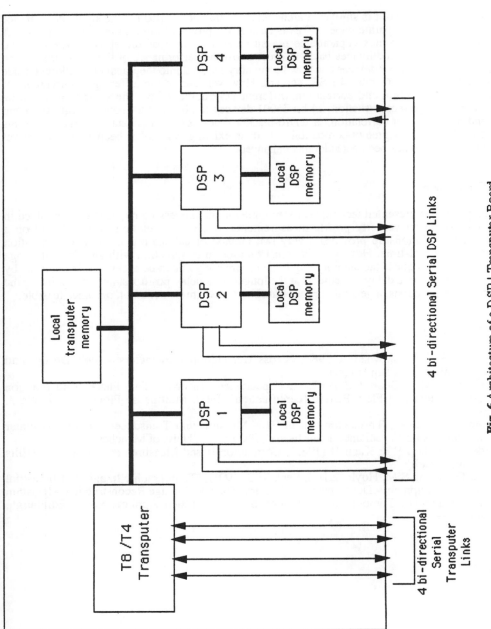

Fig. 6 Architecture of a DSP / Transputer Board

The system to be built is similar in architecture to that developed for the single capacitance imaging system (separate paper). This is basically a process farm arranged as a pipeline. A master transputer sends capacitance measurements to each of the slave processors and receives reconstructed images back. In order boost the performance of the slave processors, up to 6 Motorola DSP devices can now be memory mapped into the transputers address space as shown in figure 6 (only 4 DSPs shown). However, due to the differing requirements of image reconstruction and correlation, different DSP devices from the same family can be used. For image reconstruction, 24-bit 56001 devices can be used to reduce quantisation and rounding errors; for correlation, faster 16-bit 56116 devices are more suitable. By taking this approach, a large degree of compatibility with an existing system has been achieved and yet the performance has been considerably enhanced.

6. Conclusion

This paper has presented techniques for minimising the processing requirements involved in cross-correlation velocity profile measurements. A cross-correlation system based on a recurrence relationship provides a very fast method of calculating successive correlation functions in real-time. However, this must be used in conjunction with an efficient image buffering technique if the memory requirements are not going to be excessive. In addition, by increasing the time delay increments at the longer time-delay positions, and interpolating the correlation functions, a general purpose transputer /DSP implementation becomes feasible.

REFERENCES

Beck M S & Plaskowski A 1987, "Cross Correlation Flowmeters - their Design and Application", (Adam Hilger)

Geraets J J M & Borst J C 1987, "A Capacitance Sensor for Two-Phase Void Fraction measurement and Flow Pattern Identification", Int J. Multiphase Flow, Vol 14, No 3, pp305-320

Hammer E A 1983, 'Three Component Flow Measurement Transducers in Oil/Gas/Water Mixtures using Capacitance Transducers", Ph.D thesis, Univ. of Manchester.

Jordan J, Bishop P & Kiani B (1989),"Correlation-Based Measurement Systems", (Ellis Horwood Ltd)

Xie C G, Huang S M, Hoyle & B S, Beck M S (1991), "Tomographic Imaging of Industrial Process Equipment - Development of System Model and Image Reconstruction Algorithm for Capacitance Tomography", Int Conf. Sensors and their Applications V, Edinburgh, Sept. 1991

Acoustic Measurement of Temperature and Velocity Fields in Furnaces

A Schwarz

Institut für Meß- und Regelungstechnik, Universität (TH) Karlsruhe, Germany

ABSTRACT: In a furnace the temperature and velocity distribution of the combustion gas can be calculated by measuring the propagation time of sound waves through the measurement zone. Making some assumptions, the required distributions are reconstructed by a tomographic ART-algorithm (Algebraic Reconstruction Technique). Some simulations are presented and the effect of ray-bending is discussed.

1. INTRODUCTION

In operating industrial furnaces, temperature is an important thermodynamic parameter defining the state of the system. The temperature distribution is of interest for safety, control, efficiency and avoiding high air pollution. Usually measuring temperature in hot dust loaden gases found in furnaces is difficult and realized by suction pyrometry. This method works very slowly and allows only point measurements. A new acoustic technique (Green 1985) yields rapidly a set of measurement data, which can be used to reconstruct the temperature distribution in a plane. With the same data set it is possible to obtain the distribution of the combustion gas velocity in the same plane, which may also be of great interest for control and efficiency.

2. PRINCIPLE OF METHOD

The principle idea is an acoustic time-of-flight measurement in a moving medium, described by the local speed of sound c and the local velocity $\vec{v}$ of the medium (Braun 1991). The total speed c_{eff} of an acoustic wave traveling through this medium is a superposition of these two velocities:

$$c_{eff} \cdot \vec{t} = c \cdot \vec{t}' + \vec{v} \qquad (1)$$

$\vec{t}$ = tangent vector to the ray.
$\vec{t}'$ = tangent vector seen from the moving medium.

Assuming $|\vec{v}| << c$, the propagation time of a sound wave from a transducer A to a receiver B is approximately:

$$t_{AB} = \int_{A}^{B} \frac{1}{c} \left[1 - \frac{\vec{v}\,\vec{t}}{c} \right] ds. \qquad (2a)$$

If the sound wave travels in the opposite direction, the time is given by:

$$t_{BA} = \int_A^B \frac{1}{c} \left[1 + \frac{\vec{v}\,\vec{t}}{c} \right] ds. \tag{2b}$$

Assuming that the variation of c is much smaller than the absolute value of c, the path of a sound wave can be approximated by a straight line between transducer and receiver. Taking the sum and the difference of (2a) and (2b), one obtains:

$$t_{sum} = t_{AB} + t_{BA} = 2 \int_A^B \frac{1}{c} ds \tag{3a}$$

$$t_{dif} = t_{BA} - t_{AB} = 2 \int_A^B \frac{\vec{v}\,\vec{t}}{c^2} ds, \tag{3b}$$

which means that sound speed c and medium velocity $\vec{v}$ may be obtained from propagation times. If a set of propagation times is measured by a set of transceivers mounted in a plane, it should be possible to reconstruct the spatial distribution of c and $\vec{v}$ by a tomographic algorithm.

In hot gases the speed of sound c is related to the gas temperature T by the equation:

$$c = \sqrt{\frac{\gamma R}{M} T} \tag{4}$$

with R = universal gas constant, M = molecular weight
and γ = ratio of specific heats.

Thus the temperature distribution T in the furnace plane can be calculated by the known speed of sound.

3. THE RECONSTRUCTION TECHNIQUE ART

ART is a well-known technique to solve tomographic problems. If the problem is of scalar type, and noise is neglected, the equation to be solved is

$$\vec{p} = W \cdot \vec{x}. \tag{5}$$

$\vec{p}$ is the vector of projection data of dimension M, i.e. the number of projection rays through the measurement zone, $\vec{x}$ is the unknown image vector of dimension N, i.e. the number of pixels in the measurement zone, and W is the projection matrix of dimension MxN, containing the path length of each ray through each image pixel.   Provided W is nonsingular, the general solution of (5) is given by

$$\vec{x}^* = W^{-1} \cdot \vec{p}. \tag{6}$$

Supposed W to be quadratic (M=N), the matrix W^{-1} is given by direct matrix inversion.

In the other case, if the matrix W is not quadratic, least squares solutions for (5) exist and are defined as those vectors that minimize $(|\vec{p} - W\cdot\vec{x}|)^2$. In the overdetermined case (M>N) the solution is given by

$$\vec{x}^* = \left[W^T\cdot W\right]^{-1} \cdot W^T\cdot\vec{p} \qquad (7a)$$

and if equation (5) is underdetermined (N<M), the result is

$$\vec{x}^* = W^T\cdot\left[W\cdot W^T\right]^{-1}\cdot\vec{p} \qquad (7b)$$

where the superscript T indicates transposition.

Since $\vec{x}^*$ is directly calculated by a matrix vector multiplication, the deviation $\delta\vec{x}^*$ of the image vector $\vec{x}^*$ can be obtained by the error law if a deviation $\delta\vec{p}^*$ of the projection vector $\vec{p}^*$ is given:

$$\delta x_i^* = \sqrt{\sum_{j=1}^{N}\left[W_{ij}^{-1}\cdot\delta p_j^*\right]}. \qquad (8)$$

If the dimensions N, M are very large, equation (6) is realized by the following iterative method (Karczmarz 1937):

$$\vec{x}(k+1) = \vec{x}(k) + \lambda\cdot\frac{p_j - \hat{p}_j}{\alpha_j}\cdot\vec{W}_j \qquad (9)$$

with k = number of iteration

$$\alpha_j = \sum_{i=1}^{N} W_{ji}^2$$

$$\hat{p}_j = \sum_{i=1}^{N} W_{ji}\cdot x_i(k) \quad : \text{ projection through the reconstructed image}$$

$0 < \lambda < 2$: relaxation parameter
$\vec{W}_j$: line in projection matrix W.

If the problem is of vector type, the equation to be solved is

$$p_j = \sum_{i=1}^{N} (W_{ji}\cdot\vec{t}_j\cdot\vec{v}_i) . \qquad (10)$$

Now a modified ART-algorithm (Hauck 1990) can be applied to get the vector field $\vec{v} = (v_x, v_y)$:

$$\vec{v}(k+1) = \vec{v}(k) + \lambda\cdot\frac{p_j - \hat{p}_j}{\alpha_j}\cdot\vec{t}_j\cdot\vec{W}_j \qquad (11)$$

with $\hat{p}_j = \sum_{i=1}^{N} (W_{ji}\cdot\vec{t}_j\cdot\vec{v}_i(k)).$

It should be mentioned that the projection data only contain information about the component of the vector field $\vec{v}$ in the direction of the tangent vector $\vec{t}$ to the ray. Therefore, only the vortex distribution of the field $\vec{v}$ can be reconstructed whereas the source distribution will be suppressed.

4. SIMULATING A FURNACE

With the equations pointed out above it is possible to calculate projection data through a furnace plane if an initial temperature and gas velocity distribution and a fixed number of transducer positions is given. Then reconstruction algorithms can be tested by reconstructing these initial distributions.

The temperature perpendicular to the plane is supposed to be constant and the component of the gas velocity in this direction is neglected. It is also supposed that the distributions are averaged over the measurement time and that weak fluctuations cause a deviation error $\delta\vec{p}$ in the projection data leading to a reconstruction error $\delta\vec{x}$. The simulated plane is of quadratic shape (length L = 20.8 m) and describes the horizontal cross-section of a tangentially fired furnace in a coal fired power station (Derichs 1990).

A typical expected temperature distribution is dome shaped with a maximum in the center. The gas velocity is expected to be described by a main vortex centered in the center of the furnace accompanied by 4 smaller corner whirls (Benesch 1984). The simulated temperature distribution is of the form

$$T(x,y) = 1173 \text{ K} + 400 \text{ K} \cdot \sin(\pi \cdot x/L) \cdot \sin(\pi \cdot y/L) \tag{12}$$

and the velocity field is described by Oseen-vortecies with a tangential speed

$$v_t(r) = \frac{\Gamma_\infty}{2 \cdot \pi \cdot r} \cdot \left[1 - e^{-\left(\frac{r}{C}\right)^2} \right]. \tag{13}$$

At the furnace boundary 16 transceiver positions are given. The furnace plane was divided up into a rectangular grid of 8 x 8 pixels for reconstruction. After a set of 76 projection data was calculated (Fig. 1), the reconstruction was carried out with the iterative method and a Bezier interpolation with known boundary values was applied. Fig. 2 shows the initial and the reconstructed distributions. The reconstructed temperature agrees quite well with the initial distribution. The mean temperature was calculated to be T = 1336 K and differs from the initial mean value by 1 K. The maximum pixel error was calculated to 5 %.

The reconstructed velocity field shows the main centered whirl and the 4 corner whirls very well. While the initial maximum velocity is v = 22.5 m/s, the reconstructed maximum value is v = 18 m/s.

The structure of other simulated realistic temperature and flow fields also was in general well reproduced. The greatest deviation occured in the reconstructed vector field where the directions sometimes differ extremly from the true values.

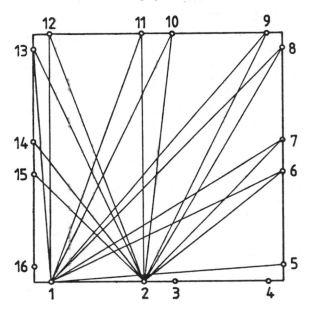

Fig. 1: Projection paths through the furnace plane
from transducer numbers one and two

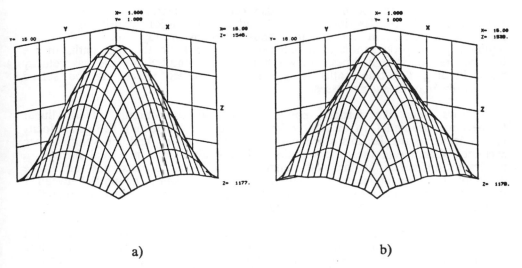

a)   b)

Fig. 2: a) Initial b) Reconstructed temperature distribution

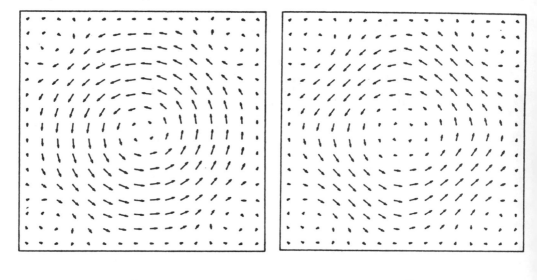

c)   d)

Fig. 2: c) Initial d) Reconstructed gas velocity field

5. THE EFFECT OF RAY BENDING

In reality there are different effects which influence the accuracy of the reconstructed fields.   As considered in (Green 1985), these are mainly the unknown exact gas composition, errors in the transit time measurement and the reconstruction algorithm.

Another effect is ray bending which also causes reconstruction errors; but this effect can easily be described and included into the ART algorithm.   Due to Fermat's principle, in an inhomogenous medium a ray follows the path minimizing the propagation time between two points. So the real paths in the furnace are not straight lines, but are bent by the temperature and gas velocity field. Finding the true paths is a variation problem which can be solved analytically only in special cases.

First, rays near the furnace boundary will be considered.   Here linear temperature gradients up to 1000 K/m can occur.   Neglecting the gas velocity $\vec{v}$, this leads to the Brachistochrone problem to be solved and the solutions are zycloides. Comparing these bent paths with a straight line in a real furnace, a maximum difference in the path length of 2 % and a maximum amplitude deviation of 2 meters is found. Superposing a flow whirl, the path between 2 transceivers splits up into 2 different paths depending on the traveling direction of the rays, but this effect can be neglected (Fig. 3).

Now rays through the center of the furnace are discussed. The bending effect is mainly caused by the flow field supposed to be a whirl with a maximum velocity of 25 m/s. Linear superposition of ray and gas velocity and a comparison to straight lines leads to a maximum difference in the path length of 0.1 % and a maximum amplitude deviation of 0.5 meters. The splitting up of the path between 2 transceivers here is the main effect whereas the path bending by temperature can be neglected. Considering more complicated temperature and gas velocity fields, in general no analytic solution describing the paths can be found and a ray tracing algorithm has to be applied.

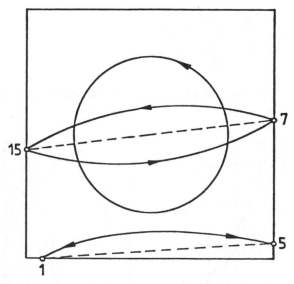

Fig. 3: Bent paths near the furnace wall and through the center

Taking into account that the furnace plane is described by a rectangular pixel grid, it is suitable to implement an algorithm using this fact. A very simple but effective algorithm is to define a ray to be straight in a pixel i and to change its direction at the boundary to the next pixel $i+1$ by a diffraction law:

$$c_{i+1} \cdot \sin(\alpha_i) = c_i \cdot \sin(\alpha_{i+1}).$$

The flow velocity $\vec{v}$ can be superposed in each pixel by simple addition. The accuracy of this algorithm depends on the resolution of the pixel grid and should be exact if the resolution tends to infinity.

To improve the simulation of a furnace, path bending by the temperature distribution was taken into account and implemented by an iterative algorithm in the following way. A more realistic set of projection data $\vec{p}$ and a better projection matrix W_I was obtained by tracing each ray through an initial temperature distribution T_I. Testing the self-consistency by reconstructing the temperature field led to T_S.

In the iterative loop a first reconstruction with the straight line projection matrix W_0 was carried out, yielding a distribution T_0. Then the ray tracing algorithm was applied on this field to obtain more realistic ray paths and an improved projection matrix W_1. After that a new temperature distribution T_1 was reconstructed. The initial temperature field was of the same form as (12), but the boundary temperature was lowered to $T = 923$ K and the amplitude was increased to $T = 750$ K to make plain the effect of path bending. An iterative ART algorithm was applied on a 8 x 8 grid while the rays were traced in a 32 x 32 temperature grid after a bezier interpolation. The results are depicted in Fig. 4 and show an improvement after this first iteration step. A good examination is possible by numerical comparison of the distributions T_S, T_0 and T_1 and the projection matrices W_I, W_0 and W_1. Here $D_T(T_1, T_2)$ is defined as

$$D_T(T_1,T_2) = \frac{\sqrt{\sum_{i=1}^{N} (T_{1i} - T_{2i})^2}}{N}$$

and SU(W) is the sum over all path lengths described by the matrix W.

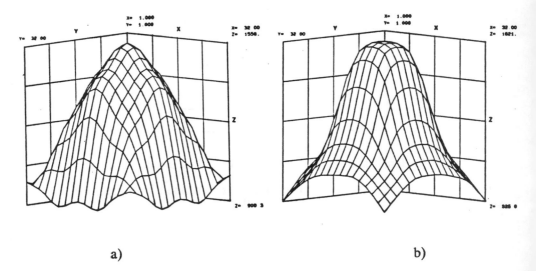

a)   b)

Fig. 4: Reconstructed temperature distribution with bent paths
    a) T_0, reconstruced with the help of projection matrix W_0
    b) T_1 after 1. iteration step, reconstructed with the help of
       projection matrix W_1

$D_T(T_S, T_0)$	:	13.8 K
$D_T(T_S, T_1)$	:	3.7 K
$SU(W_I)$	:	1598 meters
$SU(W_0)$	:	1584 meters
$SU(W_1)$	:	1594 meters

Beside that, T_0 is lowered near the furnace boundary as expected, because of the shorter path lengths in the straight line projection matrix W_0. Since the improvement is small, a second iteration step was omitted.

6. CONCLUSION

In this paper, the reconstruction of temperature and gas velocity distributions in a furnace plane by an ART-algorithm was introduced and shown to be applicable. Taking into account the effect of path bending, the results are improved.

ACKNOWLEDGEMENT

This work is financially supported by the Sonderforschungsbereich 167 of the Deutsche Forschungsgemeinschaft, 5300 Bonn 2.

REFERENCES

W Benesch (1984), *Mathematische Modellierung der Strömungs- und Mischungs-vorgänge in der Tangentialfeuerung*, Dissertation, Universität Bochum.
H Braun, A Hauck (1991), *Tomographic Reconstruction of Vector Fields, IEEE Trans. on Signal Processing*, Vol. 39, No. 2.
W Derichs (1990), *Die Schallpyrometrie - ein Meßverfahren zur Bestimmung der Temperaturverteilung in Kesselfeuerungen*, DDV-Kolloquium Aachen.
S F Green (1985), *An acoustic technique for rapid temperature distribution measurement, J. Acoust. Soc. Am.* 77 (2).
A Hauck (1990), *Tomographie von Vektorfeldern*, VDI Verlag, Reihe 8, Nr. 220.
S Karczmarz (1937), *Angenäherte Auflösung von Systemen linearer Gleichungen, Bul. Acad. Polon. Sci. Lett. A.*

Chapter 5

Preliminary Reports on Developing Concepts
for Teaching and Research Using
Tomographic Instrumentation

PERFORMANCE OF THE "SHEFFIELD" ELECTRICAL IMPEDANCE TOMOGRAPHY SYSTEM WITH RESPECT TO IMAGING BRAIN FUNCTION IN THE ADULT HEAD

D.S. Holder, Department of Physiology, University College, London WC1E 6BT, U.K.

ABSTRACT.

The suitability of the "Sheffield" Electrical Impedance Tomography (EIT) system for imaging in the adult head was assessed. In tanks filled with saline or agar, polythene rods could be localized accurately and small impedance changes could be recorded. With scalp electrodes in the rat *post-mortem*, no useful discrimination of brain contents was possible. This suggests that the system used should be suitable for imaging brain impedance changes with intracranial electrodes; improvements are needed if the more practicable goal of imaging with scalp electrodes is to be achieved.

1. INTRODUCTION.

Electrical Impedance Tomography (EIT, also termed Applied Potential Tomography, APT) is a recently developed imaging technique which enables images of the impedance distribution within a subject to be obtained from measurement with a ring of external electrodes. One potentially fruitful application of this technique lies in imaging the impedance increases of tens of per cent which occur in the brain in conditions such as cerebral ischaemia, epilepsy or spreading depression (see Holder, 1992a, Holder, 1992b, Van Harreveld and Schadé, 1962). The most desirable application would be to perform this with scalp electrodes placed in a horizontal ring around the head. It may also be possible with a similar configuration of intra-cranial electrodes. These could be placed in individual burr-holes, in which case they would sit outside the dura mater (a fibrous layer which lines the inner surface of the skull). Alternatively, the electrodes could be combined into flexible plastic strips which were then slid horizontally between the brain and skull through two or more parietal burr-holes. This would be invasive, but could be justified in exceptional circumstances; for instance, similar subdural electrodes are used at present for ambulatory recording of the EEG in patients with severe epilepsy who are being assessed for curative neurosurgery (*e.g.* Ojemann and Engel, 1987).

There is currently considerable interest in the technical development of EIT (see (Webster, 1990) for a recent review) but, to the author's knowledge, only one system, "The Sheffield EIT system", is commercially available for clinical use. Being a prototype, it has various limitations : Images can only be obtained with respect to a specified reference image; the reconstruction algorithm assumes that the electrodes are equally spaced in a circle, and that the initial resistivity of the subject is uniform. The reconstruction algorithm is relatively crude, and uses a single iteration. Its advantages are that a complete data set sufficient to produce an image can be collected in 79 ms, and image reconstruction takes about 5s. Unlike more sophisticated algorithms, the method is relatively insensitive to deviations in electrode spacing. The device is physically small - about the size of a video recorder, attached to a microcomputer - and operates at 51 kHz with an applied current of 5mA. It is therefore non-invasive and would be suitable for continuous imaging at the bedside. (See Brown and Seagar, 1987, Barber and Seagar, 1987).

Preliminary images of ECG gated changes in the adult head measured with the Sheffield EIT system (McArdle et al., 1989), and of intraventricular haemorrhage in the neonate with a different imaging system (Murphy et al., 1987) have been published. They were obtained with scalp electrodes; examples of images are shown, but their correspondence to intracranial impedance was not investigated. In a companion study to the present work, EIT images were collected during cerebral ischaemia in the anaesthetized rat. Reproducible impedance increases were observed with measurement with both cortical or scalp electrodes, but the spatial resolution within the brain was very poor when scalp electrodes were used (Holder, 1992c).

This study was therefore undertaken to assess the performance of the Sheffield EIT system for use in imaging functional activity in the human head. Initial measurements were made in saline filled tanks. This approximates to the situation in which intracranial electrodes are used to measure directly from the brain. The effects of extra-cerebral tissues - the meninges, cerebrospinal fluid, skull and scalp - were investigated by recording with scalp electrodes in the adult rat. Measurements were made either in anaesthetized animals, or *post-mortem*.

2. METHODS.

Different recording arrangements were :

1) Large cylindrical tank. Sixteen brass bolts were placed halfway up and equally spaced around a plastic cylinder, 15.3 cm in diameter and 24 cm high. They were 3 mm in diameter and projected 15 mm into the tank. All other electrodes (described below) were made of silver; exposed surfaces were chlorided.

2) Cortical electrode array and tank. A cortical electrode array, intended for measurement around the exposed brain of the rat, was constructed of blocks of silver set at regular intervals into a ring of dental acrylic about 4 mm wide. The silver blocks were connected to a flexible lead with a driven screen 12 cm in length by a solder join which was sealed into the acrylic. The acrylic ring was made to correspond to the contours of the rat brain in the plane from the frontal to occipital lobes. Its internal dimensions were 21mm in the sagittal and 13 mm in the coronal directions (termed "Y" and "X" axes respectively below). Each electrode surface was an area 3mm high and 1mm wide on the inside of the array. For tank studies, it was set in a roughly cylindrical tank, constructed so that its internal cross-section was the same as the inner dimensions of the electrode array. The walls were constructed of a rolled up flexible acrylic sheet, which was bonded to the electrode array and a perspex base with silicone rubber glue. The electrode array was placed halfway up the tank, which was 5 cm high.

3) Scalp electrodes and tank. Scalp electrodes were made of Ag wire, 0.5 mm in diameter. One end was soldered to a 12 cm length of multistranded copper wire, 1mm o.d. The solder join was insulated with silicone rubber glue, and 4 mm of wire was left exposed. For tank measurements, 16 scalp electrodes were inserted at equal intervals through holes in an acrylic plate so as to form an ellipse 21 x 16 mm along its axes. A rolled flexible acrylic sheet was glued with silicone rubber glue to the upper surface of the acrylic plate so as to form an ellipsoidal tank. This was filled with saline to a height of 3.5 cm.

The above tank measurements were made with an Ag/AgCl common mode feedback electrode which was placed at the top or bottom of the tank. The tanks were filled with saline, which consisted of 0.118 g/l (20 mMol/l) NaCl, unless otherwise stated; this had a resistivity similar to that of brain. Measurements were made at room temperature. (Temperature of saline in the tanks was not specifically controlled, but room temperature altered by less than one degree during the 30 min or less required to make any one series of measurements. This temperature difference would not have contributed significantly to baseline variability, as the impedance of saline varies by approximately -1.3% per °C (Li et al, 1968).

4) Measurements in the rat. Measurements were made either with the cortical electrode array, which was placed on exposed brain in the fronto-occipital plane, or with scalp electrodes inserted at regular intervals in the fronto-occipital plane in a direction radial to the vertex. The dimensions of the approximate ellipse formed by the mid-points of the scalp electrodes wires was about 25 and 18 mm in the sagittal and coronal directions respectively. Electrodes were connected to the front panel of the EIT device by screened leads which were 4 mm in outer diameter and 30 cm long. One EIT image was recorded each minute, and consisted of 200 complete data sets averaged to reduce noise. The temperature was monitored using a thermocouple placed in the scalp in the right parietal region. See (Holder, 1992c) for further details.

The reference phase of the phase sensitive detector in the EIT system was set at the value which gave the least variability in the EIT image when saline in tanks containing the cortical or scalp array was varied from 0.118 - 0.354% g/l of NaCl. The Sheffield EIT system is based on a four electrode method for measuring impedance, and so measures the in-phase component of the complex impedance. Below, the term "impedance" refers to this resistive component of the complex impedance.

The EIT images have been displayed as three dimensional surfaces. The X and Y axes correspond to the axes in the plane of the electrodes; the Z axis represents the change in impedance with respect to a specified reference frame. The orientation of the display is identified by a diagram of a corresponding slice through the rat's head. Only the central 812 pixels out of a 32x32 pixel matrix represent the image; surrounding pixels were set to zero.

Each pixel in *in vivo* images was corrected separately for baseline shift. The baseline was taken to be the extrapolation of the linear regression of the period of 10 min prior to carotid artery occlusion. Estimates of the blurring of objects imaged by EIT have been made by approximating Gaussian curves to impedance profiles in one or two dimensions. The standard deviation in the XY plane was calculated on this basis. A peak in the image was defined as a point where up to three pixels of equal value were greater than all of the pixels in a surrounding grid of 5 x 5 pixels, and where this was separated from any peak with a greater magnitude by a trough whose value fell to 1/e times the average of the two peaks. An estimate of the standard deviation for individual peaks was taken to be the radius of a circular area approximating to this area. The Full Width at Half Maximum (FWHM) was calculated as 1.665 times the standard deviation in the XY plane. Results are presented as mean $\pm$ S.E.

3. RESULTS.

3.1. Relationship between EIT image and variation of the resistivity of the saline in tanks.

EIT images were acquired as cortical and scalp electrode tanks were filled with saline solutions of varying concentrations. The resistivity of the saline was measured with a single channel impedance measuring device (see Holder, 1992a) using four Ag/AgCl wire electrodes set 3 mm apart in a block of araldite. Linear regression data were : $r = 0.98, 0.98$ ($p < 0.05$) and slope $= 0.94$ and 0.98 for the cortical and scalp arrays respectively. Standard errors of pixels within each image were less than 0.3%.

3.2. Baseline drift.

Baseline impedance drift was measured over a period of 10 min during resting conditions (Table 1). The standard deviation of measurements *in vivo* were about ten times greater than those made in tanks. The correlation coefficients for impedance change against time for both linear and logarithmic regression were 0.76 ± 0.19 ($n=5$ in 2 rats, $p < 0.05$ in 4 out of 5 records) and 0.83 ± 0.06 ($n=9$ in 4 rats, $p < 0.05$ in all records), for cortical and scalp records respectively.

Experimental arrangement	Electrodes	Difference in impedance measured at 0 and 10 min over whole image (%)		n
		Mean	S.D.	
Large cylindrical tank + saline	Brass bolts	-0.12±0.10	0.35±0.03	3
Tank + saline	Cortical array	0.03±0.02	0.29±0.07	3
Tank + saline	Scalp model	0.30±0.24	0.22±0.06	3
In vivo	Cortical array	-0.41±0.24	2.78±0.39	5 (2 rats)
In vivo	Scalp electrodes	-0.42±0.45	2.17±0.43	9 (4 rats)

Table 1. Changes in impedance under resting conditions in different experimental situations.

3.3. Localization of polythene rods.

The correspondence of the peak impedance change and physical position of a polythene rod suspended vertically in either the large cylindrical or cortical array tanks is shown in Figure 1.

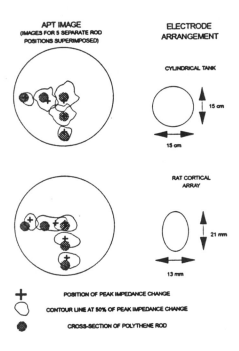

Figure 1. Localization of a polythene rod in the large cylindrical or cortical electrode array tanks. A polythene rod was suspended vertically in various positions in saline in either tank. The diameters of the polythene rods were 15 mm and 1.5 mm for the large cylindrical and cortical array tanks respectively. Each rod extended vertically more than twice the tank diameter in both directions. The peaks and boundaries of the FWHM of the image impedance change and the positions of the rods have been superimposed for several rod positions. The positions of the rod relative to the elliptical cortical electrode array are represented as a proportion of axis lengths so as to be comparable in the circular EIT image.

The difference (expressed in % of the axis dimensions of the tank) between the position of the peak impedance change in the image and the centre of the rod was $3.9 \pm 0.17\%$ (n=9, as the rod was moved in increments of 10% from X, Y coordinates of 50%, 10% to 50%, 50% to 10%, 50%) in the large cylindrical tank, and $7.4 \pm 0.35\%$ (n=9, increments of 20% from 50%, 90% to 50%, 10%, and 90%, 50% to 10%, 50%) in the cortical array tank. The ratio of the FWHM along the Y compared to the X axis was 0.99 ± 0.03 and 1.3 ± 0.03 for the large cylindrical and cortical array tanks respectively.

Under the same conditions, extrapolation from a series of images suggested that a rod placed centrally could be discriminated from a second rod when their centres were 32% or 26% apart for the large and cortical array tanks respectively (Fig. 2). The respective gaps between the rods at these points would be 22% and 18%.

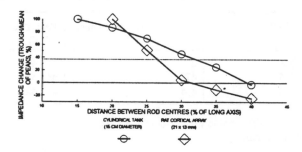

Figure 2. Discrimination of two polythene rods by EIT. One polythene rod was suspended in the centre of either the cylindrical tank or cortical array tank. Recording conditions were as in Figure 1. Images were collected as a second identical rod was approximated to the first, along the long axis in the case of the cortical array. The lowest impedance change measured along a line between two peaks corresponding to each rod, expressed as a percentage of the mean of the two peaks, has been plotted against the distance separating the centres of the two rods. The trough value falls to 1/e of the mean peak value when the rods are separated by 32% and 26% of the tank diameter in the large cylindrical and cortical array tanks respectively.

3.4. Discrimination by EIT of the cranial contents and scalp with measurement with scalp electrodes.

Post-mortem, a change in the contents of the cranial cavity from saline to air produced an approximately gaussian central increase in impedance (Figure 3). The FWHM of the increase was 27.5% of the image diameter. In reality, the cranial cavity occupied about 80% of the length of the scalp electrode array along both the X and Y axes.

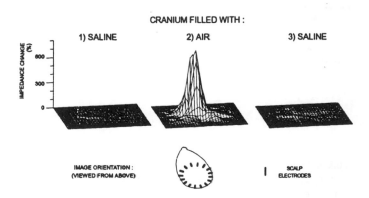

Figure 3. Sensitivity of EIT measured with scalp electrodes to replacement of cranial contents by air. Measurements were made with scalp electrodes about one hour *post-mortem*. A reference image was made with the cranial cavity filled with saline. The images shown were made 3, 12 and 13 min later, when the cranial cavity was filled successively with saline, air and saline. Quantitative measurements were :

Cranial contents	FWHM (%)	Mean impedance change under peak (%)*	Peak position (X,Y), (%)#
Saline	62.6	2.6	52, 41
Air	27.5	472.2	46, 55
Saline	52.0	4.4	43, 42

* - average of pixels with a value greater than 1/e x peak value.
\# - origin is left, occipital.

Impedance decreased reversibly by about 5% around the circumference of the EIT image when the scalp *in vivo* was selectively warmed by placing an electric light above the scalp (Fig. 4). This decrease reversed to an extent on return of the scalp temperature to its resting value.

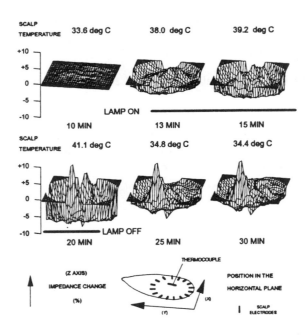

Figure 4. EIT images taken during changes in scalp temperature in the anaesthetized rat *in vivo*. Images were collected using scalp electrodes over a period of 30 min. A 60 W light bulb was placed about 10 cm above the rat's head from 10 to 20 min. The time and scalp temperature measured by a subcutaneous thermocouple are shown by each image. Images were corrected for baseline shift over the first 10 min.

An increase in impedance in the EIT image measured with scalp electrodes *post-mortem* occurred when a single polythene rod was inserted into the brain 12% of the array diameter lateral to the midline. When a second rod was added in the same position but on the opposing side of the midline, the impedance increased further, but it is not possible to distinguish two peaks separated by a trough of 1/e of their average value (Fig. 5).

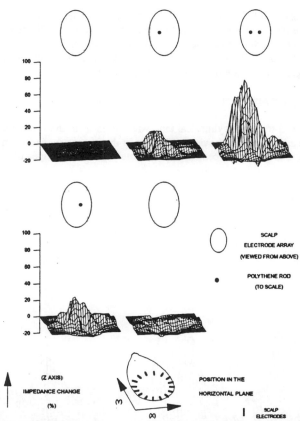

Figure 5. Imaging of intracranial polythene rods by EIT with scalp electrodes. Images were taken about 45 min *post-mortem*. The rat was supine, and the ventral surface of the brain was exposed. Polythene rods, 2.4 mm in diameter, were inserted vertically into the brain with their centres 3mm to either side of the midline in the positions shown above each image. When the left rod was removed (lower left image), the hole was filled with 0.9% saline.

3.5. Sensitivity to localized small changes in impedance.

There was a significant linear correlation between both the impedance changes and resistivity of saline solutions placed in a small central hole when the cortical tank was filled with agar. Changes of a few per cent in resistivity were detected (Fig. 6).

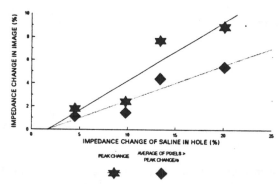

Figure 6. Detection of small localised impedance changes by EIT. The rat cortical tank was filled

with agar made from 3% agar and 0.118% saline. A vertical central hole, 2.25 mm in diameter, was made in the agar. The measurements presented were obtained from the differences between paired images obtained with 0.118% saline and test solutions in the central hole. Linear regression data (shown as lines) are : r = 0.84, 0.86, slope = 0.51, 0.30 for the peak impedance change and average change of pixels greater than the peak value /e respectively.

3.6. Effects of impedance changes out of the plane of the electrodes.

The height of saline in the large cylindrical tank was varied from the reference height of 12 cm above the electrode array to 2 cm above it. Changes in the images ranged from a toroidal increase with the largest change, and a central approximately gaussian shape for the smaller changes (Fig. 7).

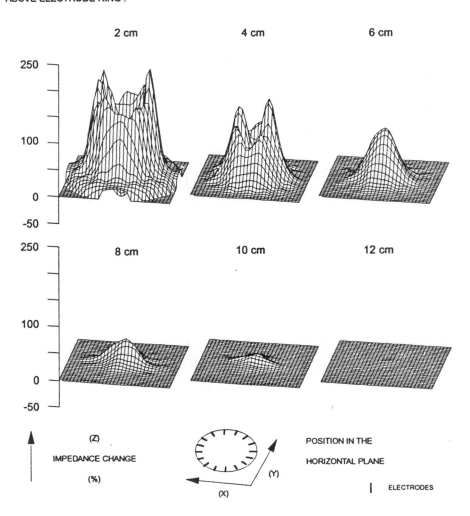

Figure 7. Effects of impedance changes out of the plane of the electrode ring on the EIT image.

Images were collected with saline at levels from 2 to 12 cm above the electrode ring in the large cylindrical tank. Images represent the change in impedance with respect to the image obtained with the saline level 12 cm above the electrode ring.

4. DISCUSSION.

From an understanding of the data collection procedure and algorithm employed by the Sheffield EIT system, it is possible to anticipate limitations in its imaging abilities :

1) Baseline shift and variability. The cause of the variation in tanks was not specifically investigated. Contributing factors include variation in temperatures of the saline, local impedance conditions at the electrodes, and drift and noise in electronic components. Only one phase signal was supplied to the phase sensitive demodulator. Data collection may therefore have been prone to errors due to variations in stray capacitance between individual channels. The magnitude of any capacitative current passing through the tissue from the recording leads would then have been influenced by electrode impedance. The following steps were taken to reduce any such effects to a minimum : i) All leads were bundled together and were not moved throughout the course of an experiment. ii) Some test EIT images were made in tanks filled with saline whose resistivities covered the ranges expected in experiments. The phase was then set to the value which gave the least variation in image pixels. Inter-pixel variation could be reduced to a standard error of less than 0.3 % in this way for resistivities corresponding to 50 - 300 % relative to brain resistivity. iii) Electrodes were chlorided before each experiment and left to stand, connected together, for 12 hours or so. This decreases variations in impedance between electrodes, as well as allowing a stable chemical equilibrium to develop (Ferris, 1974). In this way, variation in images made in tanks could be reduced to insignificant proportions.

In contrast, there was substantial variation in images *in vivo*, which affected the interpretation of results. This was presumably due to variations in tissue impedance around the electrodes. In addition, the silver chloride was friable, and it was possible that it was disturbed as the electrodes were applied, particularly in the case of the needle electrodes used in the scalp. This drift was corrected empirically. It was found that the variation in any individual pixel of the reconstructed image was linear with respect to time, so each pixel in images *in vivo or post-mortem* could be corrected for the gradient of the linear regression of its values over a resting period.

2) Spatial resolution in the electrode plane in conditions of initially uniform resistivity. Spatial resolution is likely to be best in these circumstances. The limiting factors are then the crude nature of the algorithm, and the physical limitation that current density is least in the centre of the image. Unfortunately, it is difficult to produce a test object which has a resistivity different from the initial conditions by the same amount likely to be encountered in a physiological situation. Agar containing saline of different resistivities may be used, but the test and background solutions tend to mix. Therefore the test object was a plastic rod, which has a very high resistance. The reconstruction algorithm assumes that there is a linear relation between the impedance disturbance and the potential difference change measured on the boundary (Barber and Seagar, 1987); this is only true for relatively small disturbances. The spatial resolution in practice in a biological subject with similar conditions is therefore likely to be better than that observed with a plastic object.

The immediately evident effect of a sub-optimal reconstruction algorithm is that a point impedance increase appears as a distributed disturbance in the EIT image; the degree of spread dictates the ability of the system to resolve two adjacent objects. The FWHM for a polythene rod 10 % of the array diameter in the cylindrical tank varied from about 15 % at the edge to about 25 % in the centre (Fig. 1). These figures are similar to those found by Eyuboglu et al (1989) for similar conditions with a polythene ball. This indicates that, as expected, spatial resolution is least in the centre of the image, because current density is least there. This would affect the ability of the system to discriminate two objects in the centre; the centres of two similar rods had to be more than 32 % apart to be discriminated at the centre of the tank (Fig. 2). However, the localization of the centre of a *single* object is unaffected by the degree of lateral spread of the impedance signal in the image. Spatial resolution is then determined by the pixel size, which is about 10 % of the image diameter for 16 electrodes. A polythene rod in the cylindrical tank could be well localized to about 5% of its true position on average.

The data collection hardware is sensitive to small changes in impedance. Changes of 0.1% could be measured with a cardiac gated system and averaging (McArdle et al, 1989). Small central impedance increases of 5-20% could be detected clearly. The image impedance increase bore a significant linear relation to the actual impedance increase, but the correspondence was not 1 : 1 (Fig. 6). Although the test hole was about 10% of the diameter of the test tank, it might have straddled more than one pixel. Representation of the actual impedance change as a lesser amount in the image may have been due to a partial volume effect or because sensitivity was less in the centre of the image.

Errors in representation may occur as a result of the reconstruction algorithm and filtering methods. When two or more resistive test objects were employed, as in Fig. 2, it was possible to obtain a "shadow" in the image which represented an opposite impedance change. This might be the explanation of the central impedance increase seen in Fig. 4 in the rat *in vivo* after scalp warming.

3) Distortion of the image by a non-circular electrode array. The software available for the Sheffield system assumed that the electrode array was circular. This was not possible for the planned experiments, and two test tanks were constructed, which had the approximate elliptical proportions of the cortical or scalp electrode arrays used *in vivo*. The image was distorted, but this appeared to be in a straightforward fashion. For instance, the actual relative dimensions of the cortical electrode array were 1.6:1; the ratio of the axes of the FWHM of the circular polythene rods was 1.3:1.

4) Degradation of spatial resolution by non-uniform initial resistivity. The simplest case was examined by making a reference image in a rat *post-mortem*, whose cranial contents had been replaced by physiological saline. The test image was made when the saline was replaced by air. The cranial cavity in the image was represented by a disturbance whose FWHM was 28% of the image diameter; the real dimensions of the cranial cavity compared to the electrode positions was about 80%. This supports the findings of McArdle et al (1989) that the skull is represented as a wide ring; representation of the cranial contents is compressed into a small central area. This is mainly because the algorithm assumes that the subject has uniform initial resistivity. The skull then appears far too wide, as it is represented as a layer isoresistive with brain, and of dimensions needed to produce the same resistance as the skull. Unfortunately, application of current from only two electrodes at a time is likely to worsen this effect. Even in a medium of constant resistivity, current density will be least in the centre of the subject. Shunting through the scalp and obstruction of current flow by the skull is likely to make this much worse, so it might be expected that spatial resolution of objects in the cranial cavity was degraded. It would be necessary to drive currents from multiple electrodes in order to optimize current density in the centre of an image. Progress towards this has been made by several groups (*e.g.* Fuks et al, 1991), but validation in biological subjects is still awaited.

The presence of a single polythene rod in the cranial cavity of a rat *post-mortem* could be detected on an EIT image. It was not possible to distinguish it from a second rod, placed about 25% of the electrode array diameter away in a coronal direction. This is not surprising, as two rods could only be distinguished in a tank of saline when their centres were about 30% apart. In the rat *post-mortem*, it was unfortunately not possible to produce a greater separation because rod placement was limited by the lateral limits of the skull. However, inspection of the transverse decay of the impedance disturbance in Fig. 5 suggests that spatial resolution would not have been better than about 50% of the electrode array diameter.

For comparison, an experiment was designed in which it was intended that the resistance of the scalp alone was altered. This was attempted by placing a lamp over the scalp of an anaesthetized rat. The rationale was that the scalp would warm up first, and it should have been possible to distinguish the resulting impedance change in consecutive images. A definite impedance decrease may seen in the EIT image collected 3 min after the lamp was switched on, when scalp temperature had risen by 5 °C. It forms a ring around the periphery, is about 15% of the image diameter wide, and is about -3% in amplitude. In subsequent images collected while the lamp remained it deepens, reaching an impedance decrease of about 6% when scalp temperature had increased by 7 °C. This ratio is reasonably consistent with the ratio of -1.3% per °C observed for warming of saline (Li et al, 1968). The peripheral change reversed to a large extent on scalp cooling. In the later images, a central impedance increase was observed in the EIT images. It is unclear whether this was a result of "shadowing" produced by the algorithm, or represented a cooling of the brain. Overall, it seems probable that the peripheral decrease represents scalp warming, though the precise contribution of warming of the skull or underlying brain is uncertain.

5. Contribution of off-plane impedance changes. Applied current will travel in three dimensions. Inclusion of off-plane impedance changes will therefore be a problem for all EIT systems imaging with a 2-dimensional electrode array. Because current will spread most in the centre of the image, it would be expected that sensitivity to off-plane impedance changes is greatest if they are central to the electrode ring. This is illustrated in Fig. 7. For large impedance changes, a more complex toroidal disturbance was seen. This indicates that care must be exercised in interpreting EIT images. The effect of progressively adding layers off saline to a cylindrical tank filled up to the electrode level has been reported (Rabbani and Kabir, 1991). It was observed that an extended layer of saline at a certain height from the electrode plane has a maximum effect on pixels in the image which are the same radial distance from the edge as the height of the added layer above the electrodes. Localization of an impedance disturbance can only be certain if the disturbance is known to be restricted to the image plane. It may be possible to circumvent this problem in the head by recording images at several levels; the plane in which the largest disturbance occurred could be taken to be the best guide to localization in the plane of the electrodes.

These results indicate that, at present, this EIT system would have the greatest application in localizing single, rapid impedance changes in a homogeneous medium. Even then, the spatial resolution would be about 15% of the electrode diameter, and measurement would be sensitive to off-plane events. On the other hand, it should be possible to detect small impedance changes. These conditions would best be met if EIT were used with intracranial electrodes - for instance, to localize an epileptic focus in patients being assessed for curative surgery. The images collected with scalp electrodes appear to blur the intracranial contents together and so do not seem to give more information than that obtained with single channel impedance measurement. Improvements in EIT being undertaken at present include the development of multifrequency imaging, 3-D recording, and algorithms which make no assumptions regarding initial resistivity distributions. For imaging in the head, it seems that the latter has the highest priority at present.

5. CONCLUSIONS.

The Sheffield EIT system employs a simple current drive configuration and reconstruction algorithm. It is robust with respect to inaccuracies in electrode placement, can detect small impedance changes, and permits rapid reconstruction. However, spatial resolution in the centre of the image is poor, especially if there is high initial resistance near the edge of the image (as with imaging with scalp electrodes in the head). The system should produce useful images when the assumption of the algorithm that initial resistivity is uniform is a reasonable approximation. This should be the case for imaging of brain function with cortical electrodes. Imaging of brain function with scalp electrodes will not be practicable until the system can be improved to allow for the widely differing resistivities in the extra-cerebral layers.

Acknowledgements.

Professor B.H. Brown kindly loaned the Sheffield EIT system and the single channel impedance measuring device. The author was supported by a Royal Society University Research Fellowship.

REFERENCES.

Barber D C and Seagar 1987 Fast reconstruction of impedance images Clin. Phys. Physiol. Meas. 8 Suppl. A 47-54
Brown B H and Seagar A D 1987 The Sheffield data collection system Clin. Phys. Physiol. Meas. 8 Suppl. A 91-98
Eyuboglu B M, Brown B H and Barber D C 1989 Limitations to SV determination from APT images IEEE Eng. Med. Biol. Soc. 11th Ann. Int. Conf. 442-443
Ferris C D 1974 Introduction to bioelectrodes (Plenum Publ. Corp. : New York)
Fuks LF, Cheney M, Isaacson D, Gisser DG and Newell JC 1991 Detection and imaging of electric conductivity and permittivity at low frequency IEEE Trans Biomed Eng 38, 1106-1110
Holder DS 1992a Detection of cerebral ischaemia in the anaesthetized rat by impedance measurement with scalp electrodes : implications for non-invasive imaging of stroke by electrical impedance tomography. Clin Phys Physiol Meas, 13, 63 - 76
Holder DS 1992b Detection of cortical spreading depression in the anaesthetized rat by impedance measurement with scalp electrodes : implications for non-invasive imaging of the brain with electrical impedance tomography. Clin Phys Physiol Meas, 13, 77 - 86
Holder DS 1992c Electrical impedance tomography with cortical or scalp electrodes during global cerebral ischaemia in the anaesthetized rat. Clin Phys Physiol Meas, 13, 87 - 98
Li C, Bak A and Parker LO 1968 Specific resistivity of the cerebral cortex and white matter Exp Neurol 20, 544-557
McArdle F J, Brown B H and Angel A 1989 Imaging resistivity changes of the adult brain during the cardiac cycle IEEE Eng. in Med. Biol. 11th Ann. Int. Conf. 480-481
Murphy D, Burton P, Coombs R, Tarassenko L and Rolfe P 1987 Impedance imaging in the newborn Clin. Phys. Physiol. Meas. 8 Suppl. A 131-140
Ojemann GA and Engel J 1987 Acute and chronic intracranial recording and stimulation *in* Surgical treatment of the epilepsies *ed* J Engel Jr, Raven Press : New York
Rabbani KS and Kabir AMBH 1991 Studies on the effect of the third dimension on a two dimensional electrical impedance tomography system Clin Phys Physiol Meas 12, 393-402
Van Harreveld A and Schadé J P 1962 Changes in the electrical conductivity of cerebral cortex during seizure activity Exp. Neurol. 5 383-400
Webster J G (ed) 1990 Electrical impedance tomography (Adam Hilger : Bristol, U.K.)

Application of the optical tomography for education and laboratory research.

Dr Andrzej Pląskowski, Piotr Bukalski, Tomasz Habdas,
Krzysztof Szuster

Micromath International Sp. z o.o.
Warsaw Poland

Abstract: This   paper   describes   the   original   design   and
device   of   an   optical   tomography   system   for education and
laboratory   applications.   To approach the most important idea
of tomography imaging there were used light, detectors,
measurement   turntable   and   the   reconstruction   algorithm
simply   to   understand.   Scanning   by   light   beams   of observed
area   is   the   most   important   idea   of optical tomography. The
device   was   designed   in   this   manner that it is possible to
simulate   four   kinds   of   field   patterns: parallel,   grid,
polar,   polar-grid.   The   measurements   were done for grid and
polar-grid   field   pattern. There were presented possibilities
of   choosing   numbers   of   projections   and   image accuracy of
measured   object   at   the   computer screen. The limitations of
optical   method   at   tomography imaging were described in this
paper too.

1 Introduction

Process   tomography   is   a   new   technology   which   enables to
present   in an image form phenomena occuring at the moment, at
the   particular   points,   surface,   measuring   area,   e.g.   at
laboratory or industrial installation.
To obtain data necessary to get measuring course process image
M projections and **N** measurements in each projection are made.
A   single   projection   is   understood   as   a   performance of **N**

measurements of the area in which the measuring object can be
placed.
The number of measurements and projections decide on measuring
accuracy, data collecting time and also on hardware and
software complication.
Using the visible laser light and appropriate software it is
possible to control on-line process imaging at the computer
screen and compare the images with real measured objects
location.
The quick development of tomograph systems creates necessity
of building new devices which will be helpful during works on
these systems.
.Construction of laboratory tomograph using visible light was
the Micromath International's (Warsaw Poland) idea.

2.Tomograph device construction

A new construction of optical tomograph device is presented in
this chapter.

An optical tomograph consists of six main parts which are
shown in figure 1. There are:
- turntable kit,
- moving platform kit,
- rotary mirror kit,
- main electronic board with light detectors,
- interface to PC computer,
- laser kit.
   Particular kits are mounted on the metal base plate (1). The
main electronic board (4) is mounted vertically to the base
plate (1) by the square cleats (2,3). An electronic control
circuits situated on this main board controls movement of the
platform (11), rotation of the turntable (9) and the mirror
(19) and signals from the position sensors (7). On the main
board (4) there are fixed 40 phototransistors which create the
line detector (8).
   Turntable kit consist of the table (9) fixed by two bearings
to the mandrel fixed on the base plate (1). Turntable is
driven by the reduction tooth belt gear (10) with the stepper
motor (6).
   The platform (11) shifts on the two guides (12) fixed to the
base plate (1) by the special supports (13). This platform is
driven by the stepper motor (5) and screw-nut gear (15,14)
connected by Oldham coupling (16).

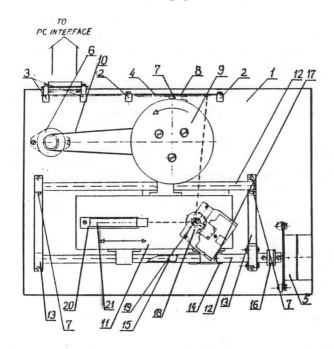

Figure 1 - The optical tomograph device.
1-base plate, 2,3-square cleats, 4-electronic main board, 5-platform stepper motor, 6-turntable stepper motor, 7-position sensor, 8-line detector, 9-turntable, 10-tooth belt, 11-platform, 12-guide, 13-special support, 14-special nut, 15-screw, 16-Oldham coupling, 17-platform guide, 18-magnetoelectronic structure, 19-flat mirror, 20-mounting plate, 21-semiconductor

The mirror kit is fixed on the platform (11). It consists of the flat mirror (19) fixed on the magnetoelectric structure coil (magnetoelectric structure (18) was taken from microammeter).
On the platform (11) there is laser kit, too. It consists of the semiconductor laser (21) and mounting plate (20) which is used to adjust light position. The light beam from laser (21) falls on the mirror (19), reflects, going through measuring space over the turntable (9) and fall on the phototransistors

(8). If there is an object across on the way of light beam it
cannot reach the detector. Alternatively, when the light beam
lightens the phototransistor it means that there are no
objects across the light way.

All signals controlling stepper motors movements, mirror
revolution and signals from position sensors are sent to and
received from the interface in a PC computer by the multi-core
wire.

The grid field pattern is created by platform shift on the
guides with the immovable mirror. The grid-polar pattern is
created by fixing the platform at one position and rotating
the mirror.

3. Measurement algorithms

The algorithm of making measurements is presented below.

The grid field pattern.

1. Commencing a program, the platform moves to the extreme
position.
2. After getting signal from a position sensor the platform
shifts to position where the light beam reaches first
phototransistors. This is the base position for the platform.
3. The stepper motor turning the turntable is switched on. The
table rotates until it reaches the base position determined by
the position sensor.
4. The stepper motor moving the platform is switched on. The
light beam moves along the detector line. For the purpose of
elimination a light reflection a signal from phototransistor
is read when the mirror is straight on this phototransistor.
5. After making one projection (40 independent elementary
measurements) the turntable rotates about one or more
elementary angle (it depend on the value of stepper motor step
angle and the transmission ratio of belt gear).
6. The platform returns. Next measurements are executed.
7. The steps above can be repeated as many times as required.

The grid-polar field pattern.

1. Starting program, the platform moves to the extreme
position.
2. After getting signal from position sensor the platform
shifts to position where the light beam goes through the

middle of the turntable (the middle of a line detector). This
is the base position for the platform.
3. The stepper motor turning the turntable is switched on. The
table   rotates   until   it   reaches base position determined by
position sensor.
4. The voltage is connected to the magnetoelectric structure
coil.   The   light   beam moves in succession along the detector
line. For the purpose of elimination of the light reflection a
signal   from phototransistor is read when the light beam falls
on this phototransistor.
5. After making one projection (40 independent elementary
measurements)   the   turntable   rotates   about   one   or   more
elementary   angle   (it   depends   on the value of stepper motor
step angle and the transmission ratio of belt gear).
6. The steps above can be repeated as many times as required.

4.Technical parameters

This   optical   tomograph allowed simulation of four kinds of
field   pattern: parallel, grid, polar and grid-polar. At each
projection   40   measurements   can   be   made.   The angle of the
turntable   stepper   motor   (6)   being   used at the constructed
device is 7.5 , but using the tooth belt gear (reduction ratio
p=3)   it   is reduced to 2.5 . So it is possible to execute 144
projections.   The   measurement   time   depend   on   the   maximum
stepper   motor   frequency and on the possibilities of reaching
phototransistors by the light beam (vibration of the mirror
on   the   magnetoelectric   structure   coil   during the platform
motion).   In   the   constructed   optical   tomograph, the single
projection   time   at   the   parallel field pattern method is 32
[sec] and at the polar is equal 5 [sec].

Technical specification:
1.Number of measurements in a single projection, max   N=40
2.Number of projections, max   M=144
3.Diameter of measuring turntable [mm]   d=100
4.Measuring time in a parallel pattern field [sec]   32
5.Measuring time in a polar pattern field [sec]   5
6.Elementary turntable angle [deg]   2.5
7.Kind of field pattern: parallel, polar, grid, polar-grid
8.Positioning sensors   optoelectronic
9.Laser type   semiconductor
10.Wavelength [nm]   670
11.Power output [mW]   1

12.Beam size [mm]   4.5x2.5
13.Dimensions (HWD) [mm]   165x366x267

5.Experimental results

Figure 2 presents sample reconstructed images obtained from
the reconstruction program. Figure 2a shows two round objects.
The field pattern is parallel. The number of casts is equal to
24 with angle step 7.5 degree. The image is created with
resolution 170x170 pixels.
The same objects reconstructed from a smaller number of
projections (4) is in figure 2b. The fidelity of
reconstruction process is reduced: the shape is not so smooth
as on the previous picture. The advantage of small number of
projections is shorter time needed for performing a
measurement as well as for reconstruction. The amount of
processed data is also small.
In figure 2c the same objects are presented again, with large
number of projections (24), but the image resolution is
reduced to 50x50 pixels. In this case the shapes of the
objects are distorted by bigger pixels. The time taken for
reconstruction is less than in case from figure 2a.
The last figure (2d) presents similar objects' configuration
with different field pattern - polar. It is noticeable, that
there are small light areas left at the image edges. This
effect appears when objects are placed close to the edge of
the tomograph's working area.

6.Application of the optical tomograph device.

The tomograph device described above is the laboratory
equipment.
It will be very difficult to apply it in the industrial
conditions, but the base role which it should perform is to
approach the principles of tomograph imaging. It means that
anybody can observe and compare changes occuring during
measurement with the computer screen images. The research
worker can change the base parameters as number of
measurements at single projection and the number of
projections to estimate projection quality.
The application of the optical tomograph can be wider than a
laboratory instrument. For instance it is possible to
construct industrial device like below - figure 3.

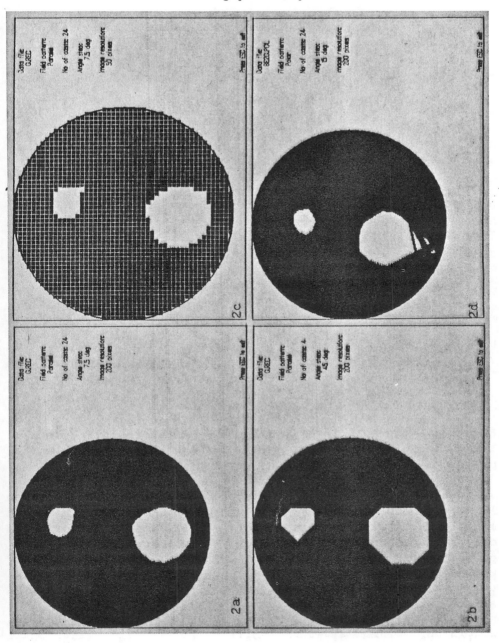

Figure 2 - Samples of reconstructed images.

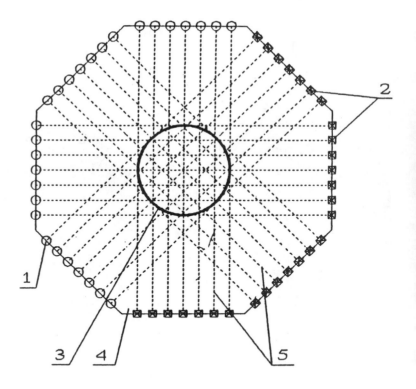

Figure 3 - The example of industrial optical tomograph model.
1-LEDiodes,   2-phototransistors,   3-measuring area,4-octagonal
prism

   At the each wall of the octagonal prism there are a few
light sources -LEDiodes (1). On the opposite side there are
light detectors - phototransistors (2) and each detector works
only with one photodiode. Of course a number of photoelements'
pairs depends on the pipe inner diameter. The number of
photoelements is limited by the prism dimension and vice
versa. · For instance to scan a 100[mm] diameter pipe the side
of a hexagon should be 100[mm] long.
   There can be reflections between the light beams from
photodiodes from different walls. So it is necessary to

multiplex pairs photodiode-phototransistor on each wall and also all walls between themselves. This device can be installed on the pipeline made of glass to measure solid particles inside it.

It should be remembered that the light application is associated with more problems and limitations which result from physic principles of optics. The most important are refractive on the edge of two materials with different refractivities, reflection and diffusion.

7.Conclusion
Successful realization of the design proved the optical ·tomography is useful for educational purpose to explain principles of tomograph imaging.

The constructed optical tomograph allows for simulation of different kinds of sensors field pattern and make maximum 144 projections.It is possible to control on-line process imaging at a computer screen and compare the images with real measuring objects location.
Measurements which were made show deviations of objects reconstruction images which were appeared for different field patterns.

INITIAL FINDINGS ON A TOMOGRAPHIC IMAGING SYSTEM FOR SEWERS

A R DANIELS, I BASARAB-HORWATH, F DICKIN, R G GREEN &
C THORNHILL

ABSTRACT

This paper describes preliminary work being carried out on a dual modality system to investigate a range of solid materials being transported in a sewer. The instrumentation techniques are based on impedance measurement, giving phase and amplitude voltages, and an infra-red sensor array. An impedance measurement circuit is described and initial results for the phase measurements are presented.

1.0 INTRODUCTION

On-line flow measurement in sewers is important if sewage treatment plants are not to be overwhelmed and the rivers protected from excessive pollution. Knowledge of flow conditions enables switching/diversions to the sewage to be made resulting in efficient use of the treatment plants. Sewers contain a very wide range of materials conveyed within a liquid phase. The three other important non-liquid components, of interest to this research, are: gross solids or faeces; paper, cloths and rags collectively known as cellulose products and rubber. This project has the long term aim of quantifying all these components using tomographic imaging methods.

There are several problems that need to be addressed when considering the most appropriate method of measuring the quantity of solids flowing in a sewer. The first is one of safety: some gasses present in sewers are potentially explosive necessitating the requirement that any equipment be intrinsically safe within this environment. Secondly: sensors should be non-intrusive otherwise soiling of these protrusions takes place leading to corruption of the data collection process. It was decided to concentrate research on two main areas:

(a)   Electrical Impedance Tomography. (EIT)
(b)   Infra-red Matrix Imaging.

Both areas are relatively new with respect to industrial process applications and their use within sewers produces its own unique set of problems. Most publications in the area of EIT have been related mainly to medical imaging techniques (1,2,3). Assumptions are made, in medical imaging, about the boundary conditions and the physical behaviour of the subject imaged that differ vastly from the situation existing within a sewer. For example, oscillator frequencies of 20-40Khz are usually chosen due to the behaviour of human body tissue at these frequencies. Optical methods (4,5) tend mostly to concentrate on two component flows such as liquid/gas or liquid/single-solid, etc. In this application there are four major components with the following physical characteristics:

(1)   Rubber: Highly resistive, very translucent.
(2)   Solids: Unknown resistivity, not translucent.
(3)   Cellulose Products: Low resistivity and unknown translucency when
        saturated with liquid.
(4)   Conveying liquid: Highly variable resistivity and very translucent.

It is due to the nature of the three major, non-fluid, components that infra-red matrix imaging and EIT have been chosen as the most suitable in order to produce a fast accurate image of sewer flows. Other methods do exist such as ultrasonic imaging, capacitance imaging and Nuclear Magnetic Resonance techniques but seem unsuitable for the purposes of this research.

2.0 PROBLEMS PRESENTED BY SEWERS

Apart from the more obvious considerations such as safety, any imaging system has to be able to cope with the changing boundaries presented by sewers. The conveying liquid will vary in depth depending on the rate and volume of flow and this is illustrated in Fig.1. All existing Tomographic imaging systems have a priori knowledge of the process boundary (6), as would be the case here if the conditions of Fig.1(a) could be guaranteed. Unfortunately this is not achievable in a typical sewer without restricting the flow in some way.

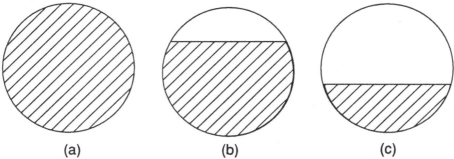

Figure 1: (a) Full sewer (b)(c) Partially full sewers illustrating the changing cross section to be imaged

Another consideration, when developing an imaging system, is the fact that the translucency and impedance of the conveying liquid will not be constant and investigations will be instigated to determine these dynamic ranges. Possible causes of these changes are:

(1)   Mineral seepage to and from surrounding strata.
(2)   Variations in temperature of the conveying liquid.
(3)   Large influxes of rain-water/mud during heavy rain.
(4)   Wide variation in discharges from factories and houses.

3.0 AIMS OF THE PROJECT

The primary aim of the project can be reduced to a series of smaller objectives in EIT hardware capable of imaging a phantom has been constructed with which it is possible to inject current via any two electrodes and measure the resultant voltage differential at any other pair of electrodes. The circuitry has been designed in a modular form avoiding the need to redesign in entirety as the project evolves and progresses. A simple back-projection method is being implemented in C++ that takes a full set of readings and ultimately produces an image of the phantoms cross- section. This will then be used to determine the effectiveness of EIT for imaging situations that closely resemble the conditions found in a sewer. If this proves positive then the complexity of the circuitry/software will be increased to produce a more accurate image. Phase measurements are also being investigated to determine whether extra information can be obtained further improving imaging accuracy. This will then allow the system to distinguish differences between the various solids. Fig.2 shows an overview of the expected final design utilising both EIT and infra- red information.

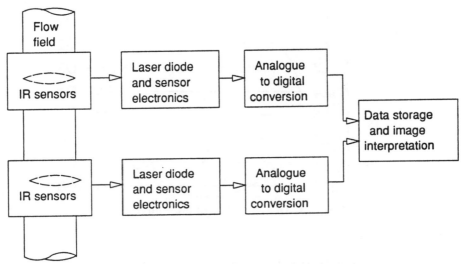

Figure 2 A system overview

Front end hardware for the infra-red imaging side still needs to be designed and this is underway. This will be based around low cost laser diodes which can be pulsed to allow higher instantaneous operating powers for short durations in a similar approach to that used by BIHE (5). An array of 8 laser diodes aligned in parallel will enable a cross-section of the flow pipe to be interrogated as shown in Fig.3. The voltages from the infra-red sensors D1-D8 can then be converted into an 8-bit word, passed via an interface to a personal computer and stored in matrix format. Information acquired from several such arrays, positioned around the flow pipe wall, can be used in reconstruction algorithms to produce an image of the flow. Fig.4 shows a possible arrangement of three such arrays.

3.1 FURTHER AREAS OF RESEARCH.

No single reconstruction method or algorithm has yet been adopted. For the purpose of initial investigation a simple back-projection method will be used as this is relatively easy to implement. At a later stage it is hoped to be able to try various reconstruction methods to discover the best way of producing the type of image required to determine the mass flow of individual components of sewage.

Some other aspects to be investigated are:

(1)   Causes and extent of the variation in resistivity of conveying liquid.
(2)   The most effective frequency for the EIT oscillator and to determine whether a multi-frequency approach would be of benefit.
(3)   Investigate the effect of variations in liquid level on sensors and reconstruction algorithms.

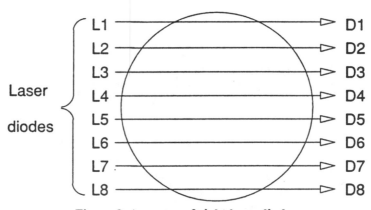

Figure 3 An array of eight laser diodes

4.0 INITIAL RESULTS

There are many areas of the project that require investigation before a coherent solution emerges. Initial measurements suggest that phase shifts in the order of 6-8 degrees do occur, at frequencies of 5-10 Khz, within a test phantom using paper, plastic and metal objects. These measurements were made using basic laboratory equipment (oscilloscope, signal generator, constant current source, buffers and a 36 electrode square phantom). It would be extremely difficult to distinguish phase shifts of this order from noise when using the conventional phase sensitive detector used in most EIT systems. However, a simple dedicated phase detection system has been designed and built, by Thornhill (7), based on an LM3189 IF demodulator I.C. The circuit block diagram is shown in Fig.5 and a typical calibration curve for input frequencies of 20 Khz, is shown in Fig.6. This demonstrates a linear relationship between measured voltage and phase change over a signal range corresponding to 30 degrees, with a sensitivity of 0.017 V/degree. This circuit will be adapted and added to the existing design in order to establish its usefulness.

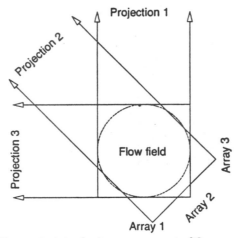

Figure 4 A typical arrangement of 3 arrays

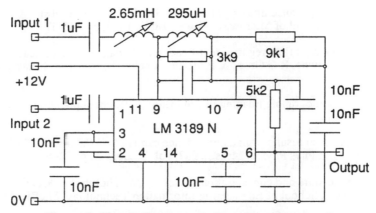

Figure 5 Circuit diagram of phase detection circuit

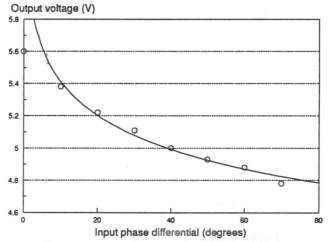

Figure 6 Phase detector performance curve

5.0 CONCLUSIONS

The project is in its early stages with the impedance system designed and implemented. This will be used to investigate the ease of imaging the major constituents of sewage using EIT. The phase detection circuitry described in the previous section will be added in the near future and if this proves unsuccessful then other methods will be investigated. Initial tests show that phase shifts can be detected and it is our aim to develop a way of incorporating these in the reconstruction process.

REFERENCES

(1)   "Imaging spatial distributions of resistivity using applied potential tomography." D C Barber, B H Browne & I L Freeston; Elec Lett, 1983, vol 19, pp 933-5

(2)   "A prototype system and reconstruction algorithms for electrical impedance technique in medical body imaging." Y Kim & H W Woo; Clin Phys Physiol Meas, 1987, vol 8, suppl A, 63-70

(3)   "Electrical impedance imaging of the thorax." Y Kim, J G Webster &
W J Tompkins; Journal of Microwave Power, 18(3), 1983, pp 245-57

(4)   "Two component flow regime identification and imaging with optical sensors."
N Saeed, M A Browne, R G Green & P Martin; Imeko IX, Houston, Texas, pp 16-21,
1988

(5)   "Infra-red tomographic imaging of fluid flows." Patent application: 9011086.7
17 May 1990

(6)   "Some physical results from an impedance camera." K Sakamoto, T J Yorkey &
J G Webster; Clin Phys Physiol Meas , 1987, vol 8, suppl A, pp 71-6

(7)   "Online moisture and concentration sensor." C M Thornhill & R G Green;
Final year project, School of Engineeirng Information Technology, Sheffield City
Polytechnic

Chapter 6

Keynote Addresses and Future Prospects
of Process Tomography

SENSORS - their Interaction with the Measurand

(SUMMARY of a Keynote Address Introducing the Session "Sensors").

F Mesch

Institut für Meß- und Regelungstechnik, Universität (TH) Karlsruhe, Germany

1: INTRODUCTION

A definite and exhaustive overview of sensors and their present state of the art does not seem feasible, since almost 10 years ago already a comprehensive survey [1] was published. Meanwhile, a large number of further sensors and sensing principles has been presented. Thus instead of a survey, some basic considerations of the interaction between the emanation used for sensing and the measurand are presented.

2. SCALAR INTERACTION
2.1 Absorption

X-rays in medicine are certainly the origin of computerized tomography (CT). The "interaction" consists of pure absorption of rays by matter, following Lambert-Beer's law, along straight rays, leading to the familiar line integrals. In the simplest case the rays are parallel. Using a linear sensor array, a one-dimensional projection is obtained, and information in the second dimension is obtained by rotation. This process is mathematically described by the Radon transform, or equivalently by the projection slice theorem using Fourier transforms, from which the well-known reconstruction formulae may be derived in a straight-forward way. A slight complication is caused by the fact that in reality divergent rays (fan beams) are used.

Absorption also occurs if ultrasonic rays are transmitted through a two-phase flow consisting of a fluid with (small) gas bubbles. By tomographic methods, the mean interfacial area of the bubbles may be determined [2].

2.2 Reflection

In an airborne radar system, all points of an object having the same distance to the aircraft contribute to the reflected wave at a certain time instant. For large distances, this means the received signal for each time instant is given by a line integral over the object reflectivity, taken along a direction perpendicular to the direction of wave propagation. If the aircraft flies a turn, i.e. a circular flight path around an object, tomographic methods may be applied to obtain a higher resolution than is possible with more conventional synthetic aperture methods [3,4].

Pure specular reflection occurs in another example pertinent to process tomography. Ultrasonic transmitters and receivers are placed around the wall of a tube containing fluid and large gas bubbles. The acoustic impedance differences between fluid and bubbles are so large that the ultrasonic rays are reflected specularly. Evaluating first, second and third echoes separately, and using elementary geometric relations, shape and position of the bubbles may be reconstructed [5].

2.3 Scattering

In medical applications of ultrasound, "weak scattering" occurs in tissues. To a first order approximation, called Born approximation, the scattered field may be described by the superposition of spherical waves emanating from single point scatterers, where these waves are induced by the ultrasonic field applied from outside. The field detected by linear or planar sensor arrays can again be described by two- or three-dimensional Fourier transforms, from which reconstruction formulae are derived. These methods are called diffraction tomography [6,7].

In reality, the stimulating field acting on any point scatterer is the superposition of the external field and the contributions from all other scatterers. This "multiple scattering problem" is very difficult to describe analytically. The Born approximation is valid only for weak scattering, and errors occurring with stronger scattering must be corrected by higher order approximations.

2.4 Impedance Tomography

The changes of capacity or resistance between a number of electrodes located around the wall of a tube are easy to measure, and so electric impedance tomography (EIT) is particularly attractive for process tomography. Theoretically, however, the method is rather complex - the fields are non-homogeneous, and moreover the fields strongly depend on the spatial distribution of particles between the electrodes. To some extent, this problem is related to the multiple scattering problem of the preceeding section.

Since the bulk of the papers presented at this meeting is devoted to EIT, no further comments are given here.

3.   VECTORIAL INTERACTION

So far, the measurands have been scalar functions of space coordinates - densities, acoustic impedances, electrical permittivities and resistivities. Now vector fields will be considered, where special consideration must be given to the type of interaction.

3.1 Time-of-Flight

An important example of vector fields is the velocity distribution of flowing gases or fluids, which might be measured by ultrasonic waves. Here it is not the amplitude but the resulting propagation velocity of the waves that is of interest. This velocity is a superposition of the sound velocity in a static medium and of the local flow velocity. If the times-of-flight between two ultrasonic transducers are measured both upstream and downstream, the sound velocity may be obtained from the sum, and the local flow velocity from the difference, of both times. It is important that only the velocity component in the direction of wave propagation is measured, which is called "longitudinal interaction". The velocity component perpendicular to the propagation direction, the "transversal interaction", might theoretically be detected from the ray deflection, but this has not yet been tried experimentally. It was shown in [8,9] by methods of field theory and vector analysis that the longitudinal interaction only yields the source free component, and the transversal interaction only the curl free component of any vector field. Thus a complete reconstruction of a general vector field is possible only if both interactions are available. In [9] the feasibility has been demonstrated of determining the vorticity of flow fields in a plane cross section of tubes by measuring times-of-flight for ultrasonic waves. For reconstruction, algorithms have been developed from those being used for scalar fields.

3.2 Schlieren

The Schlieren method is a classical optical method for the visualization of density variations in gases. Usually, the Schlieren images obtained are only qualitatively evaluated. It may be shown theoretically that the intensity variations of the image are proportional to the line integral over the gradient of refractive index in the measuring volume. Only the gradient component perpendicular to the optical rays is obtained, which corresponds to a transversal interaction.

Combining a Schlieren system with tomographic methods, temperature distributions in flames have been reconstructed [10] quantitatively.

3.3 Magnetic fields

In [11], magnetic field lines in the air gap of magnetic systems have been determined using specially wound, integrating coils together with tomographic reconstruction methods.

4. MICROSCOPY OF 3D OBJECTS

Tomograms in their original form - and according to the Greek root of the word - provide 2D cross sections through 3D objects, based on a set of 1D projections taken at varying projection angles. A more complete 3D reconstruction is approximated by repeating the procedure for a number of cross sections.

In conventional microscopy, too, 2D images are obtained, and for 3D objects with non-negligible thickness, only one plane is well in focus due to the limited depth resolution. If the complete object is of interest, the microscope is focussed to various object depths.

For many applications, an extended depth range would be desirable where all parts of a thick object are in focus in the same image. In [12], images obtained from various focus positions are combined by image processing. Essentially, this is a tomographic problem, where the focus positions replace the projection angles, and where the line integrals of conventional projections are replaced by the laws of geometrical optics for an imaging lens.

5. COMMON PROBLEMS

The analytical reconstruction formulae derived from the projection slice theorem (Sec. 2.1) or in diffraction tomography (Sec. 2.3) require ideal projections, i.e. homogeneous distribution of emanations, large sensor arrays and a large number of projections. If these requirements are not met to a reasonable approximation, algebraic reconstruction techniques (ART) must be used. This is, for example, always the case with EIT. If rays are bent, ART is also necessary to perform ray tracing corrections [13].

The most frequent limitation in practical applications is the number of sensors and the number of projections available. For severe limitations, even ART and sophisticated interpolation algorithms will not result in satisfactory reconstructions. Two ways are possible to overcome this problem.

One is based on the idea to complete the insufficient measurement data by a-priori information. An example for such a-priori information are the Navier-Stokes equations which must be fulfilled by a flow field [14].

The other approach is to renounce any reconstruction of images and to identify, instead, relevant process parameters. It seems that this idea has not yet been adequately considered in the past, and it is too thoughtless that always an image with high resolution is aimed at. Of course, tomographic images of high quality are indispensable in medicine, and also in process applications if they are required to verify process models. For field applications, however, where the data obtained serve to automatically control the process, images requiring human interpretation are useless. Here it seems by far preferable to consciously define the parameters necessary for process control, and than to restrict reconstruction to identifying these parameters.

REFERENCES

[1]   R H T Bates, K L Garden, T M Peters (1983), *Overview of Computerized Tomography with Emphasis on Future Developments*, Proc. IEEE 71, p. 356-372.

[2]   J Wolf (1988), *Investigation of Bubbly Flow by Ultrasonic Tomography*, Particle Characterization 5, p. 170-173.

[3]   D C Munson, J D O'Brien, W K Jenkins (1983), *A Tomographic Formulation of Spotlight-Mode Synthetic Aperture Radar*, Proc. IEEE 71, No. 8, p. 917-925.

[4]   D L Mensa (1981), *High Resolution Radar Imaging*, Artech House, Inc. Norwood, USA.

[5]   M A Seiraffi (1991), *Two-phase flow measurement in pipelines using ultra-sonic-tomography*, Proc. of 19th International Symposium on Acoustical Imaging in Bochum.

[6]   A C Kak, M Slaney (1987), *Principles of computerized tomographic imaging*, IEEE Press New York.

[7]   R Bamler (1989), *Mehrdimensionale lineare Systeme*, Springer-Verlag.

[8]   H Braun, A Hauck (1991), *Tomographic reconstruction of vector fields*, IEEE Trans. on Signal Processing, Vol. 39, No. 2.

[9]   A Hauck (1990), *Tomographie von Vektorfeldern*, Dissertation, Universität (TH) Karlsruhe.

[10] F Mesch, H Braun, P Deuble (1990), *Messung der Dichte- und Tempera-turverteilung in Brennräumen mit der Schlierentomographie*, Forschungs-bericht im Rahmen des Sonderforschungsbereiches 167.

[11] H Saito, K Taniguchi, M Nakajima (1991), *AC magnetic field imaging using CT technique*, XII Imeko World Congress, Beijing, China.

[12] P Schwarzmann, W Xiangchen (1989), *Nonlinear approach to the recon-struction of microscopic objects*, Proc. ECS 5, Freiburg i. Br., p. 563-568.

[13] A Schwarz (1992), *Acoustic Measurement of Temperature and Velocity Fields in Furnaces*, Proc. ECAPT-Meeting (this volume).

[14] A Wernsdörfer (1992), *Reconstruction from Limited Data with A-priori Knowledge*, Proc. ECAPT-Meeting (this volume).

DATA PROCESSING FOR TOMOGRAPHIC IMAGE RECONSTRUCTION

(SUMMARY of a Keynote Address Introducing the Session "Data Processing Mathematical Techniques and Simulation")

A R Borges

Universidade de Aveiro, Portugal

In most practical situations, the balance between required execution time, on one side, and the amount of data and complexity of the computations, on the other, places rather stringent conditions on the computer system where tomographic reconstruction algorithms are to be run. Thus, exploiting the parallel chacteristics inherent to the algorithms becomes an issue of primary importance.

In this talk, we begin by addressing the problem in a general way, presenting an overview on how the concurrency present in a given computational process may be handled and what is the absolute limit to process speed-up. Two different ways of looking at the decomposition which is performed are discussed, namely, its type and complexity level.

It is then shown how these ideas relate to the two most popular computational models nowadays in use: the MIMD (Multiple Instruction - Multiple Data) machine and SIMD (Single Instruction - Multiple Data) machine.

In the second part of the talk, two parallelization stragegies for problem decomposition in MIMD architechures are studied and its main features are presented. Figures of merit about process speed-up are in each case produced and it is also shown how in a first approximation system perfomance depends on the number of processors used.

The first strategy is suitable for data-driven solutions where independent data sets are successively processed by the same computational kernel. It consists of a combination of pipelining and data-partitioning. The basic idea is to start by splitting the processing pipe into different stages according to rules similar to those used for algorithm specification in a sequential environment. However, since the resulting organization is not usually load balanced, data partitioning is then applied to achieve spatial parallelism at the stage level.

This kind of strategy is an obvious choice for projection-driven algorithms and the filtered-backprojection algorithm is used as an implementation example to describe how this stategy maps into a planar message-passing topology.

The second stategy, on the other hand, assumes pure data-partitioning solutions where different system processors are assigned to different patches of the image matrix carrying out all the local processing. Iterative algorithms of ART-type fit rather nicely into such a decomposition model and it is also shown how they map into a planar message-passing topology.

HOW CAN TOMOGRAPHY CONTRIBUTE TO CHEMICAL PROCESS DEVELOPMENT

(SUMMARY of a Keynote Address Introducing the Session "Equipment Design and Modelling").

J C Middleton

ICI Chemicals and Polymers Ltd

A typical chemical process contains reaction, separation, purification and product presentation stages. The more efficient the reaction stage, the less expensive will be the subsequent stages and the effluent treatment stages, so attention is focused on reactor improvements. These rely on detailed knowledge of the important chemical and physical mechanisms active in the reactor, and the elucidation of these requires good measurement techniques. The complexity of the mechanisms often necessitates the use of computer models which must describe mixing and inter-phase effects alongside the chemical reactions. The adequate testing of these models also requires good measurement techniques.

Tomography offers the chance to obtain reasonably detailed 3-dimensional maps of concentrations of tracers or a dispersed phase without intrusion into the process fluid. It is therefore attractive as a laboratory technique for such measurements in research. Electrical tomography has the added attraction of relatively low cost and applicability to non-transparent vessels, so given adequate robustness may be suitable as an on-plant diagnostic tool.

Many processes involve solid particles dispersed in a fluid. These are typically reaction catalysts or products. It is often desirable to know their distribution within the equipment (vessel, pipework, centrifuge, drier, pneumatic conveying system etc), especially when there is or may be a blockage problem. Gas distribution in liquid flows can also be troublesome, for example with unexpected high pressure drops. Inspection by tomography is expected to be a useful new method of examining root causes.

Some examples are presented of the current techniques of measurement and modelling applied to process equipment as a challenge to developers of tomography instruments.

TOMOGRAPHIC APPLICATIONS FOR THE OIL INDUSTRY

(SUMMARY of a Keynote Address Introducing the Session "Process Monitoring and Control").

C P Lenn

Schlumberger Cambridge Research Ltd

The production of crude oil presents many instrumentation challenges to both the oilfield services industry and oil companies alike. Research and development in these industries is aimed at improving the efficiency and safety of recovering oil reserves.

Aspects of oilfield R & D are reviewed and areas where tomographic techniques offer possible solutions to long term problems are discussed. In particular the difficulties of the multiphase metering of oil/water/gas simultaneously are highlighted.

The measurement of the mass flowrate of three component flows requires (in theory) the determination of 9 variables. Simple assumptions can reduce this number but several metering principles need to be combined to give the flowrates of the oil/gas/water fractions emerging from oilwells.

The use of impedance methods to give component fraction information is found in many metering strategies. These methods are mixing law dependent and according to the model chosen large differences in void fraction estimation can arise due to droplet size and spatial distributions. This can be seen in the number of simple formulae such as Maxwell's that are used to relate an impedance measurement to component concentration. The use of imaging techniques provides a possible solution to these difficulties and results are shown to illustrate this.

Tomographic techniques provide powerful tools in the laboratory as well as being potential instruments for field use. The investigations of phase distributions in real time in laboratory experiments provides unique information on physical processes that could be occurring in multiphase flowmeters, pipes and associated equipment such as separators. Some images obtained from gas/oil and water/oil phase flows in Schlumberger's Cambridge research centre will show the potential of tomographic information when studying these or related process problems in other industries.

PROCESS TOMOGRAPHY - THE POTENTIAL FOR ENVIRONMENTAL APPLICATION

R B Edwards   Unilever Research, Port Sunlight Laboratory.

Process Tomography is concerned with the generation of images which provide an accurate representation of concentration profiles within a system scrutinised by externally mounted sensors. The technology offers the potential of generating detailed information on a system through the application of a relatively small number of non-invasive sensors and provides clear opportunities for industrial exploitation.

In particular, the ability of the technology to deliver both space and time variant data rapidly and efficiently gives rise to the potential for particularly beneficial application in environmental monitoring and control.

Three broad areas of interest for environmental application may be identified:

i) Process measurement and control.

Applications in this area are concerned with process measurements in heterogeneous systems where knowledge of a property distribution is essential to the measurement. A good example is the measurement of the mass flow of a single phase in a flowing multiphase system, such as solids in a liquid or gaseous effluent discharge.

ii) Process modelling.

Applications in this area are concerned with the generation of knowledge rather than 'in-process' application.

Computer based models are widely used to predict the dispersion of pollutants in the environment and there is a clear synergy between the development of such models and tomography in that their verification requires the generation of a large amount of time and space variant data which tomography can provide efficiently.

Key to successful application of tomography is the availability of appropriate sensor technology. For an application in imaging the dispersion of a gas plume one can set down requirements for the sensing technique as follows:

- must be capable of detailed spatial resolution.

- must capture data rapidly in relation to the transport processes involved.

- must be capable of sensing remote and unbounded systems.

- data is paramount, 'real time' imaging not critical.

- may be a requirement to be pollutant specific.

An interesting example of what is achievable in this respect is the use of LIDAR (Light Detection and Ranging) for imaging power station emission plumes (Bennett et al, 1992). The sensing technique essentially involves analyzing the backscatter spectrum obtained from the firing of a short laser pulse at an angle across a plume. A series of 'shots' allows the plume to be scanned and a cross sectional image to be obtained. The time required for a single 'shot' is of the order of 0.001s and a plume can be scanned in some 1.7s. The instrumentation may be sited in excess of 2km from the plume and a spatial resolution of 5m can be obtained at that distance.

iii) Environmental Monitoring.

The spatial resolution offered by tomographic imaging lends the technology to the monitoring of large areas, such as large industrial or landfill sites. Whilst there is well developed technology available for the monitoring of defined emission points at such sites the monitoring of 'fugitive emissions', which by definition may arise at any time and any point over a wide area, is more difficult.

In considering the sensor technology required for monitoring applications one can set down the following requirements:

-        must be capable of continuous application.

-        high spatial resolution of pollutant concentration gradients may not be a prime requirement. Priority may only be to deliver sufficient resolution to locate point of emission.

-        near 'real time' imaging is important so that an emission can be detected and corrective action applied without undue delay.

-        probably a greater requirement for the technique to be pollutant specific.

The potential of the technology can be illustrated by two emerging opportunities:

The first is in the monitoring of gaseous emissions from industrial sites. Spectroscopic sensing techniques are being widely applied in gaseous monitoring. One emerging piece of spectroscopic sensing technology which particularly lends itself to tomographic application is OTIM (Optical Transform Image Modulation) (Shelley,1991). Essentially this technique resolves the passive emission spectrum from a field of view to give a 'distance integrated' value of concentration of a particular pollutant. The time response of the instrument is within 1s with a distance range of the order of kilometres.

With this kind of sensor technology, coupled with tomographic imaging technology, one can in the future foresee the environmental manager of a large industrial site being able to have a near 'real time' image of the pollutant concentration profile across the facility displayed on a VDU and being able to pinpoint problems in respect of fugitive emissions as and when they occur.

The second opportunity involves the monitoring of fugitive liquid emissions which arise from loss of containment in 'in-ground' facilities such as landfill sites and effluent treatment lagoons.

Electrical Impedance Tomography has been developed as a means of tracking water flows through soils and the technology is being applied to the monitoring of 'in ground' sites such as landfill sites and effluent treatment lagoons (Tamburi,1985: Daily,1991: British Geological Survey). This may be particularly important where aquifers may be under threat and emission could be detected through the positioning of sensors around the facility or between the facility and a sensitive area.

In considering environmental applications one is struck by the realisation that the full potential of tomography will only be realised if imaging technology is linked with a wide sensor base. There is a particular challenge in linking with spectroscopic sensing techniques which are particularly important in quantitative gaseous analysis.

REFERENCES:

Bennett M, Sutton S and Gardener D R C. 'Atmospheric Environment' Vol 26A Pergamon Press 1992.

Shelley T. Eureka Journal, June 1991.

Tamburi A, Allard R and Roeper U. 2nd Canadian/American Conference on Hydrogeology. June 1985.

Daily W, Ramirez A and LaBrecque D. Journal of Water Resources Research, 1991.

British Geological Survey Publication 'Imaging Groundwater and its Pollutants'.

The Current State and Future Prospects of Process Tomography

F. J. Dickin, T. Dyakowski, R. A. Williams, R. C. Waterfall, C. G. Xie and M. S. Beck

Process Tomography Group, UMIST, P.O. Box 88, Manchester M60 1QD

ABSTRACT : The application of tomographic methods for process design, operation and control is discussed. The enabling technology is described including the current development of measurement sensors and image reconstruction algorithms. The parameters which define system performance are described, including: resolution, speed and dynamic sensitivity range. Future developments are considered, including vector velocity measurement from tomographic data process control using tomographic image data and scale-up for various sizes of process equipment.

1. INTRODUCTION

A typical process tomography system can be subdivided into three sub-systems: the sensor, the data acquisition system and the image reconstruction and display (Figure 1). As with all measurement systems the sensor is probably the most critical part. The manner in which the sensor interrogates the process, and the quality of information obtained as a result of this, has a profound effect on the reliability and accuracy of the complete system. Practical considerations place a number of constraints on the sensor. Ideally it should be compact, non-intrusive, require minimum maintenance or calibration, and in many cases also be intrinsically safe.

Sensing techniques include electrical, ultrasound, nucleonic, and optical. Most sensors can be categorised as having either a hard or a soft field. With hard field sensors, such as nucleonic, the sensor field sensitivity is not influenced by the distribution of materials in the process being imaged. However, with soft field sensors, such as capacitance and conductivity, the sensing field is altered by the component distribution and physical properties of the mixture being imaged. Although this limits the resolution compared with hard field sensors, neverthe-

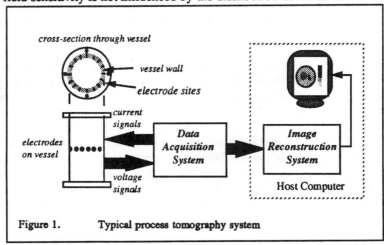

Figure 1.   Typical process tomography system

less the electronic sensing methods are often preferred for on-site process applications because of their low cost and safety.

2.   APPLICATIONS

Process tomography involves the use of instruments which provide cross-sectional profiles of the distribution of materials in a process vessel or pipeline. By analysing two suitably spaced images it will be possible to measure the vector velocity profile (Thorn et al 1991, Hayes et al 1992). Hence from this knowledge of material distribution and movement, internal models of the process can be derived and used as an aid to optimising the design of the process. This promises a substantial advance on present empirical methods of process design, often based on input/output measurements, with only a limited amount of information about the detailed internal behaviour of the process (Dickin et al 1992).

The process industry uses high capital cost plant which is often designed and operated on the basis of past experience and on models which usually assume time and space averaged parameters (e.g. 'well mixed' reactors, 'completely' fluidised beds, etc.). The measurements made in such systems are also usually based on average parameters (temperature, mean flow velocity, chemical composition, etc). In some cases it has been possible to obtain microscale data (instantaneous temperature, velocity, composition, etc) at specific points in the process. However, complex experimental approaches (e.g. laser techniques involving sensing of microscale data) are not economically or practically feasible for many process design and operation needs. For these latter cases the 'process tomography' approach using simple external sensors has much to offer.

It is envisaged that process tomography could in future be employed at the three basic stages encountered in process engineering development:

Stage 1.   Development of new process routes involving fundamentals of chemical process design (reaction kinetics, hydrodynamics etc.).

Stage 2.   Implementation of the required process route by designing efficient industrial-scale equipment.

Stage 3.   Routine process control, flow measurement and mass balancing functions, to enable operation under optimal conditions and to allow operational flexibility. Other applications exist for environmental monitoring of aqueous-based and gas-based mixtures.

At all three stages in the overall design of a process it is necessary to devise models (often based on a computational fluid dynamics approach) for the phenomena concerned, equipment characteristics and, ultimately, to simulate the entire process preferably in a dynamic sense. It is in this context that the use of tomographic techniques may offer a step-change in technology by enabling models to be verified with reference to tomographically measured internal process parameters.

Many process models have, hitherto, relied on theoretical computational fluid dynamics simulations whose model parameters are unquantifiably removed from the real process conditions, or whose predictions cannot always be adequately validated experimentally. For instance, the design of separation equipment holding concentrated solid/liquid dispersions that are optically opaque is often approached by estimating unit behaviour based on the (non-opaque) liquid phase only. The presence of multi-body particle-particle interactions often inhibits accurate prediction of the actual behaviour of the concentrated dispersion. Similarly, the modelling of process equipment frequently has to be based on empirical mass and population balance models derived from sampling the input and output streams to a given process (or so-called 'black-box' modelling). These methods can be effective, but rely upon the availability of an adequate operational data-base to describe the behaviour of similar pieces of equipment handling similar components. Consequently such methods tend to be very system specific and rarely assist in providing any understanding of the fundamental mechanisms occurring within the process equipment. The net result is that considerable caution has to be exercised in scaling-up equipment design from the laboratory or pilot plant to full industrial scale. Potentially, the use of tomography would result in a more rigorous and confident design basis for process equipment. In some cases a modified equipment design would promote: safety, cost savings in capital equipment, floor space or overall productivity. Once a plant has been installed there are some obvious benefits in having the means to 'look inside' to investigate suspected malfunctions, wall wear, or poor performance. However, and more importantly, possibilities exist to perform accurate velocity, mass and component measurements. Such information could form part of the process control strategy.

3.   ENABLING TECHNOLOGY

The availability of efficient and low-cost integrated circuit components and digital signal processing systems has provided a foundation for rapid development of new tomographic imaging systems in the late 1980's and early 1990's.

Significant projects have been carried out in UK universities, in Norway, Germany and the USA, with emergent projects in two Chinese universities and by a Polish instrument manufacturer. Related technologies associated with electrical sensors were developed for geophysical applications in the early 1980's (Dines & Lytle 1981)

3.1   Strategy for Sensor Design

Various sensing methods are needed for process tomography applications (Dickin et al 1992). In the UK a UMIST group has concentrated mainly on capacitive (section 3.1.1) and resistive (section 3.1.2) impedance sensing and on a new method of inductive sensing (section 3.1.3). Work on ultrasound sensing has been carried out at UMIST and Leeds University in the UK in association with Tianjin University in China and at Karlsruhe University in Germany (section 3.1.4). Optical sensing systems have been investigated at Bolton Institute of Higher Education, Hannover University in Germany and Micromath International in Poland (section 3.1.5). UK work on process imaging using gamma ray tomography is featured at Surrey University (Simons et al 1992). Positron based imaging is carried out at Birmingham University (Parker et al 1992). Extensive work on magnetic resonance imaging (MRI) using modified nuclear magnetic resonance (NMR) systems is being performed at Cambridge University.

A group of UK higher education establishments are collaborating on process tomography and are involved in instrumentation system modelling for solving the forward problem of field analysis, on which image reconstruction is based. It is becoming clear that process tomography instrument design could be aided by CAD packages for optimising the spatial sensitivity of the electrodes and for simulating the complete system, so that its performance can be assessed before commitment to detailed design. City University are working on CAD and they have already developed designs for capacitance tomography electrodes (Khan & Abdullah 1992).

In the following sections we will review the currently available methods which appear seem to be most suitable for providing real-time tomographic images of process equipment.

3.1.1 Capacitive impedance tomography

A capacitive tomography system for imaging oilfield pipelines is already delivering valuable images of kerosene/nitrogen flows. It uses a charge-transfer capacitance transducer working at 15 volts with a noise level as low as 0.08 fF r.m.s. and a 6" pipeline twelve-electrode system (Huang et al 1992a, Xie et al 1992a, Huang et al 1992b). It enables void fraction and the flow regime to be determined and it is the first key stage in developing a non-invasive two-component mass flow meter.

The Department of Energy in the USA are investigating the use of capacitance tomography for fluidised bed visualisation (Halow et al 1990). They use a 16-electrode system, with the electrodes energised at 500 volts to generate views of the dielectric constant of the bed.

3.1.2 Resistive impedance tomography

Resistive tomography systems for medical use have been developed during the last few years, with major contributions by the Sheffield University Hospital group (Barber & Brown 1984). A tomography system designed for process use has recently been constructed at UMIST (up to 64 electrodes, frequency 75 Hz - 150 kHz, excitation current up to 30 mA, (Wang et al 1992). It is being evaluated experimentally on process vessels, with particular attention being paid to metal walled vessels to investigate any errors due to the conductivity of the walls. There are significant differences from the medical system because the human body is never in a steady state, so the medical systems are designed on a 'difference imaging' basis to examine relative changes over a short time scale, whereas process tomography systems must give results from absolute measurements of impedance which requires more precise instrumentation and image reconstruction algorithms. A number of process applications (mixing, separator design etc) are being investigated by UMIST (Abdullah et al 1992). Rensselaer Polytechnic Institute in the USA are also making noteworthy advances in resistive impedance tomography (Isaacson 1986, Goble & Gallagher 1988), using adaptive current excitation principles.

3.1.3 Electro-magnetic tomography

This method of imaging uses a sensor system with directional sensing coils for imaging materials which affect inductive fields projected over the cross section of a process. It should enable the specific imaging of metals in the presence of substantial amounts of non-metallic materials, which is of interest in minerals processing and material recycling (Yu et al 1992).

3.1.4 Ultrasonic tomography

Ultrasonic tomography has been extensively developed for medical applications. However, these systems require operator interpretation of results and are not suitable for high-speed process tomography. A joint project between the process tomography groups at Leeds University and UMIST has resulted in the design of a system more suitable for process application, using specially developed wide-angle transmitters with transputers for image reconstruction (Gai et al 1989a&b, Weigand & Hoyle 1989). The wide angle transmitters are combined with multiple receivers, and enable the image to be obtained with a small number of transmitters being "fired" in sequence, thus speeding-up the image frame-rate compared with systems where many narrow angle transducers need to be fired in sequence. Work at Karlsruhe University has been concerned with vector tomography for velocity profile measurement (Wernsdorfer 1992), they have demonstrated the system on bubble columns. A large number of transmitters are used which enable good images to be obtained, but the frame rate is limited for the reasons given above.

3.1.5 Optical tomography

An optical tomography system using arrays of light emitting diodes and photo-detectors for each projection, has been constructed at Bolton Institute of Higher Education (Dugdale et al 1992). Optical system for investigating mixing phenomena have been developed at Hannover University (Mewes et al 1992). Future applications will employ optical techniques for calibration of other process tomography systems and in some processes it is anticipated that optical access may be possible, thus enabling higher resolution than would be achieved using conventional electrical tomography.

Optical tomography is a useful way of teaching the basic principles of tomographic image reconstruction, a demonstration system using a simple optical bench has been made in Poland (Plaskowski et al 1992).

4.   CURRENT STATUS & FUTURE CHALLENGES

Electrical field methods are emerging as robust, safe and relatively low-cost techniques for obtaining tomographic images of the contents of industrial equipment.

A capacitive impedance tomography system which can reconstruct images at 100 frames per second is now ready for further development leading to industrial use (section 3.1.1), the application being mainly to the non-conducting fluids used in the oil industry. Although the existing instrument is suitable for oil well riser applications, there is a need to improve the sensitivity and speed for applications such as measuring flame front propagation. This most demanding requirement is to capacitively image flame fronts in a cylinder head. For engines running up to 6000 rpm this would involve increasing the image speed to 36,000 frames per second and using very small electrodes.   A method of improving transducer sensitivity by the replacement of existing charge transfer techniques by stray-free capacitance bridge measurements incorporating digital signal processing is being investigated (Yang and Stott 1992). A research group in Norway is investigating the use of dedicated silicon technology to make capacitance sensors of optimal design.

The resistive impedance tomography method is suitable for use with electrically conducting systems (most chemical process applications). It forms the basis for model verification aimed to improve the design of industrial equipment. The use of impedance spectroscopy may in future provide a method for imaging specific components in a multi component mixture.

Combined capacitive and resistive impedance transducers will have to be designed for applications where the measurement zone can change between being dominated by dielectric effects or by conductivity effects. The research challenges will be to identify the fluid transition, develop electrodes and electronics suitable for conducting and non-conducting fluids and to design reconstruction algorithms suitable for imaging spaces where there are two different fluid states existing in the measurement zone.

There are a number of specific and rather fundamental challenges in process tomography which should be highlighted because their solution will need a considerable amount of research. One aspect is to define procedures for quantifying the performance of tomographic imaging systems, so far very few reports on this have been written (Seagar et al 1987, Huang et al 1992b). This leads us into considering the following challenges:

a)   *Resolution* The attainable resolution is dependent on the correct placement, sizing and shielding of impedance electrodes and energising fields. This involves solving the forward problem as part of the design method using specially adapted finite element design packages (Khan & Abdullah 1992) and is particularly important in making cost-effective tomography installations. "Empirical" approaches to electrode sizing and placement relative to guards, interfering metalwork etc. are a costly and time-consuming process.

The image resolution (and fidelity) is also influenced by the type of algorithm used to solve the inverse problem of image reconstruction. Most work so far has involved using relatively straightforward backprojection and filtered backprojection methods. However, it is postulated that variations in the position of the field equipotentials due to the spatial distribution of material in the process could be compensated for by more advanced reconstruction techniques. Investigations have started on the use of iterative reconstruction algorithms such as the modified Newton-Raphson algorithm for quantitative impedance tomography (Abdullah et al 1992).

Imaging industrial equipment with non-circular geometries will involve special challenges with electrode placement and with image reconstruction. Typical cases include plate separators and stirred tank reactors (Lyon and Oakley 1992).

b)   *Speed* Data capture rates (aperture times) of 100 frames per second have already been achieved with electrical tomography systems where the measurement frequency is high (ca. 1 MHz for capacitive and inductive sensors and ca. 50 kHz for resistive sensors). Speed increases of up to say 1000 frames per second should be attainable by parallel operation of sensing and signal processing systems, but will involve careful attention to the signal-to-noise ratio of the sensor electronics and elimination of cross-coupling by multifrequency methods. Operation at even higher speeds will probably require major developments in sensor electronics.

Data processing systems for reconstructing high-speed images fall into two general categories. For research applications it will often be sufficient to store the data and reprocess it at a lower speed. For real-time imaging concerned with some process monitoring, control and measurement applications, Transputer systems are already proving successful. Alternative configurations such as cellular array processors and the use of dedicated digital signal processing devices merit careful consideration.

c)   *Dynamic sensitivity range* This term is used to denote the ratio in the process cross-section of the maximum to minimum density (for X-rays) or specific impedance (for electrical impedance tomography). In order to form a tomographic image, the sensor radiation or the field lines from the sensors must pass through all components of the object. With a penetrating radiation such as X-rays this is not usually a problem. (However, radiation methods are often unsuitable for process tomography because of the requirements for radiation containment, high cost and slow response.) Electrical field methods are relatively straightforward for insulating mixtures (e.g. gas/oil) where electrical capacitance tomography is used, and for electrically conducting mixtures (e.g. most processes based on aqueous fluids and absorbent solids) where low frequency electrical impedance tomography is successful. The dynamic sensitivity range of the electrical methods is very wide, for example an EIT system can operate over several orders of magnitude and is fundamentally capable of imaging objects ranging from flaws in metals to conducting zones in near-insulating fluids.

Although electrical methods are suitable for very many applications, there are cases where the presently available high frequency capacitive impedance (1 MHz) and low frequency (50 kHz) resistive impedance methods may not be fully suitable. Examples include imaging of flame structure and flame front propagation in internal combustion engines, where the flame is highly ionized and electrically conducting, whereas the zone in advance of the flame front is electrically insulating. Similarly in oil industry separation process imaging, the oil-water mixture inversion means that combined capacitive and resistive impedance measurements are required. To cater for such a wide range of measurement conditions there is a need to develop multi-frequency sensor systems, measuring both resistive and reactive components.

d)   *Vector velocity* A full understanding of process behaviour requires a knowledge of the direction of material movement as well as the its distribution. The velocities can be measured by cross-correlation of the image data. This is a computer-intensive operation; especially if the direction of the velocity vector is not known. Transputer type array processors with additional digital signal processors can be used for velocity imaging. Cellular array computers and electrically reconfigurable logic arrays should enable a higher data throughput than Transputer based systems (Hayes et al 1992).

An alternative method for obtaining the velocity profiles is known as 'vector tomography'. This uses ultrasonic sensors to measure velocity data, from which the velocity profile is obtained by tomographic reconstruction. The potential of vector tomography is being investigated at Karlsruhe University (section 3.1.4).

e)   *Process control using tomographic image data* A tomographic image can provide the measurements at selected locations of internal process parameters which are critical to the optimal control of a process. Numerous opportunities for process control of plant exist and remain to be developed. For example, component control in pipelines, control of solids distribution in crystallisers, homogeneity of mixing processes, solids flow in bunkers. Thus state variables directly associated with optimal operation could be used for process control, the state being actually measured rather than estimated from other measured parameters. Such measurements for process control would be based on localised information, so simplified tomographic measurement systems could be used.

f) *Scale-up* Early applications of process tomography are to research and pilot scale plants of modest dimensions.   An advantage of electrical field methods for tomographic imaging is that they are intrinsically able to be scaled-up (and down). Indeed electrical conductivity imaging has been used on a terrestrial scale (Dines & Lytle 1981). Optical and ionising radiation methods are also amenable to scale-up. Ultrasonic methods may be more problematic because the relatively low velocity of sound results in image frame-speed limitations (section 3.1.4).

7.   CONCLUSIONS

Some process tomography systems (resistive and capacitive impedance) are available for immediate application to two-phase processes where the resolution and speed requirements are modest (say 1 in 20 of projection distance and 100 frames per second respectively). For more stringent applications, sensors having improved signal-to-noise ratios need to be developed and more accurate image reconstruction algorithms need to be implemented. This work demands using the latest methods for sensor design and construction, and for interpreting the extensive range of mathematical techniques for image reconstruction into effective signal processing algorithms.

REFERENCES

Abdullah M Z, Quick S V and Dickin F J 1992 Quantitative algorithm and computer architecture for real-time image reconstruction in process tomography *Proc. European Concerted Action on Process Tomography (Manchester) 26-29 March 1992*

Barber D C and Brown B H 1984 Applied potential tomography *J. Phys E 17 723-733*

Dickin F J, Hoyle B S, Hunt A, Huang S M, Ilyas O, Lenn C, Waterfall R C, Williams R A, Xie C G and Beck M S 1992 Tomographic imaging of industrial process equipment: techniques and applications *IEE Proc.-G 139 72-82*

Dines K A and Lytle R J 1981 Analysis of electrical conductivity imaging *Geophysics 46 1025-36*

Dugdale P, Green R G, Hartley A J, Jackson R G and Landauro J 1992 Optical sensors for process tomography *Proc. European Concerted Action on Process Tomography (Manchester) 26-29 March 1992*

Gai H, Li Y C, Plaskowski A and Beck M S 1989a Ultrasonic flow imaging using time-resolved transmission mode tomography *IEE 3rd International Conf. on Image Processing and its Applications, Warwick University*

Gai H, Beck M S and Flemons R S 1989b An integral transducer/pipe structure for flow imaging *IEEE 3rd International Ultrasonic Symposium, Montreal Canada*

Goble J C and Gallagher T D 1988 A distributed architecture for medical instrumentation: and electrical current computed tomograph *Proc. Annu. Int. Conf. IEEE Engineering in Medicine and Biology Society* **10** 285-6

Halow J S, Fasching G E and Nicoletti P 1990 from Advances in fluidisation engineering, *AlChem.E Symposium Series 276* **86** 41-50

Hayes D G, Gregory I A and Beck M S 1992 Velocity profile measurement in two-phase flows *Proc. European Concerted Action on Process Tomography (Manchester) 26-29 March 1992*

Huang S M, Xie C G, Thorn R, Snowden D and Beck M S 1992a Design of sensor electronics for electrical capacitance tomography *IEE Proc.-G* **139** 83-88

Huang S M, Xie C G, Vasina J, Lenn C, Zhang B F and Beck M S. 1992b Experimental evaluation of capacitance tomographic flow imaging systems using physical models *Proc. European Concerted Action on Process Tomography (Manchester) 26-29 March 1992*

Isaacson D 1986 Distinguishability of conductivities by electric current computed tomography *IEEE Trans.Medical Imaging* **MI-5** 91-5

Khan S.H and Abdullah F. 1992 Validation of finite element modelling of multielectrode capacitive system for process tomography flow imaging *Proc. European Concerted Action on Process Tomography (Manchester) 26-29 March 1992*

Lyon G M and Oakley J P 1992 A digital signal processor based architecture for E I T data acquisition *Proc. European Concerted Action on Process Tomography (Manchester) 26-29 March 1992*

Mewes D, Fellhölter and Renz R 1992 Measurement of mixing phenomena in gas and liquid flow *Proc. European Concerted Action on Process Tomography (Manchester) 26-29 March 1992*

Parker D J, Hawkesworth M R, Benyon T D and Bridgewater J 1992 Process engineering studies using positron-based imaging techniques *Proc. European Concerted Action on Process Tomography (Manchester) 26-29 March 1992*

Plaskowski A, Bukalski P, Habdas T and Szuster K 1992 Application of the optical tomography for education and laboratory research *Proc. European Concerted Action on Process Tomography (Manchester) 26-29 March 1992*

Seagar A D, Barber D C and Brown B H 2987 Theoretical limits to sensitivity and resolution in impedance imaging *Clin. Phys. Physiol. Meas. 8 Suppl A. 13-31*

Simons S J R, Seville J P K, Clift R, Gilboy W B and Hosseini-Ashrafi M E 1992 Application of gamma-ray tomography to gas fluidised and spouted beds *Proc. European Concerted Action on Process Tomography (Manchester) 26-29 March 1992*

Thorn R, Huang S M, Xie C G, Salkeld J A, Hunt A, and Beck M S 1990 Flow imaging for multi-component flow measurement *Flow Meas. Instrum. 1 259-268*

Wang M, Dickin F J and Beck M S, 1992 Improved electrical impedance tomography data collection system and measurement protocols *Proc. European Concerted Action on Process Tomography (Manchester) 26-29 March 1992*

Weigand F and Hoyle B S 1989 Simulations for parallel processing of ultrasound reflection-mode tomography with applications to two-phase flow measurement *IEEE Trans. Ultrasonics, Ferroelectrics & Freq. Control 36 6*

Wernsdörfer A 1992 Reconstruction from limited data with a-priori knowledge *Proc. European Concerted Action on Process Tomography (Manchester) 26-29 March 1992*

Xie C G, Huang M S, Hoyle B S, Thorn R, Lenn C, Snowden D and Beck M S 1992 Electrical capacitance tomography for flow imaging: system model for development of image reconstruction algorithms and design of primary sensors *IEE Proc.-G 139 89-97*

Yang W Q and Stott A L 1992 Low value capacitance measurements for process tomography *Proc. European Concerted Action on Process Tomography (Manchester) 26-29 March 1992*

Yu Z Z, Conway W F, Dickin F J, Xie C G, Beck M S and Xu L A.1992 Field design for electromagnetic tomography systems *Proc. ICEMI 92 Conf. Tianjin University China 20-23 October 1992*

APPENDIX 1

The ECAPT Process Tomography Information System

Richard Taylor

Adaptive Systems Engineering Group
Department of Electronics
University of York
York Y01 5DD

email : rwt@uk.ac.york.ohm
tel : (+44) 904 432351 (direct line) fax : (+44) 904 432335

Abstract

This paper describes the development and current status of the ECAPT Process Tomography Database system. The database is intended to provide a range of services, including

1. a comprehensive collection of references relating directly to process tomography theory, practice and applications;

2. the minutes of meetings held by the consortium;

3. other information held to be of use by the consortium (including references to supporting systems, conference details etc...).

4. a central facility for the distribution of database material to members of the ECAPT consortium.

1   Organisation

The database is held centrally on a MIPS RS2360, a Reduced Instruction Set Computer with a total of 1GByte of Disk space and 32 MBytes of silicon memory based at the University of York. This is connected into the JANET (and hence European Academic Network, EARN) through both a "Coloured Book" and an "Internet Protocol" connection. In practice, these two standards mean that it is possible for most computer systems used within the academic community to connect to and extract data from the database server.

The database held on the MIPS processor is the master database, all other databases distributed from the University of York are subsets of this. The system is backed up every morning at 1.00am in case of system failure, and is maintained under an 8 working hour call out scheme. In practice, this means that should the hardware fail, all data present and submitted up to the previous backup is secure, and the machine will be "on line" again within 8 working hours.

2   Contents

The database has been developed to hold information that will improve the performance of members of the ECAPT initiative. The database is therefore maintaining three distinct information bases.

- references and notes directly applicable to process tomography;
- references and notes that support process tomography (such as references to suitable computer architectures);
- published minutes of meetings held by process tomography groups.

3   Distribution

There are four means of obtaining data;

1. by sending mail to the database server, requesting complete copies of the files held by the server;
2. by logging in to the database server and making requests for specific items;
3. by requesting an IBM or Macintosh format disk with the "raw data" (similar to (1) above for those people without access to electronic mail);
4. by requesting an IBM or Macintosh format disk with the data held in a bibliographic database format called "EndNote".

Data is entered into the database in one of two ways;

1. by submission of a new entry through electronic mail (it will then be viewed, checked for accuracy and entered at York);
2. by a regular search of an online database, INSPEC.

```
%A  L Lamport
%T  LaTeX, Users Guide and Reference Manual.
%D  1986
%P  Addison Wesley
```

Figure 1: A sample of the Unix refer format

4   Database format

There is obviously a problem in standardising on a database format - that of compatibility. We have decided to make use of a combination of the Unix 'refer' and LaTeX BiBTeX formats. These both have the very great advantages that they are widely used and easily incorporated into other proprietary database formats. In addition, they are public domain and cost nothing to use. Refer is used to hold all of the "master" database, and the BibTeX database is derived from this. The BibTeX format, a more complex notation, is described completely in the reference shown in figure 1.

4.1   Refer

The refer format is made up of simple text files. In practice, this means that the file can be edited using any text editor or word processor. Each reference item is made up from a number of fields. Each field begins with a *field tag* which is a percentage sign (%) followed by a single letter identifying the kind of information in the reference field. Not all reference fields need to be present to make up a complete reference.

The complete list of reference fields recognised by the system is shown below

key	meaning
A	Author Name
B	Title of Book
C	City of Publication
D	Date of Publication
E	Editor of Book
F	Citation to insert into text
G	Government (ISBN) label
H	Header
I	Publisher (Issuer)
J	Journal Name
K	Keywords (for searching)
N	Issue Number
O	Other Information
P	Selected pages of document
Q	Corporate author
R	Technical report number
S	Series title
T	Title
U	Volume number in series
V	Volume number
W	Where it can be found
X	Abstract
Y	Series editor of book
Z	Total length of document
1	Number of characters in record
2	MSc Thesis
3	PhD Thesis

The fields 1,2 3 have been defined by the project to extend the basic database format.

5 Accessing the database through Electronic Mail

5.1 Addresses

In order to access the database in "batch" mode, you are required to submit a request to the database informing it what information you require, it then mails the results of your enquiry back. The database is currently held on a machine called *ohm* within the Electronics Department at the University of York. The full address of the information server is

```
info-server@uk.ac.york.ohm
```

if you are using a Unix based machine. Users of other machines (such as DEC VMS systems, probably the other common machine within Academia) will need to discuss how the address above translates for their machine with their local computer manager.

5.2   Formatting your requests

This information server will send out files contained in mail messages, in response to a request contained in a mail message, that you have sent it.

5.2.1   Basic Requests

Requests are of the form:

```
Request: subject Topic: topic within that subject Request: end
```

As an example suppose you want to be mailed information about tomography in the subject catalogue. You would send a message of the form:

```
Request: catalogue topic: tomography request: end
```

and the tomography information would be mailed back to you. The key words supported by the information server are: **request, topic** and **line-limit**.

These can be upper or lower case or a mixture. They are separated from the remainder of the line by tabs, spaces or : this is optional.

5.2.2   Line and Data Limits

Line-limit is for use by people who have mail systems that can only deal with small messages. Consider the following request:

```
line-limit 1000 Request: catalogue topic: tomography topic
computing request: end
```

This would mail out tomography and computing information in 1000 line chunks (Not including message header information). The line limit must lie between 1000 and 200000000. The default is send the file in 1 message. Everything after the "request end" is ignored.

Most mail systems will not handle messages of more than 100KBytes of data. All files within the system are limited so that they do not contain more than 100KBytes. In order to do this, some files have had to be split. In each case, these files are labeled "part1", "part2" etc. . . .

5.2.3   Compound Requests

Requests may be made up of a number of different topics. A complex request could look like this:

```
line-limit 2000 Request: catalogue topic: tomography topic
computing line-limit 3000 Request: computing topic: x_refs
topic:::index request: end
```

5.2.4 Top Level Requests

A list of the "top level" requests can be obtained by sending the following request to the info-server:

```
request: index topic: index request: end
```

5.2.5 Index and help information

Within a request subject, an index and also help information are available. These would be (using catalogue as the subject example).

```
request: catalogue topic: index (or help) request end
```

5.2.6 Finally

All blank lines are ignored, and the "request end" is optional, however if it is omitted and there are other lines in the message an automatic error message will be sent to you.

6   Using the 'online' database facility

This facility has been developed recently and is still being β tested. This mode of access requires that the user be able to log directly into ohm. As with section 5, it is assumed that the Unix operating system is being used. Users of other operating systems will need to refer to their system manager in order to translate these notes.

6.0.7 Logging on

Logging in can be achieved using either the **telnet** program, which is included in the Unix operating system. This is probably best achieved by referring to the database server by *Internet number*. The Internet number for ohm is 144.32.128.21. An example of using telnet is given below

```
%telnet 144.32.128.21
Trying...
Connected to 144.32.128.21.
Escape character is '^]'.


RISC/os (glenlivet)

login: tomography

*******************************************************************
* Welcome to the ECAPT Tomography Database.                       *
*                                                                 *
```

```
* Available Commands                                                 *
*   query - query database                                          *
*   help  - provides online help information                        *
*   news  - news relating to the operation of the database          *
*   quit  - exit the database                                       *
*                                                                    *
*********************************************************************

command>
```

Once logged in to the system you are placed in what is known as a 'restricted shell'. This allows you to perform four basic operations, *query*, *help*, *news* and *quit*.

6.0.8   Querying the database

The query command is extremely simple. The user is able to search the database on any of the fields described in section 4.1. Fields can be combined using both AND and OR operators. This is probably best illustrated using an example. A stop character (.) is used to terminate the search.

Suppose that we wish to search for all references with the word chicken (the system is case insensitive, CHICKEN = ChICKen = chicken).

```
command> query all chicken .

Database Query, Search : ALL, String : chicken Records found : 3

%A A Chicken
%T Salmonella, the case for.
%D June 1991
%P University of Milsquawkee
%2


%A Colonel Saunders
%T Kentucky Fried, the true story.
%D January 1991
%P A Restaurant
%O A Chicken likkin' good story


%A F Reynard
%T Twenty years of coops - or chickens unlimited.
%D July 1991
%I Hunting Press
%O No chicken this dawg

command>
```

If on the other hand we wished to find all references that contain chicken in the **Author** field, then it is necessary to conduct a selective search.

```
command> query
%A chicken


Database Query, Search : AUTHOR, String : chicken Records found : 1

%A A Chicken
%T Salmonella, the case for.
%D June 1991
%P University of Milsquawkee
%2

command>
```

Searching for all references that include the word coops in the title and are published by the Hunting Press is achieved using the AND operator, for example

```
command> query
%T coops
AND
%P Hunting Press
.


Database Query, Search : TITLE, String : coops Database Query, Search
: PUBLISHER, String : Hunting Press Records found : 1

%A F Reynard
%B Twenty years of coops.%
%D July 1991
%I Hunting Press
%O No chicken this dawg

command>
```

Full details of how to use the system are provided by the online 'help' command. As additional facilities are provided, these will be included in the help file.

7   EndNote

EndNote is a proprietary database intended for use on IBM and Macintosh microcomputers. It has been chosen as the most appropriate standard that is compatible with most popular types of microcomputer. EndNote is produced by *Niles and Associates, 200 Hearst*

St, Berkeley, CA 94709 in the United States of America, and distributed by *Cherwell Scientific Publishers* in the United Kingdom. It is an effective and comprehensive database for maintaining bibliographies, with the added advantage of interfacing with many common word processor standards.

8   Additions and Amendments to the Database

The bulk of additions to the database are through the use of general purpose, online databases. There are facilities provided however for individual users to make additions and ammendments.

Additions should be made through electronic mail, preferably in the "refer" format. Mail should be addressed to rwt@uk.ac.york.ohm with the message subject line tomography :   additions. These are then checked and incorporated into a suitable section of the database as soon as possible.

Amendments should also be submitted through electronic mail to rwt@uk.ac.york.ohm with the message subject line tomography :   amendments. These will be incorporated as soon as possible.

9   Usage

9.1   Mail Queries

In the eight months of full time operation, the database has provided 135 complete sets of references to fifteen Academic sites. Of these, only one set of references have been provided to a University outside of the United Kingdom. Twenty five sets of references have been 'repeat' requests.

9.2   Online Queries

Online queries have only been available for a very short time and have only been accessed by our β testers.

9.3   Disk distribution : Raw data

Three complete sets of 'raw' data have been provided to three academic sites.

9.4   Disk Distribution : EndNote data

Five complete sets of EndNote data, all in Apple Macintosh format have been provided to four academic sites.

10   Conclusions and further work

The bulk of the work on the database to date has been in the development of standards, procedures and software to maintain and store the tomography data. Although the total number of requests to the database have been relatively low, we expect that the introduction of an online query system, combined with the use of a personal computer based format will extend the user base.

We are currently investigating the possibility of providing a discount on the "EndNote" package through bulk purchase, and hope that this will bring the local database service to those members of the tomography community without electronic mail facilities.

APPENDIX 2

SPECIAL INTEREST GROUP ON DATA ACQUISITION HARDWARE

Introduction

An ad-hoc group of workers interested in EIT data acquisition hardware met on the evening of Thursday 26 March. The general theme of the discussion was to discover whether it would be possible to collaborate to produce a general-purpose hardware 'kit', that would form the basis of a general-purpose process tomography unit.

Requirements

Ideally, one design of instrument would be available that would be used for teaching purposes and basic investigations. Research projects often need great flexibility or performance approaching the limits of theoretical performance. On the other hand, industrial users want a turn-key operation, preferably at low-cost but certainly reliable in use. The typical process engineer is pleased to accept improved instrumentation, as long as he is convinced it will be trouble-free and produce useful results but is unlikely to be pressing for major new innovations. From this discussion, it was clear that one measurement unit would not satisfy everyone but nevertheless it was considered that the production of a basic research tool was a worthwhile goal.

Design of a flexible measurement system

It seems probable that a system would be based on digital signal processing chips (dsp's) but it is unclear whether Analog Devices, Texas Instruments or Motorola etc. produce the most suitable family. Most designers use the family with which they are most familiar and for which they have the best software and hardware support. The general conclusion was that the precise choice of components was probably secondary to factors such as 'user-friendliness'. cost and reliability.

A general purpose system should be able to measure both real and imaginary components of signals and operate across a range of frequencies. The lowest common denominator of a general purpose system could demand a very high performance design. Consideration of the approaches adopted by the Medical Tomography research groups is necessary as valuable lessons can be learned from their experience.

Providing Commonality

If possible, a manufacturer should be funded to produce a set of kits for data acquisition that could then be borrowed by research groups. In the UK, SERC have funded and administered this kind of activity previously (e.g. the Transputer Initiative). The Department of Trade and Industry might be another source of support. On the European scale, then the European Community would have to be approached via programmes such as Brite-Euram.

At a low level of activity, it might be possible to hold information of general interest on the ECAPT data-base. People with operational designs could contribute these for common use. Chris McLeod of Oxford Polytechnic volunteered some of his designs for electrode drivers, including printed-circuit board layouts, parts lists etc.

Conclusions

Everyone agreed that some form of future collaboration on data acquisition hardware was necessary and worthwhile on a European scale. It was also felt that a more intensive workshop meeting dedicated to the problems associated with the design and operation of data acquisition hardware was necessary and that this suggestion be put forward to the ECAPT management committee. Fraser Dickin agreed to contact the members of the ad-hoc group to canvas their opinions on hardware design contributions and the possibility of a separate workshop meeting.

Attendees at the meeting

Dr F J Dickin	EE & E UMIST
Mr H Grootveld	TU Delft, Netherlands
Mr A Lewis	UC London
Mr G Lyon	EE Manchester University
Dr C McLeod	Oxford Polytechnic
Dr J Oakley	EE Manchester University
Prof R Pallas-Areny	University P. Cataluña, Spain
Dr P Riu	UPC Spain
Mr J Torrents	UPC Spain
Mr M Wang	EE & E UMIST
Dr R C Waterfall	EE & E UMIST
Mr X Zhao	EE & E UMIST

R C Waterfall

APPENDIX 3

An overview of biomedical applications of Electrical Impedance Tomography.

D.S. Holder. Departments of Physiology, University College, and Clinical Neurophysiology, The Maudsley Hospital, London.

Abstract : Electrical impedance tomography is a recently developed technique in which reconstructed tomographic images of the resistive component of impedance can be made with a ring of external electrodes. Its applications in medicine and physiology are reviewed. For practical purposes, almost all results have been obtained with the "Sheffield" design. This employs 16 electrodes operating at 50 kHz and employs a simple non-iterative algorithm. Its advantages are that it is inexpensive, portable and non-invasive and so is suitable for continuous measurement at the bedside. Set against this are a relatively poor spatial resolution, sensitivity to off-plane events, and a requirement that the initial resistivity of the subject is uniform. It has been shown quantitatively to be accurate in measuring gastric emptying and total lung ventilation. Preliminary studies suggest that it might successfully be used to image gastrointestinal motility, lung ventilation and perfusion.   Other suggested uses include imaging of hyperthermia, brain function, pelvic blood congestion and fracture healing.

1. Introduction.

1.1. Scope and purpose of this review.

There is rapidly increasing interest in tomography based on electromagnetic measurement. This ranges from geophysical measurement to industrial applications and biomedical recording. This work is intended as an overview of clinical and physiological applications of electrical impedance tomography (EIT). It is intended for an audience without a biomedical background, but familiarity with common medical or anatomical terms will be assumed.

There are several areas in clinical medicine where EIT might provide advantages over existing techniques. These have been have been reviewed previously (Brown, Barber and Seagar, 1984; Dawids, 1987; Brown, 1990; Bhat, 1991). The majority of papers concerning medical EIT use have been gathered in symposium proceedings concerning all aspects of EIT design and use organised as part of a special EC initiative in EIT (Brown, Barber and Tarassenko, 1987; Brown, Barber and Jossinet, 1988; Hames, 1990; Brown and Barber, 1992).   Many publications since 1984 have addressed clinical opportunities by demonstrating that images performed on a small number of subjects are consistent with the intended applications. More recently, and especially at a recent meeting devoted solely to clinical applications of EIT in April, 1992 (Holder, *in press(a)*), there have been larger studies in which the results of EIT images have been compared objectively to results from existing methods.

This review includes findings from these more recent quantitative papers. It is intended to present the background and development of biomedical applications of EIT and address the issues : What are the limitations and advantages of current EIT systems ? In what biomedical areas does it seem that EIT could offer significant advantages over existing techniques?

1.2. Current development of biomedical EIT systems.

With impedance measurement in biological tissue below 100 kHz, the great majority of current travels in the extracellular fluid. The resistive component of the complex therefore dominates impedance measurements. As a result, all practical interest in medical impedance tomography has revolved around impedance imaging of the resistive component of the complex impedance. The term "Electrical impedance tomography" has been used to denote this; some groups have also termed it "Applied potential tomography" (APT). In this review the terms "impedance" and "resistance" will be used interchangeably.

Although other groups had published some theoretical ideas on the subject (see Iskander and Durney, 1980; Kim et al, 1983), biomedical applications started for practical purposes after 1983 when a group in medical physics at the Royal Hallamshire Hospital, Sheffield designed a prototype device which was suitable for human use (Barber, Brown and Freeston, 1983; Barber and Brown, 1984). This was demonstrated to be effective in human subjects and soon became available for the use of other groups on a commercial basis. Over thirty of these devices have now been constructed and have been used for clinical studies. There are now about twenty groups worldwide which are actively engaged in developing hardware and software for clinical application of EIT, and a further ten or so which have published clinical studies using commercially available systems. In practice, the approach used by the Sheffield group has been the only one to yield satisfactory images in human subjects. Unless otherwise stated, all the reports cited in this review have employed the original Sheffield "Mark 1" system.

This system employs 16 electrodes in a ring. Measurement is made with a "four electrode" system (Brown, 1983), as this minimizes electrode artefacts . A constant current of 5 mA or less at 50 kHz is applied sequentially to adjacent pairs of electrodes; for each driven electrode pair, 13 serial measurements of potential difference are made from all remaining adjacent electrode pairs. 208 measurements are made in about 80 msec; these constitute 104 independent measurements, as reversal of the drive and record pair for a given four electrodes provides the same information. The greatest temporal resolution is therefore 40 msec. Many images may be averaged together to reduce noise. They may also be repeatedly averaged after gating to the ECG, in order to provide pulse-related data. These 104 potential differences are reconstructed into an image on an IBM-compatible personal computer in about 5 sec. The algorithm is relatively crude but robust with respect to vagaries in electrode placement. Only differences in images are imaged : a reference frame is made at the outset of any recording and subsequent images show differences from the reference. This is termed "dynamic" imaging, in contrast to "static" imaging in which a single image of the absolute impedance is generated. The algorithm works on the basis that the measurement made with any four electrodes reflects the change in resistivity of a truncated crescent which lies between the drive and recording pairs. The borders of this volume are taken to be the isopotentials which extend from between the drive electrodes and end on the two potential recording electrodes. In reality, these lines of isopotential will be irregular and depend on the exact resistivities of the tissues within the subject. For simplicity, they are calculated on the basis that the subject has uniform resistivity. Reconstruction is achieved by weighted back-projection of all such sectors. Spatial resolution is improved by a deblurring filtering algorithm (see Barber and Seagar, 1987; Brown and Seagar, 1987; Barber (in press).

This arrangement is practicable, but clearly has certain limitations. Research is actively in progress to improve the performance of EIT systems, but the theoretical advantages of other approaches have not yet been realized in practice in human subjects. Major areas of development at present include : 1) Improved data acquisition. Use of 128 electrodes could in theory produce a spatial resolution of 1% of the diameter of the electrode array (Barber and Brown, 1984). Preliminary results with 32 electrode systems have been reported (Fuks et al, 1991). Alternative current drive arrangements should give better signal-to-noise ratios in the centre of the image, and absolute images may become possible (see Webster, 1990). 2) Improved reconstruction algorithms. The Sheffield system only uses one iteration. Superior iterative algorithms have been proposed. These require greater computing power and time, but rapid reconstruction should become possible, especially with the use of parallel computers (Paulson et al, 1990; Isaacson et al, 1992; see Webster, 1990). 3) Generation of "static" images. Improved algorithms have been developed which generate images of absolute impedance in a single measurement. Whilst this approach can produce reasonable results in a saline tank (Isaacson et al, 1990; Fuks et al, 1991; Newell et al, in press), there are not yet any satisfactory clinical images. This is largely because reconstruction is very sensitive to uncertainties in electrode positions which are unfortunately present in all clinical recordings. Other areas under development include imaging at multiple frequencies (Griffiths and Zhang, 1989, Riu et al (*in press*)) and in three dimensions (Goble and Isaacson, 1990).

The data acquisition performance of the Sheffield system has recently been improved. The principal difference is that potentials are measured with a parallel rather than a serial arrangement, and a transputer is used for image reconstruction. It is therefore possible to produce images in real time and with improved signal-to-noise ratios. This device is likely to become commercially available in the near future and will be called the "Sheffield Mark II" system (Smith et al, 1990; Sinton et al, 1992).

1.3. Advantages and limitations of current EIT systems.

The Sheffield Mark 1 and similar systems are practical but several limitations may be predicted from an understanding of their design : 1) Spatial resolution. There are 104 independent measurements and hence possible pixels in an image. This corresponds to maximum spatial resolution of about 10% of the electrode ring diameter. However, the reconstruction is unlikely to be perfect and current density will be greatest at the edges of a subject and fall off towards the centre. It might therefore be expected that spatial resolution will be worse than this, and will vary with the position within an image. 2) Off-plane impedance changes. The electrodes are in a two-dimensional ring, and images are generated on the assumption that all events occur in the electrode plane. In practice in biological subjects, current will travel out of the electrode plane in both directions, so that off-plane impedance changes will affect the image. As the algorithm does not take account of this, off-plane changes at a particular position in the electrode plane might be mapped to a different site in the image. This could be an important source of error. 3) Distortion due to assumption of initial constant resistivity. The algorithm assumes that the initial resistivity of the subject is uniform. Clearly, this is unlikely to be the case in a biological subject, and it might be expected that these effects will degrade image quality. 4) Imaging of impedance differences only. The imaging procedure has been designed to image only the difference between a specified reference image and subsequent images. 5) Assumption of a circular electrode array. It is assumed that the electrodes are equally spaced and form a circle. Any deviation from this will result in a distortion in the image. 6) It is assumed that tissues are isotropic i.e. that the impedance is independent of the direction of applied current. This is a reasonable assumption for many tissues which are composed of spherical cells, but will be untrue in tissues such as bone, muscle or white matter in the brain.

The Sheffield Mark 1 and similar systems, on the other hand, have a number of important advantages : 1) They are non-invasive. Currents used are safer than limits required by British Standards and do not damage or excite tissue. 2) The equipment is portable. The system comprises a box containing electronic circuits which is about the size of a video recorder and is attached to a microcomputer. It can be placed at the bedside or on a laboratory bench. The electronics can be made much smaller if needed. An EIT system intended for use in space consisted of a small box little larger than a pencil case which was attached to a similar sized box containing a handheld computer for data storage (Lindley et al, *in press*). 3) The system costs about £15,000 sterling at present. It is therefore far less expensive than other imaging devices such as X-ray computer tomography or Positron Emission Tomography. 4) The temporal resolution is 40 msec (25 frames may be collected per second). Temporal resolution of a few tens of microseconds could be produced by averaging after repeated stimuli; individual potential measurements could be saved in separate memory bins and combined subsequently. 5) Small impedance changes of less than 1% can be reliably discriminated (Holder, *in press(b)*). 6) Impedance changes in a characteristic way in certain physiological conditions.

EIT might therefore provide a uniquely practical imaging method in a clinical or research situation where continuous images are required over a protracted period.

2. Calibration studies in saline filled tanks.

Several factors will influence the performance of EIT systems in real measuring situations. It is difficult to insert objects of known impedance into human subjects, but EIT systems can be calibrated with the use of tanks filled with saline solution. These measurements made in tanks reproduce the important effects of the impedance of electrodes and stray capacitance, but not uncertain electrode placement or non-uniform initial resistivity. Measurements from tanks, in general, represent an upper limit for the performance of EIT systems *in vivo*.

In general, tank studies have confirmed a performance which could be predicted from an understanding of the design of the Sheffield system. Images are not true representations of the impedance in reality. Only impedance differences can be imaged; these differences are mapped to the image in a way which varies according to the position of the disturbance in the electrode plane. The same disturbance produces a smaller but more blurred impedance change towards the image centre (Eyuboglu et al, 1989; Thomas et al, *in press)*. The spatial resolution may be defined as the distance apart two objects need to be in order to discriminated apart. A suitable criterion for this is that the impedance change falls off to a value of 1/e of the average of the peaks. In the plane of the electrodes it is roughly 12% of the electrode array diameter at the edge and 20% in the centre of the image (Eyuboglu et al, 1989a; Holder, 1992a). Off-plane changes are mapped to the image in way which is unpredictable; if a given pixel in an image shows a change which is due to an off-plane event, it does not follow that the event took place vertically above or below the equivalent position in the electrode plane (Eyuboglu et al, 1989a; Holder, *in press(b)*). It therefore is most unlikely that existing systems could be applied usefully in clinical situations which required accurate true representations of the magnitude and position of impedance changes.

On the other hand, the systems can reliably detect small impedance changes of a few per cent with a good signal-to-noise ratio, as image noise is a small fraction of 1% (Sinton et al, 1992; Holder, *in press (b)*). It might therefore be expected that EIT could best be used clinically in situations where a single parameter needed to be obtained over time in a non-invasive way, and where the localization in space was of secondary importance.

3. Possible biomedical applications.

There are several areas in clinical medicine and physiology where it has been suggested that EIT could offer significant advantages over existing methods. Some reports merely propose the idea, and present relevant preliminary measurements. The majority present preliminary EIT images in a small number of subjects; more recently, other studies have addressed the quantitative accuracy of EIT imaging in statistically significant numbers of subjects. Suggested applications, and the evidence to support their use, are reviewed in this section.

Many studies employ "region of interest" analysis. This procedure can easily be performed with the software which accompanies the Sheffield systems. A series of EIT images is collected over tens of minutes. At the end of data collection, all the images are summed together. By inspection, it is usually possible to determine an area where the maximum impedance change occurred. A region of interest is defined over this area, and the sum of the impedance changes in all pixels in this area is then calculated for each image in turn. This yields a single parameter for each image which is expressed in arbitrary units. This will be termed the "region of interest integral" below. This method has the advantage that the method of measurement remains constant in any one data set, and can be optimized for individual patients. However, the criteria by which an operator selects the region are not explicitly defined, so the method is subject to observer error.

3.1. Gastrointestinal system.

An area of study where it might be expected that EIT could be useful is in measuring the regular movements of the stomach or bowel, which are an essential part of the digestive process. Broadly, these can be divided into the emptying of the stomach, which takes about half an hour, or the more rapid regular contractions of the bowel, which are termed peristalsis. Electrodes can be applied with ease around the abdomen, and there are no large bony structures likely to violate the assumption of constant initial resistivity. During gastrointestinal motor activity, there are relatively large movements of the conducting fluids within the bowel. Finally, the quantity of interest is the *timing* of activity; the absolute impedance change, and its exact location in space are of secondary importance. Timing determination can be obtained by normalizing data within each subject, so that the principal limitations of EIT of poor spatial resolution and amplitude measurement are largely circumvented.

There is a need for a non-invasive means of measuring gut motor activity, especially gastric emptying. This can be measured with radioactive tracers, radiography, dye dilution using gastric intubation, or serial blood measurement following drug administration, but all are unpleasant or invasive (see Avill et al, 1987). They are therefore unsuitable for paediatric use, or for repeated determinations over time.

EIT has been widely used for measuring gastric emptying. A test meal, usually of 200-500 ml of a conductive drink or semi-solid, is given after electrodes are placed around the upper abdomen. Images are then collected every minute or so over an hour or more. It is usually possible to identify a region of decreased impedance in subsequent analysis. This is identified manually, and a plot of the integral of impedance changes within this area is made for all images. The time to half emptying is calculated with respect to the largest change, which occurs immediately after ingestion (see, for example, Devane, *in press*). This method has been shown to compare well with other standard methods in adults, provided gastric acid secretion is suppressed by appropriate drugs (Avill et al, 1987). In infants, acid suppression has not been used. It has been shown to be qualitatively accurate in diagnosing pyloric stenosis, a serious condition in newborn babies in which muscle enlargement prevents the outflow of food from the stomach (Lamont et al, 1988). On the other hand, EIT was quantitatively inaccurate in determining absolute gastric volumes 20 min following ingestion of a test meal (Devane, *in press*).

The physiological mechanisms which give rise to the image are not entirely clear and presumably depend on the nature and volume of the test meal. Impedance in the presumed gastric area in EIT images has been shown to vary because of the physical presence of matter of different resistivity to abdominal contents (Avill et al, 1987) or because of a change in resistivity due to altered acidity (Baxter et al, 1988). All test meals reported have been digestible, so the net effect seen in EIT images is presumably due to a combination of gastric emptying, which removes stomach contents from the sensitive volume, and a change in resistivity as digestion commences. Wright et al (*in press*) have investigated the effect of ingesting different test meals without suppression of acid secretion. In all cases, the impedance determined from EIT images fell. This is surprising, as the resistivity of some of the test meals was substantially greater than that of tissues such as liver, spleen and muscle (about 5 Ω.m (Geddes and Baker, 1967)) which were presumably displaced. For example, water had a resistivity of 33 Ω.m but caused apparent impedance decreases of 2 - 20%. The most likely explanation is that the effect of conductivity was paramount; presumably the water diluted ions pre-existent in the stomach and so had the effect of filling the stomach with a conducting solution.

Gastric emptying is the only clinical area in which EIT has been used as an established method in order to obtain results. A promising diagnostic application would be in detecting pyloric stenosis, so that radiography could be avoided (Lamont et al, 1988). It has been used to implicate disordered gut motility in the nausea which occurs in chronic kidney failure (Ravelli et al, *in press*). EIT images obtained after a porridge test meal revealed delayed gastric emptying in patients with dyspepsia and gastric infection due to Helicobacter pylori. This is a bacterium which has recently been discovered to be present in a high proportion of patients with gastric ulcers, but it is unclear if it is causative of the symptoms of this condition, or is merely a consequence of the underlying disorder. A causative role was supported by the finding that gastric emptying returned to normal in one patient following antibacterial treatment (Evans et al (*in press*)). Colonic loading by voluntary suppression of defaecation for four days produced a significant decrease in gastric emptying time

(Akkermans et al, *in press*).

Normally, acid in the stomach is prevented from refluxing into the gullet by a muscular sphincter. Unlike the stomach, the gullet is not protected from acid, so that reflux causes pain and inflammation. EIT has been shown to detect episodes of reflux (Ravelli and Milla), and so might be used as a convenient and non-invasive replacement for radiological investigation. Under normal circumstances, the stomach exhibits regular contractions at a rate of about 3 min^{-1}. Using frequency analysis, similar fluctuations in region of interest integrals from EIT recordings have been observed (Smallwood et al, *in press*; Devane et al, *in press*). However, although peaks in the spectrum of EIT records matched those made with other techniques, there was clearly substantial variability in individual traces. It remains to be determined if this could be sufficiently accurate to be used diagnostically. The migrating motor complex is a period of increased peristaltic activity lasting some tens of minutes which propagates from the stomach to the small bowel at intervals of about 100 min. The times of onset but not the durations, estimated from EIT region of interest integrals, have been shown to correlate significantly to records of pressure measured with swallowed radiotelemetry capsules (Wright and Evans, 1990).

EIT might also be used as a non-invasive index of gastric acid production if it could be ensured that gastric volume remained constant over the period of measurement.   Acid secretion following a drink of sherry has been measured by this method (Baxter et al, 1988). It is possible that EIT could be used routinely to replace direct gastric sampling in standard clinical tests for acid production (Baxter et al, 1988). However, although a significant correlation has been shown between EIT region of interest integrals and acid production after acid stimulation by pentagastrin, it is evident that there is a wide scatter in measurements around the best fit line (Baxter et al, 1988).   The diagnostic accuracy of such an application remains to be determined.

An ingenious possible application of EIT is in measurement of the time it takes for a bolus of food to be swallowed. There is a clinical need for such studies in patients with muscular or nervous weakness affecting the pharynx; liquid may be inhaled into the lungs and cause pneumonia. At present screening with X-rays is employed, but the dose of X-rays prevents repeated examination which is desirable over the course of an illness (Liu et al, 1992). Electrodes were placed around the neck and images were acquired during swallowing of a conductive solution. Substantial movement artefacts were reduced by subtracting images made whilst water was swallowed. The pharyngeal transit time may be calculated from the region of interest integral and fell within expected limits (Liu et al, 1992; Liu et al, *in press*), but no data directly comparing this method with other techniques are yet available.

3.2. Pulmonary function.

Lung pathology can be imaged with great precision by conventional radiography, X-ray computed tomography or magnetic resonance imaging, but there are clinical situations where it would be desirable to have a portable means of regional imaging which could, if necessary, generate repeated images over time. The impedance of lung tissue varies with inspiration, as air has a far higher resistivity than lung tissue itself. In dogs, the lung resistivity measured at 100kHz increased from 7.3 to 23.6 Ω.m on inspiration (Witsoe and Kinnen, 1967). The magnitude of impedance change might therefore be expected to be detected by EIT systems with a high signal-to-noise ratio. In humans, mean impedance determined from region of interest integrals increased by 250% on inspiration (Harris et al, 1987).   Unlike the abdomen, current applied by EIT systems will have to pass between the ribs. There are movements of the ribcage and thoracic tissues during respiration. The "thickness" of the volume to which EIT systems are sensitive is unknown, but significant amounts of current may pass into the abdomen if electrodes are placed around the lower thorax. Any images produced from a ring of electrodes placed around the thorax will therefore be a complex result of lung impedance changes and movement of tissues. No studies have addressed the contribution of these factors in EIT images, but current flow in the thorax has been extensively studied with respect to the older technique of impedance pneumography in which respiration is monitored using single channel impedance measurement. Although single channel impedance has been shown to be linearly related to diaphragmatic or chest wall respiration, it appears that the great majority of current passes around the lungs, and changes in chest geometry contribute significantly to the observed impedance changes (see (Baker, 1989) for a recent review).

Several investigators have obtained EIT images during respiration from electrodes placed in a ring around the chest at various levels. Usually, a reference image is obtained during breath holding at a particular level, and then other images are produced as the subject holds their breath at other levels. Harris et al (1988) modified the Sheffield APT system so that a single value from a defined region of interest could be calculated in real time. The change in this value during normal breathing could then be extracted off-line to give an index of ventilation. EIT images obtained during respiration with breath holding reveal two kidney shaped areas of impedance change either side of the midline if electrodes are placed around the 5-7th intercostal space anteriorly. The impedance change resembles an transverse hourglass if electrodes are placed higher. A localized impedance change of opposite polarity is usually seen in the central part of the image (Harris et al, 1987; Holder and Temple, *in press*). There is a good linear correlation between region of interest integrals and overall ventilation measured with a spirometer (Harris et al, 1988; Holder and Temple, *in press*). It therefore seems reasonable to assume that these changes represent lung ventilation, but it should be emphasized that there is no direct evidence to support or quantify this view. The origin of the opposite impedance change in the central image is unknown; it might represent compression of the mediastinum (Holder and Temple, *in press*). The magnitude of the impedance changes is larger centrally. This is presumably because current flow out of the plane of the electrodes will yield a larger signal towards the centre of the chest.

EIT might provide a useful non-invasive bedside method for monitoring during various bedside therapeutic procedures. An example is draining of a pleural effusion. This is a collection of fluid at the lateral bases of the lungs which can occur after inflammation or as a result of heart failure. It is usually aspirated with the aid of a needle inserted through the chest wall. Aspiration with a syringe is usually performed until no more fluid comes out. However, it may be that the needle is wrongly positioned, and fluid remains at a different site. These effusions can be easily seen on X-rays, but it is clearly impracticable to make these continuously. In practice, one is performed before and after the aspiration. As aspiration may need to be performed many times, this can lead to large doses of X-rays. It would be of considerable assistance if a non-invasive index of the success of the intervention were available at the bedside on a continuous basis (Morice et al, *in press*). Two preliminary studies have been encouraging : In cases of pleural effusion, lobar pneumonia and pneumothorax (air in the space between the lungs and chest wall) there were qualitative correspondences between EIT images and X-rays (Morice et al, *in press*). EIT abnormalities in a patient with a large lung cavity were consistent with the known abnormality (Harris et al, 1987). In contrast, Holder and Temple (*in press*) imaged ventilation in 30 normal and four abnormal subjects by placing electrodes at the 2nd or 7 ribs anteriorly in all subjects. The variation between normal subjects was such that the only patient whose EIT image could be clearly distinguished from the normals had absent ventilation in one entire lung due to obstruction of the main bronchial tube by a tumour. EIT images from patients with medium sized ventilation defects due to tumour, pulmonary embolus (blood clots in the lungs) or pleural effusion could not be distinguished from normals.

On the basis of existing evidence, it seems possible that EIT could be a useful method for monitoring changes in ventilation in the same patient during a procedure, or for measuring regional ventilation over protracted periods, perhaps in an intensive care unit. The variations between patients make it unlikely that it could be used for "once-off" diagnosis in individual patients in the near future.

A related possible application would be to monitor pulmonary oedoema over time in individual patients at risk of left heart failure or fluid overload. A clear fall in the region of interest integral determined from the presumed lung areas has been shown after the intravenous infusion of saline (Harris et al, 1988; Campbell et al, *in press*). There was considerable variation in both inter-

and intra-subject measurements, so it is not yet clear if this method will be sufficiently accurate to be of practical use.

3.3. EIT imaging of changes in blood volume.

The resistivity of blood is about 1.5 Ω.m, which is approximately one third of that of most intrathoracic tissues (see Geddes and Baker, 1967). It therefore seems possible that EIT images related to blood flow could be imaged. In practice, these are likely to be small : the imaged quantity will be the change in impedance due to replacement of tissue by blood (or vice versa) as a result of the pulse. This may be relatively large in the ventricles, but will be small in the peripheral lung fields, and is likely to be near the contrast resolution of EIT systems.

Thoracic EIT images synchronised to the pulse may be obtained with the Sheffield Mark 1 system. The frame rate is increased to 25 per second and noise is reduced by repeated averaging after triggering from the ECG. With this method, images represent the difference between two stages of the cardiac cycle. The heart comprises four main chambers. Blood returns from the body and from the lungs to the right and left sides of the heart, respectively. It first enters the low pressure atria and is pumped by them into the larger and more muscular ventricles. During "diastole" the ventricles are relaxed, and fill up with blood; during "systole" the ventricles contract and expel blood. The valves between the ventricles and atria are closed during this phase. Therefore at end-diastole the ventricles are full and the atria are empty. At end systole the reverse is true; the atria are full and the ventricles have emptied.

Reproducible impedance changes of 1-3% can be observed in various parts of the image if electrodes are placed around the chest (Killingbeck et al, *in press*). In an image showing the difference between end-systole and end-diastole, it would therefore be expected that impedance was increased in the area of the ventricles, and decreased in other areas corresponding to the atria, aorta, pulmonary arteries and lung fields. Such changes have been observed and appear to have the expected timing (Eyuboglu et al, 1987). In ten normals impedance reproducible mean peak impedance changes of +1.9%, -2.7%, and -0.8% were observed in areas respectively attributed to the ventricles, atria and lungs (Eyuboglu et al, 1989b). Similar reproducible changes have been observed in other studies (McArdle et al, 1988; Killingbeck et al, *in press*). It certainly appears reasonable that such changes are due to changes in blood volume within various vascular organs, but, as for pulmonary ventilation, there is no direct evidence to support this assertion. In an elegant indirect study, McArdle et al (*in press*) demonstrated that the impedance change visible in the presumed area of the heart is probably a mixture of changes of opposite polarity. This was achieved by comparing the images obtained normally, when atrial and ventricular volumes change in opposite directions, to those obtained when drugs were used to diminish the total amount of blood in the heart, when they change in the same direction. As the atria and ventricles are in reality less than 10% of the diameter of the chest apart, it is not surprising that the changes are blurred together, given that the spatial resolution of the system is likely to be worse than 15% of the electrode array diameter.   The physiological mechanisms which give rise to changes in EIT images have not been investigated directly, but studies of current flow have been undertaken with respect to the technique of impedance cardiography. With this method, cardiac output is estimated from single channel impedance measurements made with four electrodes, usually placed around the mid-thorax and neck. Contributions from the lungs, atria, aorta and ventricles can all contribute to impedance measured in this way(see (Patterson, 1989) for a recent review). Pulse related changes in EIT images are presumably due to the changes in blood volume, but may also be affected by movement of organs such as the ventricles during the cardiac cycle. A further contributing factor may be the rate of blood flow. As this increases, the poorly conducting red blood cells tend to line up along the centre of vessels, so that the impedance may decrease by up to 15% (Sakamato and Kanai, 1979).

An important possible use of EIT could be to diagnose pulmonary embolism. This is a condition in which blood clots form in leg or pelvic veins. They may break off into the venous circulation and then block the heart or lung vessels, with very serious consequences. Correct diagnosis is important, as treatment with anticoagulants is then mandatory. This is usually achieved by imaging pulmonary ventilation and perfusion with the use of inhaled or injected radioactive tracers. This is expensive and invasive; there is usually a wait of some days before it can be organized. If EIT could detect such changes, diagnosis could be performed at the bedside in a rapid and non-invasive way. In three patients with chest abnormalities, McArdle et al (1988) observed qualitative similarities between EIT and radiological images. EIT electrodes were positioned at the appropriate level with the benefit of the radiological data. In contrast, Holder and Temple (*in press*) produced pulse gated EIT images with electrodes at the 2nd or 7th rib anteriorly in 30 normal subjects and four with intrathoracic abnormalities. The variation in normals was such that the only abnormal subject whose EIT image could be distinguished from normal had absent perfusion in one entire lung; a moderately large pulmonary embolus could not be differentiated. Further studies may find ways of improving inter-subject variability, but the present evidence suggests that this is too great to permit accurate diagnosis of pulmonary embolism in a single subject in whom images had not been acquired previously under normal conditions.

Pulmonary embolism is often caused by deep venous thrombosis in the calf. This is usually diagnosed by venography : a radioopaque dye is injected into veins in the foot and serial X-rays are made to detect its passage through leg veins. This is uncomfortable and invasive, and also, in practice, takes several days to arrange. Preliminary data is available regarding two approaches which might provide a practical alternative using EIT : In one subject, Brown et al (1992) observed a peak impedance decrease of 3% in the forearm after intravenous injection of 10 ml of saline; this was followed 45 s later by a decrease of 0.4%. These were attributed respectively to saline passing through the arms veins and then through the radial artery after passing through the circulation. Kim et al (1989) obtained EIT images after placing 16 electrodes around the calf. The image was obtained after occlusion of venous return by inflation of a cuff; the reference was taken with no cuff inflation. Images were reconstructed with an iterative algorithm which took about 10 min on an IBM 4381 superminicomputer. A central impedance change was clearly observed. This was attributed to blood pooling in central veins, but it is unclear why a signal from peripheral veins could not be seen as well. The cuff inflation technique would be difficult to apply elsewhere than on a limb, but the saline injection technique might be used to improve signal discrimination of thoracic blood flow. Impedance decreases of 4% were observed in the ventricular region of thoracic EIT images following saline injection into a peripheral vein (Brown et al, 1992). This application is certainly attractive, but it remains to be determined if the resolution of EIT will be sufficient to give clinically useful images of peripheral venous drainage.

3.4. Hyperthermia.

Malignant tumours may be treated by artificially increasing temperature by microwave radiation or lasers. It is essential to monitor tissue temperature so that normal tissue is not heated, and malignant tissue is heated to the desired temperature of about 43 °C. At present, this is achieved by inserting thermocouples into the tumour. This is practicable for superficial tumours, but difficult for deep ones. There is therefore an urgent need for an accurate non-invasive thermometry method, especially for deep tumours. In principle, EIT might be suitable for this, because there is a linear relation between temperature and impedance change of about 2%/°C (Griffiths and Ahmed, 1987). Unfortunately, this requires a high degree of both spatial and contrast resolution. Calibration studies have been performed in tanks and by infusing warmed liquids into the stomachs of volunteers. They indicated a largely linear relation between region of interest integrals and temperature, but these varied according to position in the tank and between subjects (Möller et al, *in press*; Conway et al, 1992). Single images in the thigh (Griffiths and Ahmed, 1987) and over the shoulder blade (Conway, 1987) of human subjects during warming showed substantial artefacts, and it has also been demonstrated in normal volunteers without warming that baseline variability would produce impedance changes which were equivalent to temperature changes of several degrees (Liu and Griffiths, *in press*).

The clinical requirement is for a method which could be applied to a new patient and produce accurate temperature measurements. Prior calibration would require the use of inserted thermocouples, which would defeat the purpose of using a non-invasive technique. Given the uncertainty in calibration *a priori*, and the baseline variability *in vivo*, it seems that EIT is unlikely to be of practical use in this respect unless there are substantial improvements in EIT system performance.

3.5. The central nervous system (CNS).

There are at present excellent ways of imaging structural abnormalities in the nervous system, by X-ray computed tomography and magnetic resonance imaging. However, these methods are expensive and immovable. They require the patient to be transported to them and, from a practical point of view, are in great demand so that they are usually only suitable for imaging at single sessions. There is a need in some situations for a diagnostic system which could operate at the bedside and produce images of the head continuously over protracted periods. The cost, portability and non-invasive nature of EIT would make it suitable for this purpose. A particular application of this type would be its use in detecting intraventricular haemorrhage in premature babies. This is a condition where brain blood vessels burst and leak blood into the fluid filled ventricles which lie deep in the cerebral hemispheres. There is a high risk of this; early diagnosis can lead to improved treatment. Blood has a higher resistivity than cerebrospinal fluid which occupies the ventricles, so in theory EIT could be used for this purpose. Neonatal skull is not calcified, so it might present less of an obstacle to current flow than adult skull. A single preliminary image has been obtained during intraventricular haemorrhage in a neonate, using 16 electrodes and a reconstruction algorithm based on a sensitivity matrix (Murphy et al, 1987).

Other possible applications of EIT lie in imaging functional changes in the central nervous system. Functional impedance changes over minutes may occur through two main mechanisms : 1) In conditions such as stroke, epilepsy or hypoglycaemia, cells outrun their energy supplies and so swell. At the frequencies employed in EIT current passes almost entirely in the extracellular space, because cells are surrounded by a lipid membrane with a high impedance. As a result, tissue impedance is determined by the extracellular space. This decreases as fluid enters cells during swelling, so that tissue impedance rises by tens of per cent (Holder, 1992a; Holder, 1992b) with a time course of the duration of the pathological condition - usually minutes or tens of minutes. The impedance change can be completely reversed if normal conditions recur. 2) During normal functional activity, brain impedance increases by a few per cent (Adey et al, 1962). This is probably due to changes in blood flow (Holder, *in press(c)*). Both these types of events can be imaged by Positron Emission Tomography. EIT might offer practical advantages in imaging continuously at the bedside. A particular application where it could prove to be of substantial benefit is in locating the cerebral focus in patients with intractable epilepsy who require surgical excision of the abnormal area of the brain. Evidence to support these proposals is at present circumstantial : EIT images with good signal to noise ratios have been acquired during cerebral ischaemia in rats (Holder, 1992a), and it has been shown that cerebral impedance increases of about 4% occur in humans during epilepsy (Holder et al, *in press(d)*). Unfortunately, the assumption of uniform initial resistivity is violated if EIT is performed with scalp electrodes, because of the high resistance of the skull (Holder, 1992a). For the time being, any clinical applications in the brain will have to be performed with intracranial electrodes. As epilepsy surgery patients already have these electrodes inserted for localization by electroencephalography, it has been proposed that EIT images could be ethically obtained in these patients with a ring of electrodes slid inside the skull (Holder et al, *in press*).

Functional activity in the nervous system is produced by depolarization of nerve cells. The impedance of nerve membranes decreases by a factor of forty during depolarization; the impedance of active neural tissue should therefore also decrease. The precise size of this change is uncertain; it is likely to be less than one per cent (see Holder, *in press*(c)). It may therefore be possible to use EIT to generate images of neuronal activity with a high temporal resolution. If possible, this will provide a very substantial advance in neuroscience technology.

3.6. Pelvic congestion.

Pooling and congestion of blood in the pelvis is a poorly understood phenomenon which is thought to be the cause of pelvic discomfort in women. Thomas et al (1991) investigated the possible use of EIT in its diagnosis, on the basis that abnormal pooling would produce impedance changes. EIT images were collected with a ring of electrodes around the pelvis in the horizontal and vertical positions using a tilt table. A central area of impedance change was observed in both normals and subjects with pelvic congestion diagnosed on venography. A significant difference in the ratio of the areas anterior and posterior to the coronal midline and greater than 10% of the peak impedance change was observed. Venography is an invasive procedure, so EIT would provide a welcome alternative. The physiological origin of these changes has not been clarified, although it has been shown that they are at least plausible by comparison with EIT images made in tanks with saline filled tubing (Thomas et al, *in press*). This is an intriguing and potentially valuable application, but larger prospective studies will be needed before its use can be established.

3.7. Other possible applications.

Using a 16 electrode system operating at 10 kHz and an algorithm similar to that of the Sheffield system, Kulkarni et al (1990) were able to produce EIT images in long bones. Areas of increased resistivity could be identified in the normal subject and 16 weeks after fracture, whilst a similar region showed lower resistivity in another subject, 4 weeks after fracture. It remains to be determined if such results could be used effectively to monitor fracture healing. However, fractures can at present be assessed with great accuracy by X-ray. EIT might offer an advantage if repeated measurement was needed for follow-up, but it is unlikely that it could offer appropriate spatial resolution.

Other proposed applications have included EIT imaging of cell death, bladder filling, imaging of breast tumours, body fat and water, lean-to-fat ratios, limb plethysmography and apnoea monitoring (Dawids, 1987; Skidmore et al, 1987; Brown, 1990; Bhat, 1991) but no direct evidence is yet available to assess these possibilities.

4. Conclusions.

Clinical impedance imaging effectively commenced with the construction of the Sheffield EIT system just under a decade ago. It has clear limitations in terms of spatial resolution and ill-defined sensitivity to off-plane events and deviations from initial uniform resistivity in the subject. On the other hand, it is portable, safe, inexpensive and robust with respect to inaccuracies in electrode placement which are inevitable if electrodes are to placed on live subjects. There is no doubt that it produces reproducible reconstructed images in saline filled tanks with a spatial resolution of about 15% of the electrode diameter. The spatial resolution is likely to be worse than this in living subjects, but no direct data has yet been obtained in this respect.

Its use has only been validated quantitatively in measuring gastric emptying and pulmonary ventilation. Other areas where it has theoretical advantages over existing methods and where preliminary studies are encouraging include measurement of gastrointestinal motility, swallowing, pulmonary perfusion and regional ventilation, peripheral venous return, normal and abnormal function in the brain and pelvic congestion. If absolute measurements in space or of the amplitude of the impedance change are required, then the accuracy suffers because of uncertainties in mapping of three dimensional events to the image. This is the greatest problem if performance rests on accurate measurements made "blind" in individual subjects. It is therefore unlikely that the existing Sheffield system could be used effectively to measure temperature changes in hyperthermia, where the temperature change needs to located accurately in space, or in diagnosing pulmonary embolism in naive patients, as inter-subject variability appears to be substantial. In general, it is much more effective at measuring impedance changes which are relative in both amplitude and position within the image. These conditions are best met if a single variable can be defined using a region of interest and then followed in an individual subject. Measurement of gastric emptying is the best example of this to date.

References.

Adey WR, Kado RT, Didio J. 1962. Impedance measurements in brain tissue of animals using microvolt signals. Exp Neurol 5, 47-66.

Akkermans LMA, Tekamp FA, Smout AJPM, Roclofs JMM, Weigant VM (*in press*). The effects of stress on gastric emptying measured by Electrical Impedance Tomography (EIT) In Clinical and physiological applications of Electrical Impedance Tomography, Holder DS (ed), UCL Press : London.

Avill R, Mangnall F, Bird NC, Brown BH, Barber DC, Seagar AD, Johnson AG, Read NW. 1987. Applied potential tomography. A new non-invasive technique for measuring gastric emptying. Gastroenterology 92, 1019-1026..

Baker LE. 1989. Applications of the impedance technique to the respiratory system. IEEE EMBS Magazine 8, 50-52..

Barber DC (*in press*). An overview of EIT image reconstruction. In Clinical and physiological applications of Electrical Impedance Tomography, Holder DS (ed), UCL Press : London.

Barber DC, Brown BH, Freeston IL. 1983. Imaging spatial distributions of resistivity using applied potential tomography. Electronic Lett 19, 933-935.

Barber DC & Brown BH. 1984. Applied potential tomography. J Phys E : Sci Instrum 17, 723-733.

Barber DC & Seagar AD. 1987. Fast reconstruction of impedance images. Clin Phys Physiol Meas 8, Suppl A, 47-54.

Baxter AJ, Mangnall YF, Loj EH, Brown B, Barber DC, Johnson AG, Read NW. 1988. Evaluation of applied potential tomography as a new non-invasive gastric secretion test. Gut 29, 1730-1735.

Bhat S. Clinical applications. In Electrical Impedance Tomography, Webster JG, (ed), Adam Hilger: Bristol.

Brown BH. 1983. Tissue impedance methods. In Imaging with non-ionizing radiations, Jackson DF, (ed), Surrey University Press, pp 85-110.

Brown BH. 1990. Overview of clinical applications. In Proc 3rd European Community workshop on Electrical Impedance Tomography (Copenhagen), Hames TK, (ed), EC concerted action on EIT, pp. 29-35.

Brown, B.H., Barber, D.C. and Seagar, A.D. 1985. Applied potential tomography : possible clinical applications. Clin Phys Physiol Meas 6, 109-121.

Brown BH & Barber DC. 1992. Electrical impedance tomography. Clin Phys Physiol Meas 13, Suppl. A.

Brown BH, Barber DC, Tarassenko L. 1987. Electrical impedance tomography - applied potential tomography. Clin Phys Physiol Meas 8, Suppl. A.

Brown BH, Barber DC, Jossinet J. 1988. Electrical impedance tomography - applied potential tomography. Clin Phys Physiol Meas 9, Suppl. A.

Brown BH, Leathard A, Sinton A, McArdle FJ, Smith RWM, Barber DC. 1992. Blood flow imaging using electrical impedance tomography. Clin Phys Physiol Meas 13, Suppl A, 175-179.

Brown BH & Seagar AD. 1987. The Sheffield data collection system. Clin Phys Physiol Meas 8, Suppl A, 91-98.

Campbell JH, Harris ND, Zhang F, Morice A, Brown BH (*in press*). The monitoring of changes in intrathoracic fluid volumes with APT. Clinical and physiological applications of Electrical Impedance Tomography, Holder DS, (ed), UCL Press : London.

Conway J. 1987. Electrical impedance tomography for thermal monitoring of hyperthermia treatment: an assessment using in vitro and in vivo measurements. Clin Phys Physiol Meas 8, Suppl A, 141-146.

Conway J, Hawley M, Mangnall Y, Amasha H, Van Rhoon GC. 1992. Experimental assessment of electrical impedance imaging for hyperthermia monitoring. Clin Phys Physiol Meas 13, Suppl A, 185-189.

Dawids SG. 1987. Evaluation of applied potential tomography : a clinician's view. Clin Phys Physiol Meas 8, Suppl A, 175-180.

Devane SP (*in press*). Application of EIT to gastric emptying measurement in the premature baby unit - validation against residual volume method. Clinical and physiological applications of Electrical Impedance Tomography, Holder DS, (ed), UCL Press : London.

Devane SP, Bisset WM, Ravelli A, Milla PJ (*in press*). Simultaneous measurement of gastric emptying and antral motor activity using EIT. Clinical and physiological applications of Electrical Impedance Tomography, Holder DS, (ed), UCL Press : London.

Evans DF, Wright JW, Benson MJ, Logan R (*in press*). Gastric emptying studies on patients with Helicobacter pylori. Is delayed emptying cause or effect ? Clinical and physiological applications of Electrical Impedance Tomography, Holder DS, (ed), UCL Press : London.

Eyuboglu BM, Brown BH, Barber DC, Seagar AD. 1987. Localisation of cardiac related impedance changes in the thorax. Clin Phys Physiol Meas 8, Suppl A, 167-173.

Eyuboglu BM, Brown BH, Barber DC. 1989a. Limitations to SV determination from APT images. IEEE EMBS 11th Ann Int Conf, 442-443.

Eyuboglu BM, Brown BH, Barber DC. 1989b. In vivo imaging of cardiac related impedance changes. IEEE EMBS Magazine 8, 39-45.

Fuks LF, Cheney M, Isaacson D, Gisser DG, Newell JC. 1991. Detection and imaging of electric conductivity and permittivity at low frequency. IEEE Trans Biomed Eng 38, 1106-1110.

Geddes LA & Baker LE. 1967. The specific resistance of biological material - a compendium of data for the biomedical engineer and physiologist. Med Biol Eng 5, 271-293.

Goble J and Isaacson D. 1990. Fast reconstruction algorithms for three-dimensional electrical tomography. Proc 12th Ann Int Conf IEEE Biology Soc 10, 285-286.

Griffiths H, Ahmed A. 1987. Applied potential tomography for non-invasive temperature mapping in hyperthermia. Clin Phys Physiol Meas 8, Suppl A, 147-153.

Griffiths H, Zhang Z. 1989. Dual frequency electrical impedance tomography in vitro and in vivo. IEEE EMBS 11th Ann Int Conf, 476-477.

Hames TK (ed) 1990 Proc 3rd European Community workshop on Electrical Impedance Tomography (Copenhagen). EC concerted action on EIT.

Harris ND, Suggett AJ, Barber DC, Brown BH. 1987. Applications of applied potential tomography (APT) in respiratory medicine. Clin Phys Physiol Meas 8, Suppl A, 155-165.

Harris ND, Suggett AJ, Barber DC, Brown BH. 1988. Applied potential tomography: a new technique for monitoring pulmonary function. Clin Phys Physiol Meas 9, Suppl A, 79-85.

Holder DS. 1992a. Electrical impedance tomography with cortical or scalp electrodes during global cerebral ischaemia in the anaesthetized rat. Clin Phys Physiol Meas 13, 87-98.

Holder DS.1992b. Detection of cortical spreading depression in the anaesthetized rat by impedance measurement with scalp electrodes:implications for non-invasive imaging of the brain with electrical impedance tomography. Clin Phys Physiol Meas 13, 77-86.

Holder DS (ed) (*in press* (a)). Clinical and physiological applications of Electrical Impedance Tomography, UCL press: London.

Holder DS (*in press*(b)). Performance of the Sheffield electrical impedance tomography system with respect to imaging brain function in the adult head. In Proceedings of EC action in Process

Tomography, Manchester, Holder DS (*in press(c)*). Opportunities for EIT imaging in the nervous system   In Clinical and physiological applications of Electrical Impedance Tomography, Holder DS, (ed), UCL Press : London.
M. Beck (ed).

Holder DS, Binnie CD, Polkey C (*in press*) The possible application of EIT to imaging epileptic foci. In Proc COMAC in Biomagnetism, Cambridge, Fenwick P, (ed).

Holder DS & Temple AJ (*in press*). Effectiveness of the Sheffield EIT system in distinguishing patients with pulmonary pathology from a series of normal subjects   In Clinical and physiological applications of Electrical Impedance Tomography, Holder DS, (ed), UCL Press : London.

Isaacson D, Newell JC, Goble JC, Cheney M. 1990. Thoracic impedance changes during ventilation. Ann Int Conf IEEE EMBS 12, 106-107.

Isaacson D, Cheney M and Newell JC. 1992. Comments on reconstruction algorithms. Clin Phys Physiol Meas 13 Suppl A, 83-89.

Iskander MF & Durney CH. 1980. Electromagnetic techniques for medical diagnosis : a review. Proc IEEE 68, 126-132.

Killingbeck ALT, Zadehcoochak M, Blott BH, Hames TK (*in press*). Pulmonary ventilation, pulmonary perfusion and ventricular ejection profile studies with EIT. In Clinical and physiological applications of Electrical Impedance Tomography, Holder DS, (ed), UCL Press : London.

Kim Y, Webster JG, Tomkins WJ. 1983. Electrical impedance imaging of the thorax. J Microwave Power 18, 245-257.

Kim Y, Woo H, Luedtke AE. 1989. Impedance tomography and its application in deep venous thrombosis detection. IEEE EMBS Magazine 8, 47-49.

Kulkarni V, Hutchison JMS, Ritchie IK, Mallard JR. 1990. Impedance imaging in upper arm fractures. J Biomed Eng 12, 219-227.

Lamont GL, Wright JW, Evans DF, Kaplia L. 1988. An evaluation of applied potential tomography in the diagnosis of infantile hypertrophic pyloric stenosis. Clin Phys Physiol Meas 9, Suppl A, 65-69.

Lindley EJ, McArdle FJ, Brown BH, Wilson AJ, Knowles R, Mangnall Y (*in press*). Development of a portable APT system for gastric emptying measurement In Clinical and physiological applications of Electrical Impedance Tomography, Holder DS, (ed), UCL Press : London.

Liu P, Griffiths H, Wiles CM, Nathadwarawala KM, Stewart W. 1992. Measurement of pharyngeal transit time by electrical impedance tomography. Clin Phys Physiol Meas 13, Suppl A, 197-200.

Liu P, Griffiths H (*in press*). Limitations to the sensitivity of EIT in monitoring tissue temperature in hyperthermiaIn Clinical and physiological applications of Electrical Impedance Tomography, Holder DS, (ed), UCL Press : London.

Liu P, Hughes TAT, Griffiths H, Wiles CM, Nathadwarawala KM (*in press*). The effect of bolus volume on pharyngeal transit time as measured by EIT. In Clinical and physiological applications of Electrical Impedance Tomography, Holder DS, (ed), UCL Press : London.

Möller PH, Tranberg K-G, Blad B, Henriksson PH, Lindberg L, Weber L, Persson BRR (*in press*) Electrical impedance tomography for measurement of temperature distribution in laser thermotherapy (laserthermia) In Clinical and physiological applications of Electrical Impedance Tomography, Holder DS, (ed), UCL Press : London.

McArdle FJ, Suggett AJ, Brown BH, Barber DC. 1988. An assessment of dynamic images by applied potential tomography for monitoring pulmonary perfusion. Clin Phys Physiol Meas 9, Suppl A, 87-91.

McArdle FJ, Turley A, Hussain A, Hawley K, Brown BH (*in press*(a)) An in-vivo examination of cardiac impedance changes imaged by cardiosynchronous averaging In Clinical and physiological applications of Electrical Impedance Tomography, Holder DS, (ed), UCL Press : London.

Morice AH (*in press*). APT in the investigation of chest disease In Clinical and physiological applications of Electrical Impedance Tomography, Holder DS, (ed), UCL Press : London.

Murphy D, Burton P, Coombs R, Tarassenko L, Rolfe P. 1987. Impedance imaging in the newborn. Clin Phys Physiol Meas 8, Suppl A, 131-140.

Newell JC, Isaacson D, Cheney M, Saulnier GJ, Gisser DG, Goble JC, Cook RD. (*in press*). In-vivo static images using trigonometric current patterns In Clinical and physiological applications of Electrical Impedance Tomography, Holder DS, (ed), UCL Press : London.

Patterson RP. 1989. Fundamentals of impedance cardiography. IEEE EMBS Magazine 8, 35-38.

Paulson K, Breckon W, Pidcock M. 1990. Concurrent EIT reconstruction. Proc 3rd European Community workshop on Electrical Impedance Tomography (Copenhagen).

Ravelli A, Bisset WM, Milla PJ.(*in press*). Gastric emptying and motility in children with chronic renal failure (CRF). In Clinical and physiological applications of Electrical Impedance Tomography, Holder DS, (ed), UCL Press : London.

Ravelli AM & Milla PJ (*in press*(a)). Detection of gastro-oesophageal reflux by Electrical Impedance Tomography. In Clinical and physiological applications of Electrical Impedance Tomography, Holder DS, (ed), UCL Press : London.

Riu PJ, Rosell J, Lozano P, Palls-Areny R (*in press*) A broadband system for multifrequency static imaging in EIT. Clin Phys Physiol Meas.

Sakamoto K & Kanai H. 1979. Electrical characteristics of flowing blood. IEEE Trans Biomed Eng BME-26, 686-695.

Sinton AM, Brown BH, Barber DC, McArdle FJ, Leathard AD. 1992. Noise and spatial resolution of a real-time electrical impedance tomograph. Clin Phys Physiol Meas 13, Suppl A, 125-130.

Skidmore R, Evans JM, Jenkins D and Wells PNT. 1987. A data collection system for gathering electrical impedance measurements from the human breast. Clin Phys Physiol Meas 8, Suppl A, 99-102.

Smallwood R, Nour S, Mangnall Y, Smythe A (*in press*). Impedance imaging and gastric motility In Clinical and physiological applications of Electrical Impedance Tomography, Holder DS, (ed), UCL Press : London.

Smith RWM, Brown BH, Freeston IL, McArdle FJ. 1990. Real time electrical impedance tomography. Proc 3rd European Community workshop on Electrical Impedance Tomography (Copenhagen), 212-215.

Thomas DC, McArdle FJ, Rogers VE, Beard RW, Brown BH. 1991. Local blood volume changes in women with pelvic congestion measured by applied potential tomography. Clin Sci 81, 401-404.

Thomas DC, Siddall-Allum JN, Sutherland IA, Beard RW (*in press*). The use of electrical impedance tomography to assess blood volume changes in the female pelvis. In Clinical and physiological applications of Electrical Impedance Tomography, Holder DS, (ed), UCL Press : London.

Webster JG. 1991. Electrical Impedance Tomography. Adam Hilger: Bristol.

Witsoe DA, Kinnen E. 1967. Electrical resistivity of the lung at 100kHz. Med Biol Eng 5, 239-248.

Wright JW, Evans DF. 1990. Applied potential tomography (APT): a non-invasive method of detecting the migrating motor complex (MMC). Proc 3rd European Community workshop on Electrical Impedance Tomography (Copenhagen), 270-275.

Wright JW, Evans DF, Bush D (*in press*). The effect of nutrient and non-nutrient meals on gastric emptying (GE) as measured by EIT. In Clinical and physiological applications of Electrical Impedance Tomography, Holder DS, (ed), UCL Press : London.

First International Conference on:
CLINICAL AND PHYSIOLOGICAL APPLICATIONS OF ELECTRICAL IMPEDANCE TOMOGRAPHY

The Royal Society, London
22-24 April 1992

EC Concerted Action in
Electrical Impedance Tomography

Programme

EIT TECHNOLOGY AVAILABLE FOR CLINICAL USE

Overview

Review of EIT systems available for medical use.
BH Brown

Overview of EIT image reconstruction methods.
DC Barber

Recent Developments

In-vivo static images using optimal current patterns (experience with the Rensselaer Polytechnic EIT system).
JC Newell, D Issacson, M Cheney, GJ Saulnier, DG Gisser, JC Goble and RD Cook

Development of a portable APT system for gastric emptying measurement.
EJ Lindley, FJ McArdle, BH Brown, AJ Wilson, R Knowles and Y Mangnall

Dependence of thorax imaging on the reconstruction route.
M Zadehcoochak, BH Blott and TK Hames

The NIBEC electrode harness
ET McAdams, J McLaughlin, FJ McArdle and B Brown

Image Analysis

Statistical comparison of reconstructed images - experience with Positron Emission Tomography.
C Frith

GASTROINTESTINAL APPLICATIONS

The effect of nutrient and non-nutrient meals on gastric emptying as measured by EIT.
DF Evans and JW Wright

The effects of stress on gastric emptying.
LMA Akkermans

Application of EIT to gastric emptying measurement in premature infants - validation against residual volume method.
SP Devane

Simultaneous measurement of gastric emptying and antral motor activity using APT.
SP Devane, A Ravelli, WM Bisset and PJ Milla

Can APT detect the distribution of testmeal within the proximal and distal stomach during gastric emptying? A comparison with gamma scintigraphy.
JW Wright and DF Evans

Gastric emptying in chronic renal failure.
A Ravelli, WM Bisset and PJ Milla

Gastric emptying studies on patients with *Helicobacter pylori*. Is delayed emptying cause or effect?
DF Evans, MJ Benson and R Logan

Measurement of gastric motility in neonates with APT.
S Nour, Y Mangnall and R Smallwood

Assessment of dysphagia with EIT.
P Liu, H Griffiths, M Wiles, TAT Hughes and KM Nathadwarawala

Gastro-oesophageal reflux can be detected by APT.
A Ravelli and PJ Milla

POSSIBLE APPLICATIONS OF EIT IN THE CENTRAL NERVOUS SYSTEM

Opportunities for EIT imaging in the nervous system.
DS Holder

Cardiosynchronous images of impedance change within the adult head.
FJ McArdle, BH Brown and A Angel

Physiological constraints to EIT brain imaging with scalp electrodes.
DS Holder

The Keele approach to EIT in the neonatal head.
R Gadd, P Record, F Vintner and P Rolfe

OTHER APPLICATIONS - HYPERTHERMIA AND PELVIC BLOOD VOLUME

Will EIT provide effective temperature mapping in hyperthermia?
H Griffiths, P Liu

Electrical impedance measurement of temperature distribution in laser thermotherapy and hyperthermia (laserthermia).
BRR Persson, KG Tranberg, B Blad, PH Moller, J Rioseco and L Weber

An assessment of pelvic blood volume changes in women, using APT.
DC Thomas, J Siddall-Allum, I Sutherland, R Beard

EIT AND THE THORAX

Imaging of Ventilation

APT in the investigation of lung disease.
AH Morice, ND Harris, F Zhang, J Campbell and BH Brown

Lung impedance imaging with and without positive airways pressure.
FJ McArdle, ND Harris, A Hussain and BH Brown

The monitoring of changes in intrathoracic fluid volumes with APT.
JH Campbell, ND Harris, Z Zhang, A Morice, and BH Brown

EIT measurements and lung volume: a study in pigs.
LAW Smulders and A van Oosterom

Imaging of Blood Flow

An in-vivo examination of cardiac impedance changes images by cardiosynchronous averaging using APT
FJ McArdle, A Turley, A Hussain and K Hawley

Cardiovascular imaging of injected saline.
A Leathard and L Caldicott

Concurrent Imaging of Ventilation and Blood Flow

Effectiveness of the Sheffield EIT system in distinguishing patients with pulmonary pathology from a series of normal subjects.
DS Holder and AJ Temple

Pulmonary ventilation and perfusion.
ALT Killingbeck, M Zadehcoochak and BH Blott

LIST OF PARTICIPATING ORGANISATIONS - March 1992

France
  Elf Oil
  Observatoire de Grenoble
Germany
  University of Hannover
  University of Karlsruhe
Netherlands
  TU Delft
Norway *
  Chr Michelsens Institute
  University of Bergen
 Poland *
  Micromath, Warsaw
  Warsaw Technical University
Portugal
  University of Aveiro
Spain
  University Polytechnic of
  Catalunya
Sweden *
  Lund University
U.S.A. *
  Du Pont (Engineering)

United Kingdom
  Bolton Institute
  British Gas Research
  British Nuclear Fuels plc
  City University, London
  Harwell Laboratory
  ICI Polymers & Chemicals
  Oxford Polytechnic
  Rolls Royce
  Royal Hallamshire Hospital
  S.E.R.C.
  Schlumberger Cambridge Research
  Sheffield Polytechnic
  UMIST
  Unilever Research, Port Sunlight
  University College, London
  University of Birmingham
  University of Leeds
  University of Manchester
  University of Surrey
  University of York

(* invited EFTA-affiliated or non-EC participant)

LIST OF PARTICIPANTS

Dr F Abdullah   City University   Tel: +(44) 071 253 4399
                     Department of EEIE   Fax: +(44) 071 490 0719
                     Northampton Square
                     London EC1V 0HB
                     United Kingdom

Mr M Z Abdullah   UMIST   Tel: +(44) 061 200 4786
                     Department of Electrical Engineering   Fax: +(44) 061 200 4789
                     and Electronics
                     PO Box 88
                     Manchester M60 1QD
                     United Kingdom

Dr T Allen   E I Du Pont de Nemoirs & Co   Tel: +(1) 302 366 2154
                     Engineering Department   Fax: +(1) 302 366 4889
                     PO Box 6090
                     L13W52
                     Newark DE 19714
                     USA

Mr M Bair   University of Manchester   Tel: +(44) 061 275 4534
                     Department of Electrical Enginering   Fax: +(44) 061 275 4512
                     Oxford Road
                     Manchester M13 9PL
                     United Kingdom

Dr I Basarab   Sheffield City Polytechnic   Tel: +(44) 0742 533276
                     School of EIT   Fax: +(44) 0742 533306
                     Pond St
                     Sheffield S1 1WB
                     United Kingdom

Prof M S Beck   UMIST   Tel: +(44) 061 200 4785
                     Department of Electrical Engineering   Fax: +(44) 061 200 4789
                     and Electronics
                     PO Box 88
                     Manchester M60 1QD
                     United Kingdom

Mr R Bidin   Sheffield City Polytechnic   Tel: +(44) 0742 533276
                     School of EIT   Fax: +(44) 0742 533306
                     Pond St
                     Sheffield S1 1WB
                     United Kingdom

Prof A R Borges · Universidade de Aveiro · Tel: +(351) 34 25085
Departamento de Electronica e · Fax: +(351) 34 381128
Telecomunicaoes
3800 Aveiro
Portugal

Mr R Brant · UMIST · Tel: +(44) 061 200 4784
Department of Electrical Engineering · Fax: +(44) 061 200 4789
and Electronics
PO Box 88
Manchester M60 1QD
United Kingdom

Dr R Brassington · UMIST · Tel: +(44) 061 200 4784
Department of Electrical Engineering · Fax: +(44) 061 200 4789
and Electronics
PO Box 88
Manchester M60 1QD
United Kingdom

Prof K Brodowicz · Warsaw Technical University · Tel: +(48) 22 259757
00-665 Nowowiejska 25 · Fax: +(48) 22 250565
Warsaw
Poland

Mrs Q Chen · University of Leeds · Tel: +(44) 0532 332056
Department of Electronic and · Fax: +(44) 0532 332032
Electrical Engineering
Leeds LS2 9JT
United Kingdom

Mr W Conway · UMIST · Tel: +(44) 061 200 4784
Department of Electrical Engineering · Fax: +(44) 061 200 4789
and Electronics
PO Box 88
Manchester M60 1QD
United Kingdom

Dr A A da Rocha · Universidade de Aveiro · Tel: + (351) 34 25085
Departamento de Electronica e · Fax: + (351) 34 381128
Telecomunicaoes
3800 Aveiro
Portugal

Dr L Desbat · Observatoire de Grenoble · Tel: +(33) 76 51 47 87
Cermo BP 53X · Fax: +(33) 76 44 88 21
38041 Grenoble Cedex
France

Dr F J Dickin	UMIST Department of Electrical Engineering and Electronics PO Box 88 Manchester M60 1QD United Kingdom	Tel: +(44) 061 200 4791 Fax: +(44) 061 200 4789
Mr P Dugdale	Bolton Institute of Higher Education School of Engineering Deane Road Bolton BL3 5AB United Kingdom	Tel: +(44) 0204 28851 Fax: +(44) 0204 399074
Dr T Dyakowski	UMIST Department of Chemical Engineering PO Box 88 Manchester M60 1QD United Kingdom	Tel: +(44) 061 200 4373 Fax: +(44) 061 200 4399
Mr E Dykesteen	Chr Michelsens Institute Department of Science and Technology Fantoftvegen 38 N-5036 Fantoft Bergen Norway	Tel: +(47) 5 74000 Fax: +(47) 5 74001
Mr R B Edwards	Unilever Research Port Sunlight Laboratory Quarry Road East Bebington Wirral L63 3JW United Kingdom	Tel: +(44) 051 645 2000 x3109 Fax: +(44) 051 645 3249
Mr E Etuke	UMIST Department of Electrical Engineering and Electronics PO Box 88 Manchester M60 1QD United Kingdom	Tel: +(44) 061 200 4783 Fax: +(44) 061 200 4789
Dr R Green	Sheffield City Polytechnic School of EIT Pond St Sheffield S1 1WB United Kingdom	Tel: +(44) 0742 533276 Fax: +(44) 0742 533306

Mr H Grootveld   TU Delft   Tel: +(31) 15 78 3725
                      Chemical Process Technology Department   Fax: +(31) 15 78 4452
                      Particle Technology Group
                      Julianalaan 136
                      2628 BL Delft
                      Netherlands

Dr E Hammer   University of Bergen   Tel: +(47) 5 21 27 61
                      Department of Physics   Fax: +(47) 5 31 83 34
                      Allegaten 55
                      N-5007 Bergen
                      Norway

Dr A Hartley   Bolton Institute of Higher Education   Tel: +(44) 0204 28851
                      School of Engineering   Fax: +(44) 0204 399074
                      Deane Road
                      Bolton BL3 5AB
                      United Kingdom

Dr M Hawkesworth   University of Birmingham   Tel: +(44) 021 414 4708/9
                      School of Physics and Space Research   Fax: +(44) 021 414 6709
                      Birmingham B15 2TT
                      United Kingdom

Mr D Hayes   UMIST   Tel: +(44) 061 200 4792
                      Department of Electrical Engineering   Fax: +(44) 061 200 4789
                      and Electronics
                      PO Box 88
                      Manchester M60 1QD
                      United Kingdom

Dr P Henriksson   Lund University   Tel: +(46) 46 17 31 10
                      Radiation Physics Department   Fax: +(46) 46 12 71 63
                      Lasarettet
                      S-221 85 Lund
                      Sweden

Dr D Holder   University College, London   Tel: +(44) 071 387 7050
                      Department of Physiology   Fax: +(44) 071 383 7005
                      Gower Street
                      London WC1E 6BT
                      United KIngdom

Dr B Hoyle   University of Leeds   Tel: +(44) 0532 332056
                      Department of Electronic and   Fax: +(44) 0532 332032
                      Electrical Engineering
                      Leeds LS2 9JT
                      United Kingdom

Dr S M Huang Schlumberger Cambridge Research Ltd Tel: +(44) 0223 325224
      PO Box 153   Fax: +(44) 0223 315486
      Cambridge CB3 0HG
      United Kingdom

Mr Ø Isaksen University of Bergen   Tel: +(47) 5 21 27 61
      Department of Physics   Fax: +(47) 5 31 83 34
      Allegaten 55
      N-5007 Bergen
      Norway

Dr R Jackson Bolton Institute of Higher Education Tel: +(44) 0204 28851
      School of Engineering   Fax: +(44) 0204 399074
      Deane Road
      Bolton BL3 5AB
      United Kingdom

Mr S Keningley Unilever Research   Tel: +(44) 051 645 2000
      Port Sunlight Laboratory   Fax: +(44) 051 645 3249
      Quarry Road East
      Bebington
      Wirral L63 3JW
      United Kingdom

Dr S Khan City University   Tel: +(44) 071 253 4399
      Department of EEIE   Fax: +(44) 071 490 0719
      Northampton Square
      London EC1V 0HB
      United Kingdom

Dr J Landauro Bolton Institute of Higher Education Tel: +(44) 0204 28851
      School of Engineering   Fax: +(44) 0204 399074
      Deane Road
      Bolton BL3 5AB
      United KIngdom

Mr M Lee UMIST   Tel: +(44) 061 200 4369
      Department of Chemical Engineering Fax: +(44) 061 200 4399
      PO Box 88
      Manchester M60 1QD
      United Kingdom

Dr C Lenn Schlumberger Cambridge Research Ltd Tel: +(44) 0223 325224
      PO Box 153   Fax: +(44) 0223 315486
      Cambridge CB3 0HG
      United Kingdom

Dr A Lewis	University College, London Department of Physiology Gower Street London WC1E 6BT United Kingdom	Tel: +(44) 071 387 7050 x ? Tel: +(44) 071 383 7005
Mr G Lyon	University of Manchester Department of Electrical Enginering Oxford Road Manchester M13 9PL United Kingdom	Tel: +(44) 061 275 4534 Fax: +(44) 061 275 4512
Dr P Martin	Harwell Laboratory EPED Building 404 Oxfordshire OX11 0RA United Kingdom	Tel: +(44) 0235 434411 Fax: +(44) 0235 432313
Mr F McArdle	I.B.E.E.S. Lodge Moor Hospital Redmires Road Sheffield S10 4LH United Kingdom	Tel: +(44) 0742 630324 Fax: +(44) 0742 630326
Mr S McKee	UMIST Department of Chemical Engineering PO Box 88 Manchester M60 1QD United Kingdom	Tel: +(44) 061 200 4369 Fax: +(44) 061 200 4399
Dr C McLeod	Oxford Polytechnic School of Engineering Headington Oxford OX3 0BP United Kingdom	Tel: +(44) 0865 819508 Fax: +(44) 0865 819673
Prof F Mesch	University of Karlsruhe Institut fur Mess und Regelungstechnik Postfach 6980 7500 Karlsruhe 1 Germany	Tel: +(49) 721 608 2334 Fax: +(49) 721 66 18 74
Prof D Mewes	University of Hannover Institut Fur Verfahrenstechnik Callinstrasse 36 D-3000 Hannover Germany	Tel: +(49) 511 7623638 Fax: +(49) 511 7623031

Dr J Middleton	ICI Chemicals and Polymers Ltd PO Box 8 The Heath Runcorn WA7 4QD United Kingdom	Tel: +(44) 0928 513707 Fax: +(44) 0928 581178
Dr J E Nordtvedt	University of Bergen Department of Physics Allegaten 55 N-5007 Bergen Norway	Tel: +(47) 5 21 27 61 Fax: +(47) 5 31 83 34
Dr J Oakley	University of Manchester Department of Electrical Enginering Oxford Road Manchester M13 9PL United Kingdom	Tel: +(44) 061 275 4534 Fax: +(44) 061 275 4512
Dr J Oliveira	Universidade de Aveiro Departamento de Electronica e Telecomunicaoes 3800 Aveiro Portugal	Tel: + (351) 34 25085 Fax: + (351) 34 381128
Prof R Pallas -Areny	University Polytechnic de Catalonya Departament D'Enginyeria Electronica PO Box 30002 Barcelona 08080 Spain	Tel: +(34) 3 401 6766 Fax: +(34) 3 401 6801
Dr D Parker	University of Birmingham School of Physics and Space Research Birmingham B15 2TT United Kingdom	Tel: +(44) 021 414 4605 Fax: +(44) 021 414 6709
Mr S Quick	UMIST Department of Electrical Engineering and Electronics PO Box 88 Manchester M60 1QD United Kingdom	Tel: +(44) 061 200 4792 Fax: +(44) 061 200 4789
Dr P Riu	University Polytechnic de Catalonya Departament D'Enginyeria Electronica PO Box 30002 Barcelona 08080	Tel: +(34) 3 401 6766 Fax: +(34) 3 401 6801

Dr J Rogers	Rolls Royce plc GP2-5 Filton Bristol BS12 7QE United Kingdom	Tel: +(44) 0272 797083 Fax: +(44) 0272 797644
Mr A Schwarz	University of Karlsruhe Institut fur Mess und Regelungstechnik Postfach 6980 7500 Karlsruhe 1 Germany	Tel: +(49) 721 608 2334 Fax: +(49) 721 66 18 74
Dr D Scott	Du Pont Science and Engineering Labs Building 357 Experimental Station PO Box 80357 Wilmington Delaware 19880-0357 USA	Tel: +(1) 302 695 4883 Fax: +(1) 302 695 2747
Dr S Simons	University of Surrey Department of Chemical and Process Engineering Guildford Surrey GU2 5XH United Kingdom	Tel: +(44) 0483 300 800 x2192 Fax: +(44) 0483 303807
Dr L Stott	UMIST Department of Electrical Engineering and Electronics PO Box 88 Manchester M60 1QD United Kingdom	Tel: +(44) 061 200 4727 Fax: +(44) 061 200 4789
Mr P Szuster	Micromath Co Ltd Al Stanow, Zjednoczonych 51 03-965 Warsaw Poland	Tel: +(48) 22 106705 Fax: +(48) 22 133346
Mr D Tallantire	Science and Engineering Research Council 2 Crouch Hall Gardens Redbourn St Albans Herts AL3 7EL	Tel: +(44) 058 2792239

Mr W Tang	UMIST Department of Electrical Engineering and Electronics PO Box 88 Manchester M60 1QD United Kingdom	Tel: +(44) 061 200 4787 Fax: +(44) 061 200 4789
Dr R Taylor	University of York Department of Electronics York YO1 5DD United Kingdom	Tel: +(44) 0904 432351 Fax: +(44) 0904 432335
Dr J Torrents	University Polytechnic de Catalonya Departament D'Enginyeria Electronica PO Box 30002 Barcelona 08080 Spain	Tel: +(34) 3 401 6766 Fax: +(34) 3 401 6801
Prof G Van Weert	Delft University of Technology Faculty of Mining and Petroleum Engineering Mijnbouwstraat 120 2628 RX Delft Netherlands	Tel: +(31) 15 781606 Fax: +(31) 15 784891
Mr M Wang	UMIST Department of Electrical Engineering and Electronics PO Box 88 Manchester M60 1QD United Kingdom	Tel: +(44) 061 200 4786 Fax: +(44) 061 200 4789
Dr R Waterfall	UMIST Department of Electrical Engineering and Electronics PO Box 88 Manchester M60 1QD United Kingdom	Tel: +(44) 061 200 4727 Fax: +(44) 061 200 4789
Mr L Wei	University of Leeds Department of Electronic and Electrical Engineering Leeds LS2 9JT United Kingdom	Tel: +(44) 0532 332056 Fax: +(44) 0532 332032

Mr A Wernsdorfer   University of Karlsruhe   Tel: +(49) 721 608 2334
                    Institut fur Mess und Regelungstechnik   Fax: +(49) 721 66 18 74
                    Postfach 6980
                    7500 Karlsruhe 1
                    Germany

Dr R Williams   UMIST   Tel: +(44) 061 200 4346
                    Department of Chemical Engineering   Fax: +(44) 061 200 4399
                    PO Box 88
                    Manchester M60 1QD
                    United Kingdom

Dr J Winterbottom   University of Birmingham
                    School of Chemical Engineering
                    Birmingham B15 2TT
                    United Kingdom

Dr C G Xie   UMIST   Tel: +(44) 061 200 4791
                    Department of Electrical Engineering   Fax: +(44) 061 200 4789
                    and Electronics
                    PO Box 88
                    Manchester M60 1QD
                    United Kingdom

AUTHORS' INDEX

Proceedings of a Workshop sponsored by the Commission of the European Communities, Directorate-General for Science, Research and Development, under the Brite/Euram Industrial Technologies R&D programme (1989-1992), held in Manchester, 26-29 March, 1992

TOMOGRAPHIC TECHNIQUES
FOR PROCESS DESIGN
AND OPERATION

TOMOGRAPHIC TECHNIQUES FOR PROCESS DESIGN AND OPERATION

Edited by:

M.S. Beck* E. Campogrande** Margaret Morris*
R.A. Williams* R.C. Waterfall*

*University of Manchester Institute of Science and Technology,
Manchester, U.K.

**Commission of the European Communities, Brussels, Belgium.

Computational Mechanics Publications
Southampton UK and Boston USA

M.S. Beck, Margaret Morris, R.A. Williams & R.C. Waterfall
University of Manchester Institute of Science and Technology (UMIST)
P.O. Box 88
Manchester M60 1QD
UK

E. Campogrande
Commission of the European Communities
Brussels
Belgium

*The texts of the various papers in this volume were set individually
by typists under the supervision of each of the authors concerned.*

Computational Mechanics Publications
Ashurst Lodge, Southampton, SO4 2AA, UK
Tel: 44 (0)703 293223 Fax: 44 (0)703 292853
Email: CMI@uk.ac.rl.ib

For USA, Canada and Mexico:
Computational Mechanics Inc
25 Bridge Street, Billerica, MA 01821, USA
Tel: 508 667 5841 Fax: 508 667 7582

British Library Cataloguing-in-Publication Data

A Catalogue record for this book is available
from the British Library

ISBN 1-85312-246-7 Computational Mechanics Publications, Southampton
ISBN 1-56252-170-5 Computational Mechanics Publications, Boston

Library of Congress Catalog Card Number 93-70678